The Dr. Barbara O'Neill's Herbal Remedies & Natural Medicine Encyclopedia

A Self-Healing Collection of 500+ Naturopathic Recipes and Holistic Secrets So Revolutionary That Big Pharma Wants Them Buried

LADY VERITAS

Table of Contents

Introduction

I stumbled into the world of natural healing very differently from how others do. I was recruited out of college to join an agency that will remain unnamed. At first, the opportunity seemed to match my values—solving food shortage issues, researching food quality and consumption standards, and building a healthier world.

What I was to discover is that, that's not the way it works in a world where medicine and food collide. The statistics and instructions we were given as researchers often didn't meet up with the agency's promise to bring safe, clean foods to people, and worse, much of our funding was received by big pharma organizations that had one agenda—keep people on the brink of illness: All the time!

This sinister symbiotic relationship between food industries and big pharma is well-known, but is often dismissed as conspiracy theory. Even I shunned the notion that my food was making me sick when I was first confronted with it. But, as the months and years rolled on, I could no longer shy away from an undeniable truth:

We were all being poisoned for the sake of profit!

I believed the diagnosis that I had received, "Autoimmune, POTS, and health anxiety," and it never occurred to me that the one thing I needed to sustain and nourish me was also the thing that was keeping me hooked on low-dose chemotherapy to keep my autoimmune disease under control.

Of course, I was knowledgeable, I studied this, and at first, I was ashamed of how naive I had been. The research was in front of me with the instruction to skew it and I knew what I had to do.

And when I stopped all Western treatment... When I chose to make what I knew was healthy and what my body needed a priority? My diagnosed ailments suddenly disappeared. I was healthier, happier, and stronger than I had been in years.

Natural medicine has been around for thousands of years. Our ancestors relied on plants, herbs, and other natural remedies to treat our ailments and remain healthy long before Western medicine came to be. It's fascinating to see how different cultures across the globe developed their own unique approaches to healing using local plants and herbs.

Recently, there's been a resurgence of interest in natural medicine with people realizing that sometimes, the best solutions can be found right in our own backyards. I've even heard stories of folks growing their own insulin—yes it is possible.

While many will argue that this resurgence is as a result of the soaring cost of healthcare, I would say that people are waking up to the same truth I was exposed to—that nature has the answer and that our bodies know how to heal themselves!

We are no longer looking for solutions that alleviate our symptoms or that fix our problems as they arise—we want to prevent issues before they take place and live a naturally healthy and holistic life without the profiteering of big pharma driving us into fear and isolation.

Yes, natural medicine can be incredibly helpful when we do get sick or experience various ailments but it's the power of holistic healing and the recipes in this book that will truly unlock our body's true potential. We need to seek balance and that balance comes from embracing what nature has to offer us while understanding that we are pawns in a profiteering racket of global proportions.

This means eating plenty of whole, natural foods, staying hydrated, getting enough rest, and moving our bodies regularly but it also means being mindful of what we put into our bodies and why. And it's this balanced life that I have kept in mind when creating this Self-Healing Collection of 500+ Naturopathic Recipes and Holistic Secrets So Revolutionary That Big Pharma Wants Them Buried—a curation of natural recipes to heal you when you're ill and help you thrive through life.

Each chapter is divided into topical treatments, herbal brews and drinks, and recipes you can use to help nourish and heal your body, now and in your newly natural life. And, in making the choice to heal your body and mind naturally with this book, you will gain access to an exclusive video course. Available after our chapter on colds and flu remedies, your access includes never-been-seen before footage of how to create herbal recipes and medicines, dosage instructions, and insightful tips and tricks on fostering health and well-being.

For now though, let's begin with your self-healing recipes using *The Doctor Barbara O'Neill Herbal Remedies & Natural Medicine Encyclopedia.*

Discover Time-Honored Herbal Wisdom with Exclusive Access to Video Recipes

Are you looking for a natural way to support your health and well-being? Are you sick and tired of being sick and tired?

The Barbara O'Neill Herbal Remedies & Medicine Encyclopedia is your comprehensive guide to harnessing the power of medicinal herbs, and now, you have access to this timeless wisdom through a never-been-seen-before transformative video course.

By gaining exclusive access, you will be introduced to:

- Detailed profiles of common healing herbs, including their traditional uses and modern applications.
- Step-by-step instructions for preparing some of the herbal teas, tinctures, salves, and other natural remedies featured in The Babara O'Neill Herbal Remedies & Natural Medicine Encyclopedia.
- Guidance on using herbs safely and effectively to address common health concerns including dosages.
- Fascinating insights into what herbs can do for you and your well-being.
- In-depth video tutorials demonstrating advanced herbal preparation techniques.
- Simply scan the QR code below to unlock your access to a time-honored wisdom and tradition.

Whether you're a beginner exploring herbal remedies for the first time or a seasoned herbalist seeking to deepen your knowledge, The Barbara O'Neill Herbal Remedies & Natural Medicine Encyclopedia and bonus video course will empower you to take control of your health naturally now and in the future.

Don't miss this opportunity to tap into the profound wisdom of medicinal herbs.

Antioxidant Boosting

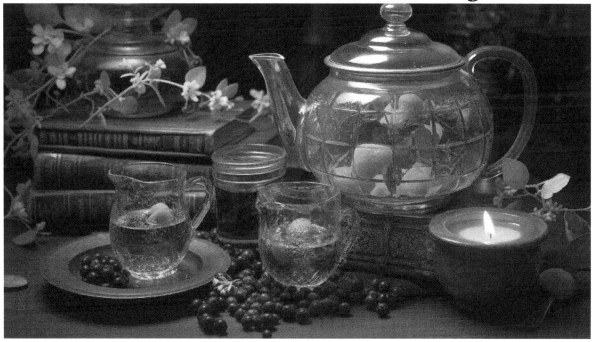

"Let food be thy medicine and medicine be thy food." — Hippocrates

Our bodies are constantly bombarded by free radicals, oxidative stress, and the ravages of modern living and it's no wonder that many of us are turning to nature for support. From barefoot grounding to antioxidant-rich herbs and natural foods, Mother Nature provides us with everything we need to help fortify our body's defenses and promote optimal well-being.

Topical Treatments

Antioxidant Bath Soak

Ingredients:

- 1 cup Epsom salt (also known as magnesium sulfate)
- 1/2 cup baking soda
- 10 drops of lavender essential oil
- 1 tablespoon dried lavender buds (optional, for added fragrance and visual appeal)
- Purple or blue food coloring (optional, for aesthetic purposes)

Directions:

1. In a mixing bowl, combine the Epsom salt and baking soda. Stir well to ensure they are evenly mixed.
2. Add the lavender essential oil to the salt mixture. If using dried lavender buds, add them to the mixture as well.
3. If desired, add a few drops of food coloring to the mixture. Stir until the color is evenly distributed.
4. Transfer the mixture to a sealable glass jar or container.
5. Close the lid tightly and shake the container gently to further mix the ingredients.
6. Label the jar with the date and name of the bath salts.
7. To use, add a generous spoonful (about 1/4 cup or 60 ml) of the bath salts to warm running bathwater.
8. Stir the water to dissolve the salts before soaking in the bath for at least 20 minutes to enjoy the relaxing benefits of lavender.

Antioxidant Face Mask for Glowing Skin

Ingredients:

- 1/4 cup mixed berries (e.g., strawberries, blueberries, and raspberries)
- 1 tablespoon honey
- 1 tablespoon yogurt

Directions:

1. Mash the mixed berries in a bowl until smooth.
2. Add honey and yogurt to the mashed berries, mixing well.
3. Apply the mixture to your clean face, avoiding the eye area.
4. Leave the mask on for 15-20 minutes.
5. Rinse off with lukewarm water and pat your face dry.

Antioxidant Brews and Drinks

Cinnamon and Apple Spiced Tea

Ingredients:

- 2 cups (480 ml) filtered water
- 1/2 cup (120 ml) unfiltered fresh pressed apple cider or apple juice
- 2 Ceylon cinnamon sticks (plus extra for serving, if desired)
- 1 teaspoon whole cloves
- 1 star anise
- 2 rooibos tea bags
- Apple slices for serving (optional)
- Maple syrup or sweetener of choice, to taste

Directions:

1. In a medium saucepan, combine water, apple cider or juice, and spices.
2. Bring the mixture to a simmer, then reduce the heat, cover, and let it simmer for 10 minutes.
3. Turn off the heat, add the tea bags, cover, and let them steep for 5 minutes.
4. Remove the tea bags and strain the spices from the mixture.
5. Stir in maple syrup or sweetener of choice to taste.
6. Serve the tea in mugs, optionally garnished with thinly sliced apples and a cinnamon stick for stirring.

Minty Matcha Morning Brew

Ingredients:

- 1 teaspoon matcha latte powder
- 1 teaspoon loose-leaf peppermint tea
- 1/2 cup (120 ml) hot water
- 3/4 cup (180 ml) non-dairy milk

Directions:

1. Steep the loose-leaf peppermint tea in 1/2 cup of hot water for 5-7 minutes to allow the mint to infuse its invigorating essence into the water.
2. While the mint tea is steeping, gently warm the non-dairy milk in a saucepan or microwave until warm but not boiling.
3. In a separate cup or bowl, sift the matcha powder to ensure a smooth texture when mixed.
4. Gradually add a small amount of warm milk to the matcha powder and whisk vigorously to create a smooth, vibrant green paste.
5. Once the matcha paste is smooth, gradually pour in the remaining warm milk while continuing to whisk, ensuring the matcha is fully incorporated.
6. Remove the mint tea leaves or tea bag from the steeped water and discard.
7. Pour the infused mint tea into the matcha-milk mixture.
8. If desired, add your preferred sweetener to the mint matcha and stir until dissolved.
9. Pour your Mint Matcha into your favorite cup, sit back, and take a moment to relish the revitalizing aroma.

Rooibos and Almond Tea

Ingredients:

- 6 oz (177 ml) milk or almond milk
- 2 oz (59 ml) water
- 1 tablespoon rooibos tea (such as David's Tea Alpine Punch)
- 1/2 teaspoon vanilla extract
- 1 teaspoon maple syrup

Directions:

1. In a small saucepan, combine the milk (or almond milk) and water.
2. Add the rooibos tea to the saucepan.
3. Heat the mixture over medium heat until it begins to simmer.
4. Reduce the heat to low and let the mixture steep for 5 minutes.
5. Remove the saucepan from the heat and strain out the tea leaves.
6. Stir in the vanilla extract and maple syrup.
7. Pour the vanilla rooibos latte into a mug and enjoy its comforting warmth.

Citrus and Berry Warm Brew Tea

Berry Syrup **Ingredients:**

- 1 cup raspberries
- 1 cup blueberries
- 1 cup blackberries
- 1 1/2 cups sugar
- 4 cups water

Iced Tea **Ingredients:**

- 8 cups water, divided
- 6 black tea bags
- 1/4 teaspoon baking soda

Directions:

Berry Syrup:

1. In a saucepan, combine the raspberries, blueberries, blackberries, sugar, and 4 cups of water.
2. Bring the mixture to a boil over medium heat, stirring occasionally.
3. Once boiling, reduce the heat to low and let it simmer for about 15-20 minutes, or until the berries have broken down and the liquid has thickened slightly.
4. Remove the saucepan from the heat and strain the mixture through a fine-mesh sieve to remove the berry solids, pressing down gently to extract as much syrup as possible.
5. Allow the syrup to cool before transferring it to a jar or bottle for storage. Store in the refrigerator for up to two weeks.

Iced Tea:

6. In a large saucepan or kettle, bring 4 cups of water to a boil.
7. Once boiling, remove from heat and add the black tea bags. Allow them to steep for 5 minutes.
8. In a pitcher, combine the remaining 4 cups of water and the baking soda.
9. Remove the tea bags from the hot water and pour the brewed tea into the pitcher with the water and baking soda mixture.
10. Stir well to combine.
11. Serve the tea warm or chilled tea over ice, sweetening each glass with a drizzle of homemade berry syrup according to taste.

Ginger Detox Tea

Ingredients:

- 1 teaspoon fresh grated ginger
- 1 lemon wedge
- 1 cup hot water
- 2-3 teaspoons raw honey

Directions:

1. Boil water in a kettle.
2. Use a large coarse grater to shave fresh ginger into a mug. Place a wedge of fresh lemon in the mug. You can place both in a tea infuser to strain the tea if you like.
3. Pour boiling water into the cup and let the lemon and ginger steep for 5 minutes before serving.
4. Add honey to taste if drinking for enjoyment.

Antioxidant-Rich Recipes

Rich Berry Smoothie

- 1/2 cup frozen blackberries
- 1/2 cup frozen raspberries (or substitute strawberries)
- 1/4 cup frozen blueberries (preferably wild blueberries)
- 1 frozen banana
- 2 cups organic spinach
- 1 tablespoon flaxseed meal
- 1 tablespoon almond butter (or your preferred nut butter)
- 1/2 cup plain Greek yogurt (whole, 2%, or fat-free)
- 1/2 cup unsweetened almond milk, plus more as necessary
- Optional: 1 tablespoon hemp seeds

Directions:

1. In a large high-powered blender, combine all ingredients.
2. Blend on high for 1-2 minutes or until all ingredients are well combined and smooth.
3. If the smoothie is too thick, add more almond milk to achieve your desired consistency.
4. Pour into a glass and enjoy immediately.

Walnut and Chia Seed Breakfast Pudding

Ingredient:

- 2 1/2 cups unsweetened almond milk
- 3 tablespoons pure maple syrup
- 1/2 cup chia seeds
- 1/4 cup walnuts, chopped

Directions:

1. In a jar or container, combine the almond milk, maple syrup, and chia seeds. Stir well or shake the jar to ensure thorough mixing.
2. Seal the jar/container and refrigerate overnight to allow the chia seeds to absorb the liquid and create a pudding-like consistency.
3. In the morning, stir the pudding. If the consistency is not thick yet, return it to the refrigerator for another hour or so.
4. Preheat the oven to 375°F (190°C). Spread the chopped walnuts on a baking sheet.
5. Roast the walnuts for 5 to 8 minutes, or until they are slightly browned and toasted. Keep an eye on them to prevent burning.
6. To serve, pour the chilled pudding into bowls or glasses. Top each serving with the roasted walnuts and an additional drizzle of maple syrup, if desired.

Avocado, Spinach, and Strawberry Salad

Ingredients:

- 8 cups baby spinach or salad blend with spinach
- Salt and pepper, to taste
- 8 large strawberries, hulled and quartered
- 1 avocado, sliced
- 1/3 cup sliced almonds

Strawberry Vinaigrette Dressing Ingredients:

- 5 large strawberries
- 2 tablespoons extra virgin olive oil
- 2 tablespoons fresh lemon juice
- 1/4 teaspoon ground ginger
- 1/8 teaspoon white pepper

Directions:

1. In a large bowl, place the baby spinach or salad blend and season with salt and pepper.
2. Add the quartered strawberries, sliced avocado, and sliced almonds to the bowl.
3. In a blender, combine all the ingredients for the strawberry vinaigrette dressing: strawberries, extra virgin olive oil, fresh lemon juice, ground ginger, and white pepper. Blend until smooth.
4. Serve the salad with the strawberry vinaigrette dressing on the side or drizzled over the top.

Antioxidant Defense

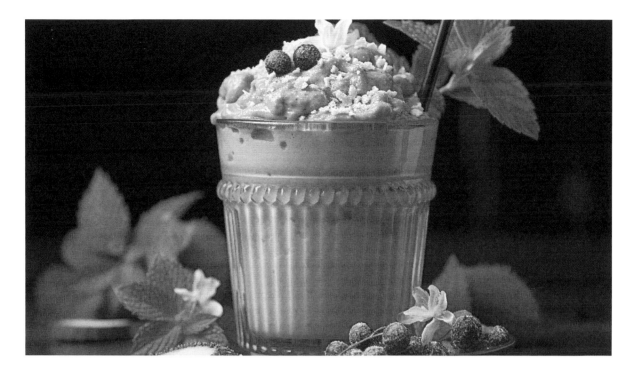

"Antioxidants are the silent warriors that protect our cells from the ravages of time and the chaos of oxidative stress." –Dr. Amara Noor

Our bodies are constantly defending against a barrage of free radicals, oxidative stress, and environmental toxins. These damaging effects can wreak havoc on our cells, leading to premature aging, chronic diseases, and a host of other health issues. Antioxidants provide us with a natural arsenal to help defend against free radicals and oxidative stress.

Antioxidant Defense Topical Treatments

Black Pepper and Turmeric Gel Caps

Ingredients:
- Turmeric powder
- Fresh ground black pepper
- "oo" gelatin or vegan capsules

Equipment:
- Gloves
- Glass dish with a flat bottom
- Spoon

Directions:

1. Put on your gloves for protection.

2. In a glass dish with a flat bottom, mix the turmeric with black pepper using a spoon. Use a ratio of approximately 2/3 cup of turmeric to about 2 teaspoons of black pepper.

3. Open a capsule and use the larger segment to push it down into the turmeric mixture. You will feel the pressure indicating that the capsule is full.

4. Slide the shorter segment of the capsule onto the filled segment until it is snug and secure.

5. Repeat the process with the remaining capsules until all are filled.

6. Store the filled capsules in a bottle or container for future use.

7. Take 1 capsule with food. Do NOT take on an empty stomach.

Herbal Body Rinse

Ingredients:

- 3 tablespoons liquid castile soap
- 3 tablespoons raw honey
- 2 tablespoons oil (e.g., 1 tablespoon each of castor oil and olive oil)
- 10 drops citrus essential oil of your choice (adjust to preference)

Directions:

1. Carefully mix all ingredients by hand using a spoon in a glass liquid measuring cup. Avoid using a blender, whisk, or hand mixer as this may create bubbles, making it difficult to pour into a container.
2. Once thoroughly mixed, pour the body wash into a preferably glass container for storage.
3. Use the homemade body wash in the shower as a luxurious and nourishing cleanser for your skin.
4. For application, consider using a natural sea sponge.

Basil and Lemon Body Rinse

Ingredients:

- 1 small handful of fresh basil leaves (torn into large pieces)
- 1 lemon, sliced
- 1-inch piece of ginger, sliced or shaved
- 2 cups water

Directions:

1. In a large pitcher, add the torn basil leaves, lemon slices, and ginger slices or shavings.
2. Using a large wooden spoon, gently muddle the basil, lemon, and ginger. Lightly press down on the ingredients to start releasing their oils.
3. Add as much water into the pitcher as desired to fill it up.
4. Place the pitcher in the refrigerator for at least a couple of hours to allow the oils to infuse into the water.
5. When ready to use, warm the water to just above room temperature, pouring the pitcher over your body in the shower or bath.

Honey and Flaxseed Hand and Face Mask

Ingredients:

- 1 tablespoon honey
- 1 tablespoon flaxseeds (soaked overnight)
- 2 teaspoons lemon juice

Method:

6. Begin by soaking the flaxseeds overnight to soften them.
7. The next day, grind the soaked flaxseeds to a paste-like consistency.
8. In a small bowl, combine the ground flaxseeds with honey and lemon juice. Mix well to form a smooth mixture.
9. Apply the mixture evenly onto your clean face, avoiding the eye area.
10. Allow the mask to dry for approximately 30 minutes.
11. After the mask has dried, gently wash it off with lukewarm water.
12. Pat your face dry with a clean towel.
13. Follow up with your favorite moisturizer to lock in hydration.

Herbal Brews and Drinks

Ginger, Cinnamon, and Lemon Shots

Ingredients:

- 1/4 cup (24g) fresh ginger, chopped
- 1/2 inch fresh turmeric
- 1 lemon, peeled, seeded, and chopped
- 2 oranges, peeled, seeded, and chopped
- A dash of ground cinnamon
- A dash of cayenne pepper
- A dash of freshly cracked black pepper

Directions:

1. Add all of the ingredients to a blender and blitz until mostly smooth.
2. Place a fine-mesh strainer over a measuring cup or bowl and pour the mixture into the strainer.
3. Use a spoon to help strain the liquid from the pulp. Discard the pulp.
4. Pour 1 oz. (30ml) of the strained liquid into a small glass and enjoy as a shot.
5. Store the remaining mixture in a glass jar in the refrigerator for future use.

Iced Green Tea and Pomegranate

Ingredients:

- 8 Green Tea Bags
- 8 cups Boiling Water
- 2 cups Pomegranate Juice
- 1 cup Pomegranate Arils
- 1 cup Sliced Strawberries

Directions:

1. Place the green tea bags in a large heatproof pitcher and pour boiling water over them.
2. Allow the tea to steep and cool to room temperature.
3. Use 2 cups of the brewed tea to make ice cubes.
4. Once the tea has cooled, add the pomegranate juice to the pitcher and stir well.
5. Refrigerate the tea until thoroughly chilled.
6. To serve, add the homemade green tea ice cubes to glasses and pour the chilled pomegranate berry tea over them.
7. Garnish each glass with a handful of pomegranate arils and sliced strawberries.

Hibiscus and Rosehip Iced Tea

Ingredients:

- 4 tablespoons rosehips
- 4 tablespoons hibiscus
- 1/2 cup raw honey
- 2 to 3 lemons
- Ice

Directions:

1. Bring 3 to 4 cups of water to a boil in a kettle or pot.
2. While the water is heating, add the rosehips and hibiscus to a metal strainer or infuser pot.
3. Once the water is almost boiling, pour it over the rosehips and hibiscus.
4. Let the tea steep for 15 minutes to allow the flavors to infuse fully.
5. After steeping, pour the tea into a large pitcher.
6. Add the raw honey to the pitcher, stirring until it dissolves completely.
7. Juice the lemons and add the lemon juice to the pitcher, stirring well to combine.
8. Add several cups of ice to the pitcher to cool down the tea and dilute it to your desired strength.
9. Stir the tea once more to ensure the ingredients are evenly distributed.
10. Serve the iced tea in glasses over ice cubes.

Beet and Carrot Shots

Ingredients:

- 1 medium beet, peeled and quartered
- 4 large carrots, washed and scrubbed or peeled
- 2 oranges, peeled
- 1 1/2-inch pieces of fresh ginger, peeled

Directions:

1. Prepare all of the juicing ingredients. Peel and quarter the beet. Wash and scrub or peel the carrots. Peel the oranges and ginger, and cut them to fit into the juicing chute.
2. Add all of the ingredients to a juicer and run them through.
3. Once juiced, pour the mixture into glasses.
4. Serve immediately and enjoy the vibrant and refreshing flavors of this beet, carrot, orange, and ginger juice!

Antioxidant Defense Recipes

Pineapple and Spirulina Breakfast Smoothie

Ingredients:

- 1 cup baby greens (spinach, kale, arugula, etc.)
- 3/4 cup frozen mango chunks or pineapple
- 1/2 cup frozen banana
- 1/2 cup cucumber or frozen zucchini
- 1/4 cup frozen avocado chunks
- 1 kiwi
- 1 tablespoon ground flaxseed
- 1/2 – 1 teaspoon spirulina powder
- 1 cup unsweetened almond milk or water

Directions:

1. Combine all ingredients in a high-powered blender.
2. Blend until smooth and creamy, ensuring all ingredients are well incorporated.
3. Pour the smoothie into glasses or a bowl.
4. Enjoy!

Walnut, Avocado, and Basil Pesto Salad

Ingredients:

- 1 ripe avocado
- 1/3 cup basil, lightly packed
- 1/4 cup raw walnuts
- 2 tablespoons grated parmesan cheese, plus extra for topping
- 2 tablespoons lemon juice
- 1 tablespoon extra virgin olive oil
- 1 clove garlic, mashed
- 1/4 - 1/2 teaspoon salt, or more to taste

Directions:

1. In a food processor, combine all ingredients. For a more textured pesto, reserve the walnuts to be added later.

2. Add walnuts toward the end of processing and pulse until they are well-incorporated and finely chopped to add some texture to the pesto.

3. Process until creamy or until the desired texture is reached.

4. Eat immediately or freeze for later use.

5. This recipe is not refrigerator-stable for more than 24 hours.

Mixed Berry Compote

Ingredients:

- 12 ounces (340g) fresh strawberries, hulled and chopped
- 12 ounces (340g) fresh blueberries
- 12 ounces (340g) fresh raspberries
- 3 tablespoons honey or stevia
- Juice of 1 lime (optional, you can start with juice of 1/2 lime)

Directions:

1. Combine the strawberries, blueberries, and raspberries in a medium saucepan or pot.

2. Add the honey or stevia and lime juice.

3. Toss to combine.

4. Bring the mixture to a boil over medium-high heat, stirring occasionally, for about 5 minutes.

5. Once the berry mixture is boiling, reduce the heat to low (the lowest setting on your stovetop).

6. Allow the berries to simmer for about 15 to 20 minutes, stirring often, until the fruit has softened considerably and the compote has reduced by about half in volume.

7. Remove the pot from the heat. At this point, you can use the back of a fork or a potato masher to mash the fruit further, if you prefer a smoother compote.

8. Taste to adjust sweetness, adding more honey or stevia if necessary.

9. Let the berry compote cool for about 15 to 30 minutes before serving. It will continue to thicken as it cools.

Anxiety Relief

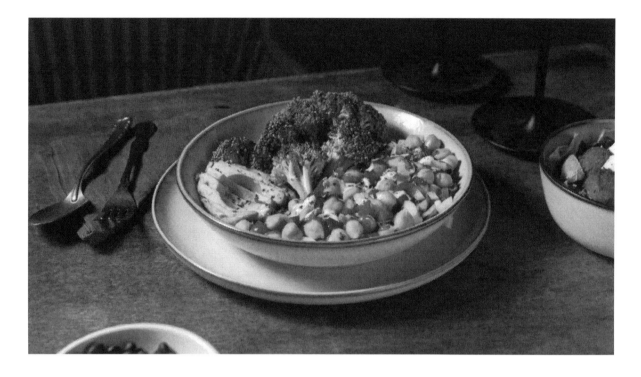

"In the midst of life's turbulent storms, let nature's gentle embrace be your anchor of tranquility." –Aria Summers

Anxiety has become an all-too-familiar companion for people but nature has provided us with everything we need to help balance our fight-or-flight response. For centuries, herbs have been revered as nature's apothecary, offering solace and comfort to those of us gripped by anxiety.

Topical Treatments

Herbal Infusion Massage Oil

Ingredients:

- 3.5 ounces (100g) Arnica and St. John's Wort flowers mixed
- 13.5 fluid ounces (400ml) Organic oil (olive, sesame, or sun-

flower)

Equipment:

- A clean and dry jar

Directions:

1. Fill a clean and dry jar with Arnica and St. John's Wort flowers.
2. Pour the organic oil (olive, sesame, or sunflower) over the flowers until they are fully submerged.
3. Seal the jar tightly and label it with the contents and date.
4. Place the jar in a dark, warm spot for 2-3 weeks to allow the flowers to infuse into the oil.
5. Shake the jar gently every day to help the infusion process.
6. After 2 to 3 weeks, strain the flowers from the oil using a fine mesh strainer or cheesecloth.
7. Store the infused oil in a dark and cool place, preferably in a glass container to preserve its quality.
8. Use a small amount of the infused oil to gently massage your body, avoiding broken skin.

Calming Bath Soak

Ingredients:

- 1/4 cup Epsom salt
- 1 tablespoon of Dead Sea salt (or pink Himalayan salt)
- 5 drops of lavender essential oil
- 5 drops of chamomile essential oil

Directions:

1. Fill a basin or foot tub with warm water.
2. Add the Epsom salt and the Dead Sea salt (or pink Himalayan salt) to the water.
3. Drop in the lavender and chamomile essential oils.
4. Stir the mixture gently to ensure the salts and oils are well combined.
5. Soak your feet in the warm foot bath for 15-20 minutes, allowing the calming properties of the lavender and chamomile to relax your senses and soothe your feet.
6. After soaking, pat your feet dry with a towel and moisturize if desired.

Anxiety Relief Balm

Ingredients:

- 45 mL (1.5 fl oz) lavender-infused coconut oil or olive oil (or a mixture of both)
- 3.5-4.5 g (0.12 -0.16 oz) beeswax
- 14 drops total of calming essential oil(s) of choice:
- Lavender
- Neroli
- Sweet orange
- Vetiver
- Sweet basil
- Lemon verbena
- German chamomile
- Rose geranium
- Rose otto
- Metal salve tins

Directions:

1. Over low heat, warm coconut and/or olive oil in a double-boiler reserved specifically for cosmetic projects.
2. Add the beeswax, warming until just melted.
3. Remove the double boiler from heat.
4. Add the calming essential oils, stir well, and swiftly pour the mixture into tins before it hardens.
5. Label the tins accordingly and let them cool completely.
6. Apply the balm to your temples as needed.
7. Take a deep breath and feel the relaxing effects of this soothing balm wash over you.

Soothing Oatmeal Mask

Ingredients:

- Whole rolled oats
- Whole or 2% milk
- Cinnamon (optional)

Recipe:

8. Measure 1 tablespoon of whole rolled oats into a mixing bowl.
9. Add 2 tablespoons of milk.
10. Sprinkle in 1/4 teaspoon of cinnamon (optional).
11. Stir well until the mixture is smooth and even.

How To Apply:

12. Wash your face, neck, and décolleté with warm water and an oil-free cleanser to remove makeup and open pores.
13. Apply the oatmeal mixture to your face, neck, and décolleté, spreading it evenly.
14. Let the mask sit for twenty minutes to allow the ingredients to work their magic.
15. After twenty minutes, wash off.

Passionflower Gel Caps

Ingredients:

- Passionflower powder
- "00" gelatin or vegan capsules

Equipment:

- Gloves
- Glass dish with a flat bottom
- Spoon

Directions:

1. Put on your gloves for protection.
2. In a glass dish with a flat bottom, pour your passionflower powder.
3. Open a capsule and use the larger segment to push it down into the passionflower mixture.
4. Continue filling the capsule until the powder is compacted into it. You will feel the pressure indicating that the capsule is full.
5. Slide the shorter segment of the capsule onto the filled segment until it is snug and secure.
6. Repeat the process with the remaining capsules until all are filled.
7. Store the filled capsules in a bottle or container for future use.
8. Take 1 capsule with food. Do NOT take on an empty stomach.

Herbal Brews

Lavender and Chamomile Tea

Ingredients:

- 1 teaspoon dried chamomile or 1 tablespoon fresh chamomile
- 1/2 teaspoon dried lavender or 1 1/2 teaspoons fresh lavender
- 1/2 teaspoon dried mint or 1 1/2 teaspoons coarsely chopped fresh mint
- 1 cup boiling water

Directions:

1. Combine the chamomile, lavender, and mint in a teapot or heatproof pitcher.
2. Pour the boiling water over the herbs.
3. Let the mixture steep for 15 minutes to allow the flavors to infuse.
4. Strain the tea into cups or mugs, discarding the herbs.
5. Serve and enjoy the soothing and relaxing herbal tea.

Passionflower and Mint Tea

Ingredients:

- 8 ounces (240ml) of boiling water
- 1 teaspoon of dried passionflower leaves (or 1 tablespoon fresh)
- 1/2 teaspoon dried mint

Directions:

1. Place the dried passionflower leaves (or fresh leaves, if using) in a muslin bag or tea infuser.
2. Pour the boiling water over the passionflower leaves and add the dried mint to the hot water.
3. Let the mixture steep for about five minutes to allow the flavors to infuse.
4. Remove the muslin bag or tea infuser containing the herbs.
5. Enjoy this herbal tea about an hour before bedtime.
6. Limit yourself to one cup within a 24-hour period.

Rose and Lavender Iced Tea

Ingredients:

- 1/2 cup (120ml) water
- 1/3 cup honey
- 1 teaspoon fresh lavender
- 2 black tea bags
- 1/2 teaspoon rose water

Directions:

1. In a pot, combine water, honey, and fresh lavender.
2. Bring to a boil and simmer for about 8-10 minutes until the mixture has reduced.
3. Remove from heat and let cool until thickened, approximately 15 minutes.
4. Boil 2 cups of water in a pot.
5. Add rose water and black tea bags to the boiling water.
6. Steep until the tea is dark and fully infused.
7. Add one tablespoon of lavender syrup to the bottom of your glass.
8. Pour 1 cup of brewed black tea over the syrup.
9. Stir well and enjoy immediately.

Peppermint Calming Tea

Ingredients:

- 1/2 cup dry peppermint leaf
- 3 - 4 cups very hot water
- 2 - 3 tablespoons honey

Directions:

1. Boil about 3 or 4 cups of water in a kettle or pot.
2. Once the water reaches a boil, turn off the heat.
3. Add the peppermint leaves to the hot water.
4. Let the tea steep for about 5 minutes to infuse the flavor.
5. Pour the tea through a tea strainer to remove the peppermint leaves.
6. Stir in honey to sweeten, adjusting to taste.
7. Pour the tea into cups and serve immediately.

Anxiety Relief Recipes

Omega-3 Rich Smoothie

Ingredients:

- 2 cups purchased unsweetened almond milk
- 1/2 medium banana
- 1 tablespoon maple syrup, plus more to taste
- 2 cups mixed berries, frozen
- 1 teaspoon chia seeds
- 1 teaspoon ground flaxseeds
- 1 teaspoon shelled hemp seeds
- 1/4 teaspoon ground cinnamon, plus more to taste

Directions:

1. Pour 2 cups of unsweetened almond milk into a blender.
2. Add 1/2 medium banana and 1 tablespoon of maple syrup.
3. Blend until the mixture swirls easily inside the blender.
4. Add 2 cups of frozen mixed Driscoll's Berries.
5. Blend until the mixture swirls easily inside the blender.
6. Add 1 teaspoon of chia seeds, 1 teaspoon of ground flaxseeds, 1 teaspoon of shelled hemp seeds, and 1/4 teaspoon of ground cinnamon.
7. Blend until smooth and well combined.

Grounding Ashwagandha Smoothie

Ingredients:

- 1 medium banana
- 300 ml (10 fl oz) plant milk of choice
- 2 teaspoons ashwagandha powder
- 1 teaspoon maca powder
- 1/4 teaspoon cinnamon powder
- Pinch of ginger powder
- 1 tablespoon almond butter
- 1 heaped teaspoon apricot puree (made from dried apricots)
- 2 tablespoons gluten-free oat flakes

Directions:

1. Soak a handful of dried apricots overnight in enough water to cover them.
2. Without draining, blend the soaked apricots in a blender to form a paste.
3. Store the apricot puree in the fridge for up to a week.
4. Pour the plant milk into a blender or smoothie maker.
5. Add the banana, ashwagandha powder, maca powder, cinnamon powder, ginger powder, almond butter, apricot puree, and gluten-free oat flakes.
6. Blend until smooth and well combined.
7. Serve immediately and enjoy this nutritious and energizing smoothie.

Warm Brussel Sprouts Salad

Ingredients:

- 3 tablespoons olive oil
- 3 tablespoons fresh lemon juice
- 1-2 teaspoons pure maple syrup
- 1 teaspoon Dijon mustard
- 1 clove garlic, minced
- 1/2 teaspoon salt
- Freshly ground black pepper
- 1/2 cup raw hazelnuts, chopped (raw pecans or almonds would

also work well)

- 1 tablespoon olive oil
- 1 pound Brussels sprouts, washed, stems removed, and roughly chopped or shredded

- 1/2 cup shaved Parmesan cheese
- Optional: 1/3 cup dried cranberries, dried cherries, or dried blueberries

Directions:

1. In a medium bowl, whisk together the olive oil, lemon juice, maple syrup, Dijon mustard, minced garlic, salt, and freshly ground black pepper. Set aside.

2. Place a large skillet over medium-low heat. Add the chopped hazelnuts and toast for 2-3 minutes until golden brown and fragrant. Remove from the skillet and set aside.

3. Add 1 tablespoon of olive oil to the skillet and increase the heat to medium-high. Stir in the Brussels sprouts and sauté for a few minutes until they begin to turn golden brown.

4. Reduce the heat to low and add the prepared dressing, shaved Parmesan cheese, and cooked bacon to the skillet with the Brussels sprouts. Stir well to combine and cook for a few more minutes until the cheese melts and the flavors meld together.

5. Serve the Brussels sprouts salad immediately and enjoy!

Anxiety-Relieving Quinoa Avocado Salad

Ingredients:

- 1 1/2 cups cooked quinoa (red or tricolor)
- 2 small avocados diced
- Juice of 1 lime
- 2 mini cucumbers, diced
- 1/3 cup chopped cilantro

- 1/3 cup chopped red onion
- 1 jalapeño, thinly sliced with seeds
- 1 teaspoon extra virgin olive oil
- 1/4 teaspoon kosher salt, plus more to taste

Directions:

1. Combine all the ingredients together in a bowl and eat right away.

2. Taste for salt and lime juice, and adjust as needed.

3. If meal prepping, combine all the ingredients except for the avocado, and add when ready to eat.

4. Multiply the recipe for more servings.

Auto-Immune Support

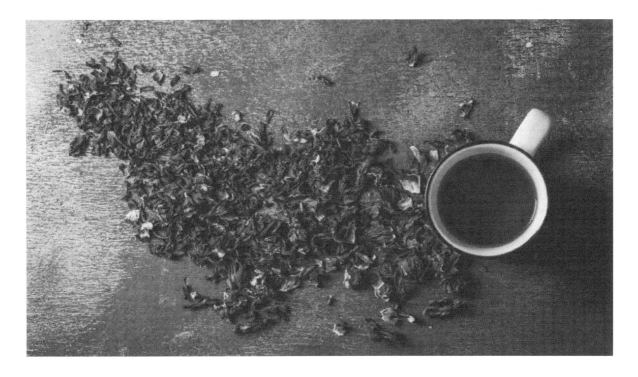

"In the tapestry of life, our immune system is the thread that weaves resilience and vitality into every cell. When this delicate balance falters, nature's herbal allies stand ready to gently guide us back to harmony." –Ava Woodley

The immune system defends our bodies from external threats and illnesses, helping to not only fight off harmful pathogens but also set off the healing process within us. For some though, the immune system can become misguided, turning it on the body that houses it. Auto-immune disease is on the rise, especially in a world that is filled with triggers and stressors. We need to find ways to balance our defensive systems, directing them toward balance using nature's gifts.

Topical Treatments

Thyme Body Wash

Ingredients:

- 1/3 cup (80 ml) liquid castile soap
- 1/3 cup (113 g) raw honey
- 1/3 cup (79 ml) carrier oil (such as olive oil, jojoba oil, refined avo-cado oil, fractionated coconut oil, or sweet almond oil)
- 30-60 drops of thyme essential oil

Directions:

1. Combine all ingredients in a bowl and mix thoroughly until well combined. Alternatively, place ingredients in a blender and blend until thoroughly mixed.
2. Pour the mixture into a squeeze-top or pump-top soap dispenser.
3. Shake the bottle well before each use.
4. Dispense a small amount onto a soft natural sponge, loofah sponge, or washcloth.
5. Use the body wash as you would any commercial body wash, lathering and cleansing your skin thoroughly.

Soothing Green Tea Facial and Skin Mist

Ingredients:

- 6 ounces (177 ml) distilled water
- 1 teaspoon loose green tea leaves or 1 green tea bag
- 3 drops lavender oil
- 3 drops aloe vera gel

Directions:

1. Brew a 6-ounce (177 ml) cup of strong green tea and let it cool. For UK measurements, brew a cup with approximately 170 grams of distilled water.
2. Once cooled, add 3 drops of lavender essential oil and 3 drops of aloe vera gel to the tea. Stir well using a sterile instrument.
3. Transfer the mixture into a sterilized spray bottle. Remember to shake well before each use.
4. Store the bottle in the refrigerator to maintain freshness. Optionally, you can include a drop of vitamin E oil for added preservation.

Anti-Inflammatory Comfrey Balm

Ingredients:

- 10 drops German chamomile (Matricaria recutita) essential oil
- 10 drops peppermint (Mentha piperita) essential oil
- 4 drops lavender (Lavandula angustifolia) essential oil
- 7 tablespoons comfrey-infused oil
- 1 to 2 tablespoons beeswax pastilles or flakes (use the greater amount for a firmer balm)
- One 4-ounce dark glass or plastic jar

Directions:

1. In a very small saucepan over low heat or in a double boiler, combine the comfrey-infused oil with the beeswax.
2. Warm the mixture until the beeswax is just melted.
3. Remove from heat and allow to cool for 5 minutes, stirring occasionally.
4. Add the German chamomile, peppermint, and lavender essential oils to the mixture.
5. Stir thoroughly to blend all ingredients evenly.
6. Slowly pour the liquid balm into the 4-ounce jar.
7. Securely cap the jar, label it, and set it aside for 30 minutes to allow it to thicken.
8. No refrigeration is necessary. Store the balm at room temperature, away from heat and light. Use within 1 year.

Whipped Magnesium Body Butter

Ingredients:

- 1/4 cup (60 ml) coconut oil
- 1/2 cup (120 ml) shea butter or cocoa butter (mango butter can also be used)
- 1/4 cup (60 ml) magnesium oil
- 15 drops lavender essential oil
- 5 drops frankincense essential oil

Directions:

1. Measure the coconut oil and shea butter (or cocoa butter) into a double boiler. If you don't have a double boiler, you can use a heat-safe bowl placed over a pot of simmering water.
2. Gently heat the oils until they are melted, ensuring not to overheat and damage the oils.
3. Once melted, remove the mixture from the heat source. Let it cool at room temperature until it starts to become cloudy.
4. Add the magnesium oil and the essential oils (you can use any essential oils of your preference).
5. Transfer the mixture to a stand mixer or whip it by hand.
6. Place the mixture in the refrigerator until it reaches a semi-solid state. It should still be soft enough to press your finger into but not completely solid or runny.
7. Once the mixture reaches the desired consistency, whip it again using a stand mixer until it becomes super fluffy and soft.
8. Scoop the whipped body butter into a container for storage. A mason jar with a sealing lid works well to keep it fresh.
9. If your home is warm and the body butter begins to soften too much, store it in the refrigerator to maintain its fluffy texture. Otherwise, it can be kept at room temperature.

Herbal Brews

Parsley and Ginger Health Shots

Ingredients:

- 1 piece of fresh ginger, approximately 4-5 cm long
- Juice of 1 lime
- 1 kiwi
- 20 spinach leaves
- 1 handful of flat parsley leaves (adjust to taste)
- 1 teaspoon honey
- 1 pinch of black pepper

Directions:

1. Prepare all the ingredients. If possible, opt for organic products. Roughly chop the ginger. Wash the spinach leaves and parsley.
2. In a blender, combine the chopped ginger, lime juice, peeled kiwi, spinach leaves, parsley, honey, and a pinch of black pepper.
3. Blend the ingredients for about 30 seconds or until a smooth and homogeneous liquid is obtained. If the mixture is too thick, you can add a little water or more lime juice for those who enjoy extra tanginess.
4. Once blended, strain the mixture using a fine sieve or cheesecloth placed over a container to collect the liquid.
5. Your parsley and ginger shot is now ready to be enjoyed!

Matcha Anti Inflammatory Tonic

Ingredients:

- 475 ml (2 cups) water, plus 30 ml (2 tablespoons), divided
- 4 sprigs fresh thyme
- 1 (5 cm) piece of ginger, peeled and sliced
- 1 teaspoon turmeric powder
- 45 ml (3 tablespoons) honey
- 15 ml (1 tablespoon) apple cider vinegar
- 60 ml (¼ cup) fresh lemon juice
- 2-3 teaspoons matcha, sifted
- 355 ml (1 ½ cups) chilled sparkling water
- Ice

Directions:

1. In a small saucepan over medium heat, combine 475 ml (2 cups) of water, thyme, ginger, turmeric, honey, apple cider vinegar, and lemon juice.
2. Allow the mixture to simmer for 5 minutes, then remove from heat.
3. Let it cool to room temperature.
4. In a small bowl, combine the sifted matcha with the remaining 30 ml (2 tablespoons) of water.
5. To a tall glass, add 120 ml (½ cup) of the cooled lemon mixture. Add ice to the glass.
6. Pour the chilled sparkling water over the ice in the glass.
7. Top the drink with the matcha shot.
8. Stir well before enjoying.
9. Serve and enjoy your sparkling turmeric-ginger matcha lemonade for gut health!

Lemon and Turmeric Shot

Ingredients:

- 3 large lemons*
- 22 ml (3/4 fl oz) fresh turmeric (approximately 3 inches)
- 60 ml (1/4 cup) water
- 1/4 teaspoon ground peppercorn

Directions:

1. Squeeze the lemons to extract the juice, then pour the juice into a blender.
2. Add the fresh turmeric, water, and ground peppercorn to the blender with the lemon juice.
3. Blend the ingredients until everything is fully combined and smooth.
4. Pour the mixture into a shot glass.
5. Consume one shot daily before breakfast.
6. Store any remaining shots in a bottle in the refrigerator for up to 5 days.
7. Adjust the amount of lemon juice according to the size and juiciness of the lemons.

Rosehip Tea

Ingredients:

- ½ cup (A handful of) rosehip
- 5 or 6 cups of water
- 1 tablespoon honey

Directions:

1. Pour water into a saucepan with a lid or a teapot. Add the rosehips to the water.
2. Place the lid on the saucepan or teapot.
3. Bring the water to a boil, then reduce the heat to medium-low. Let it simmer for 15-20 minutes or until the tea has a nice color and taste.
4. Serve the rosehip tea in cups, sweetened with a little honey.
5. If you prefer to drink it cold, pour the tea into a jug, mix in the honey, and chill it in the refrigerator until cold.
6. Enjoy your refreshing rosehip tea hot or cold!

Peppermint Green Tea

Ingredients:

- 120 ml (1/2 cup) fresh mint leaves
- 3 green tea bags
- 2 tablespoons honey
- 960 ml (4 cups) boiling water
- 4 stalks lemongrass, for garnish

Directions:

1. In a large heatproof pitcher or container, combine the fresh mint leaves, green tea bags, honey, and boiling water.
2. Allow the mixture to steep for 5 minutes. Then, remove the tea bags.
3. Refrigerate the tea until chilled.
4. Once chilled, divide the tea among 4 large ice-filled glasses.
5. Garnish each glass with a stalk of lemongrass.
6. Serve and enjoy your refreshing peppermint iced green tea!

Autoimmune Foods

Functional Food Smoothie

Ingredients:

- 240 ml (1 cup) unsweetened almond milk
- 1 frozen banana, sliced
- 1/4 inch piece of fresh ginger (peeled and sliced)
- 1/4 inch piece of fresh turmeric (peeled and sliced)
- 1/4 teaspoon ground cinnamon
- 1/2 teaspoon chia seeds
- 1/2 teaspoon flax seeds
- 240 ml (1 cup) fresh baby spinach

Directions:

1. Place all ingredients in the blender.
2. Blend for several minutes until very smooth.
3. Pour into a glass and drink up.
4. Enjoy your nutritious and delicious anti-inflammatory smoothie!

Greens and Berries Smoothie

Ingredients:

- 3 small bananas
- 120 ml (1/2 cup) milk
- 1–2 handfuls of spinach
- 140 g (1 cup) frozen berries (blueberries, blackberries, etc.)
- 60 g (1/2 cup) bran cereal such as All Bran original
- 15-30 ml (1–2 tablespoons) sweetener (honey or agave)
- Ice cubes (optional)

Directions:

1. Blend bananas and milk until smooth.
2. Add spinach and blend on a high setting until most of the spinach has been broken down into small pieces.
3. Add the frozen berries and blend until the smoothie mixture is all one color.
4. Add the bran and sweetener; blend until desired consistency.
5. Add ice cubes and blend again until smooth (optional – I usually don't).
6. Enjoy

Lemon and Asparagus Chicken Skillet

Ingredients:

- 680 grams (1 ½ pounds) chicken breast (2 to 3 large chicken breasts)
- Kosher salt
- Black pepper
- 1 tablespoon homemade Italian seasoning (or quality store-bought)
- 1 teaspoon sweet paprika
- 65 grams (½ cup) all-purpose flour, or more as needed
- Extra virgin olive oil
- 454 grams (1 pound) fresh asparagus, hard ends trimmed, cut on the diagonal into 2-inch pieces
- 4 garlic cloves, minced
- 120 ml (½ cup) white wine
- 1 lemon, juiced
- 120 ml (½ cup) homemade chicken broth (or low-sodium store-bought)

Directions:

1. Place each chicken breast half on a cutting board.
2. Place your non-dominant hand on top of the chicken to keep it from moving.
3. Using a good chef's knife, carefully slice the chicken horizontally down the middle so that you end up with two thinner chicken cutlets. (If the chicken is still uneven, you can pound it briefly until you have cutlets that are about ¼-inch thick).
4. Season the chicken on both sides with Italian seasoning, sweet paprika, and a big pinch of salt and pepper.
5. Place the flour in a shallow dish.
6. Turn the chicken in the flour to lightly coat on both sides.
7. Give it a gentle shake to remove excess and set it aside for now.
8. In a large pan with a lid, heat about 2 tablespoons of olive oil over medium-high until shimmering.
9. Add the asparagus and season with a big pinch of salt and pepper.
10. Sauté, tossing occasionally, until just tender, 3 to 5 minutes.
11. Use a pair of tongs to transfer the asparagus to a plate for now.
12. To the same pan over medium-high, add a drizzle more olive oil.
13. When it's fully shimmering, add the chicken and sear until golden.
14. Flip and sear until the other side is golden, about 3 minutes per side.
15. Add the garlic and push it around until fragrant, about 30 seconds.
16. Add the white wine and allow it to reduce by about half, then add the lemon juice and chicken broth.
17. Turn the heat down to low and cover the pan.
18. Cook for about 7 to 8 minutes, or until the chicken is cooked through.
19. Turn the heat off and tuck the asparagus in between the chicken pieces to allow it to warm through.
20. Serve immediately.

Sweet Potato Popper Snacks

Ingredients:

- 454 grams (1 pound) sweet potatoes, peeled and cut into large pieces
- 60 ml (1/4 cup) unsweetened plant milk, such as almond, soy, cashew, or rice
- 60 ml (1/4 cup) nutritional yeast
- 30 ml (2 tablespoons) white wine vinegar
- 1/2 teaspoon ground turmeric
- Sea salt, to taste
- Freshly ground black pepper, to taste
- 7 fresh jalapeño chiles, halved lengthwise and seeded (keep stems attached)

Directions:

1. Preheat oven to 200°C (400°F).
2. Line a baking sheet with parchment paper.
3. Place sweet potato pieces in a steamer basket in a large saucepan. Add water to just below the steamer basket. Bring to a boil. Steam, covered, for about 10 minutes or until sweet potatoes are very tender. Transfer sweet potatoes to a bowl. Let cool and mash.
4. In a small saucepan, whisk together milk, yeast, vinegar, and turmeric. Bring to a boil. Cook for 1 minute or until the mixture thickens.
5. Transfer the milk mixture and mashed sweet potatoes to a blender. Blend until smooth. Season with salt and black pepper.
6. Spoon sweet potato mixture into jalapeño halves.
7. Place on the prepared baking sheet.
8. Bake for 30 minutes or until lightly browned on the edges.
9. Enjoy your delicious sweet potato poppers!

Vegan AIP Chocolate Moose

Ingredients:

- 1 ripe avocado
- 470 ml (2 cups) coconut cream, or the thick part of a can of full-fat coconut milk
- 3 tablespoons cacao powder
- 60 ml (1/4 cup) pure maple syrup, + more if you like it really sweet!
- Raspberries
- Coconut cream

Directions:

1. Combine all of the ingredients in a large bowl.
2. Use a hand mixer to beat everything until stiff peaks form.
3. Divide the mixture between 4 ramekins.
4. Top with coconut cream, raspberries, and chocolate shavings.
5. Enjoy your delicious paleo vegan chocolate mousse!

Blood Health

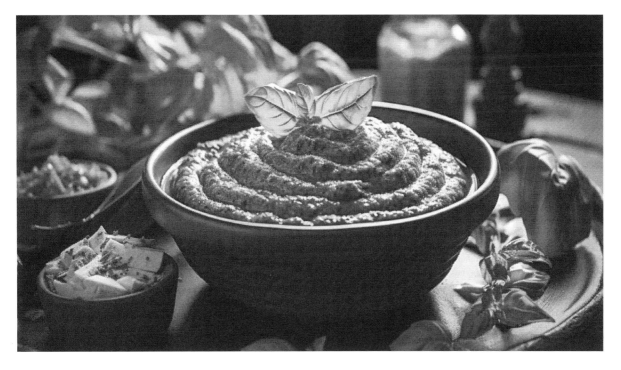

"In the vibrant river of life that flows within us, our blood holds the key to nourishment, vitality, and the very essence of our being." –Dr. Amara Noel

Our blood is the life-giving elixir that courses through our veins, carrying nourishment, oxygen, and vital essence to every cell in our bodies. Modern processed foods, environmental toxins, and the stresses of daily life, however, reduce our optimal blood health, leaving us feeling depleted and out of balance. While herbs alone cannot improve our blood health, adding natural remedies to our daily diets and cutting out processed foods can restore us to health and well-being.

Topical Treatments

Circulation Bath Soak

Ingredients:

- 60 ml (1/4 cup) red clay
- 240 ml (1 cup) Epsom salt
- 240 ml (1 cup) baking soda
- 60 ml (1/4 cup) sweet almond oil
- 10 drops juniper berry essential oil
- 1 small carnelian gemstone (optional)

Directions:

1. Put all the ingredients except for the carnelian gemstone in a bowl and mix with a wooden spoon.
2. Add the carnelian gemstone to the mixture to infuse into the salt (optional).
3. Store the mixture in a glass jar with a lid and label.
4. To use your bath soak, draw a warm bath, placing a handful of the mixture into the water to dissolve, leaving the gemstone in the jar.
5. Soak for 20 minutes.
6. Keep in mind that pigmented clays can stain white towels, robes, and rugs, so plan accordingly.
7. Gently pat your skin dry.

Garlic and Hot Pepper Pulse Balm

Ingredients:

- 120 ml (1/2 cup) olive oil (garlic infused)
- 30 ml (2 tablespoons) cayenne powder (or 15 grams)
- 14 grams (1/2 ounce) beeswax
- 4-ounce tins or jars

Directions:

1. Begin by combining the cayenne and olive oil in a double boiler or a pan on very low heat.
2. Heat the oil and cayenne until it is warm, turn off the heat, and let it sit (warmly) for about 20 minutes, then turn the heat on again.
3. Repeat this process for at least one hour to a couple of hours.
4. Once the cayenne and olive oil have been infused, strain off the powder through a cheesecloth.
5. Reserve the infused oil.
6. Heat the beeswax until it is melted.
7. Stir in the infused oil until the beeswax and oil have been thoroughly melted together and combined.
8. Immediately pour this mixture into jars or tins.
9. Let it cool and then label it.

Rosemary and Lime Foot Soak

Ingredients:

- 3 sprigs Rosemary, fresh or dried
- 2 Limes, sliced
- 120 grams (1/2 cup) Epsom Salt
- 120 grams (1/2 cup) Baking Soda

Directions:

1. Bring a large pot of water to a boil.
2. Add in rosemary and allow it to boil for 5 minutes, allowing the rosemary to infuse into the water.
3. Remove from heat.
4. In a large container big enough to fit your feet into, layer sliced limes onto the bottom.
5. Then, sprinkle in Epsom salt and baking soda.
6. Pour the hot water with rosemary into the container and allow it to cool enough so you can put your feet into the container without burning them.
7. Soak your feet in the mixture for 15 – 30 minutes.
8. Enjoy your relaxing and detoxifying foot soak with rosemary and lime!

Herbal Brews

Warm Ginger and Cayenne Pepper Tea

Ingredients:

- Juice of half a lemon
- 15 ml (1 tablespoon) honey
- 1/4 teaspoon cayenne pepper (can use up to 1/2 tsp if you want the heat)
- 1 tablespoon fresh ginger
- 240 ml (1 cup) water

Directions:

1. Boil water.
2. Peel and chop ginger into fine pieces.
3. Add lemon juice, honey, cayenne pepper, and ginger to a mug.
4. Top with boiling water and let steep for five to ten minutes, until the ginger is strong and aromatic.
5. Stir well and enjoy while flipping through your favorite magazine

Hawthorn Berry Herbal Tincture

Equipment:

- Rolling pin
- Large ziplock bag
- Glass jar
- Fine mesh sieve
- Muslin
- Dark glass bottle
- Funnels
- Dropper bottles

Ingredients:

- 240 ml (1 cup) fresh hawthorn berries or 177 ml (3/4 cup) dried
- 473 ml (2 cups) Vodka (40-50% alcohol)

Directions:

1. Pick the red berries from hawthorn trees in autumn. Choose plump red berries in an area away from traffic. Alternatively, purchase fresh berries.

2. Remove the leaves and brittle stems and rinse the berries to remove dust and other impurities. Allow to drip dry in a strainer or sieve. They can still be a little moist for the next step.

3. Place the berries in a ziplock bag and then roll over them with a rolling pin. This opens the berries but doesn't crush the seeds inside. You should avoid crushing the seeds when making hawthorn tincture.

4. Empty the crushed hawthorn berries into a glass jar. Pour the vodka over them, seal tightly with a lid, then shake for about a minute.

5. Store the jar in a dark and cool (to room temperature) place such as a kitchen cupboard. Leave it to infuse for two to four weeks. Shake the jar every couple of days. As the soluble components of hawthorn extract into the vodka, the berries lose their color.

6. After the allocated time has passed, strain the hawthorn tincture through a muslin laid over a fine mesh strainer to remove the berries.

7. Get every last drop of tincture that you can from the berries. Gather the muslin up and squeeze as much liquid out as you can. Afterward, discard the berries.

8. Pour the tincture through a funnel and into a dark glass bottle. Label it with the type of tincture and the date made, and store it in a cool to room temperature place out of direct sunlight. It has a shelf-life of about two years.

Dosage: Adults typically use 2 ml (a few drops) daily.

Gold Milk Evening Drink

Ingredients:

- 480 ml (2 cups) milk (dairy or dairy-free)
- 5 ml (1 teaspoon) ground turmeric
- 1.25 ml (1/4 teaspoon) ground cinnamon

  Optional:
- 7.5 ml (1/2 tablespoon) coconut oil
- Additional spices or flavors such as ginger, cardamom, or vanilla

- Pinch of black pepper
- 15 ml (1 tablespoon) maple syrup or honey

  extract

Directions:

1. Add all ingredients to a saucepan over medium heat and bring to a simmer.

2. Simmer for 10 minutes to let the flavors meld.

3. Pour the golden milk into a cup and enjoy.

Turmeric Zinger Shots

Ingredients:

- 120 ml (1/2 cup) unsweetened cherry juice
- 120 ml (1/2 cup) apple cider vinegar
- 1 thumb-sized piece of ginger, sliced

- 15 ml (3 teaspoons) turmeric dried spice
- 2.5 ml (1/2 teaspoon) cayenne, or to taste

Directions:

1. Place everything in a blender and blend until smooth.

2. Pour into a small mason jar with a lid. The ginger and spice tend to separate, so give it a shake before your morning shot.

3. Take about an ounce after your morning coffee and morning practices, a few minutes before breakfast.

4. Enjoy your invigorating turmeric zinger shots!

Beet Berry Juice

Ingredients:

- 1 medium beet
- 1/4 of a lemon, peeled
- 1/2 inch piece of fresh ginger, peeled

- 480 ml (2 cups) kale, chopped
- 170 grams (6 ounces) blueberries

Directions:

1. Cut the leafy tops off 1 medium beet and scrub it clean, but do not remove the peel.

2. Cut the beet into quarters and place it into the juicer hopper.

3. Add 1/4 of 1 peeled lemon.

4. Add a ½-inch piece of peeled fresh ginger.

5. Add 2 cups of chopped kale.

6. Add 1 package (6 ounces) of blueberries.

7. Juice the ingredients into a tall drinking glass.

8. Serve immediately.

9. Enjoy your refreshing beet berry juice!

Blood Health Food

Nut and Seed Trail Mix

Ingredients:

- 180 grams (1 1/2 cups) raw nuts (e.g., almonds, pecans, cashews, peanuts, etc.)
- 140 grams (1 cup) raw seeds (e.g., sunflower seeds, pumpkin seeds, etc.)
- 140 grams (1 cup) of unsweetened, unsulphured dried fruit
- Fun stuff (amounts vary) e.g., 70 grams (1/2 cup) of chopped dark chocolate
- 1/4 teaspoon sea salt
- 1/2 teaspoon cinnamon
- Pinch of nutmeg (optional)

Directions:

1. Preheat the oven to 175°C (350°F).
2. Combine all ingredients in a large bowl and mix well.
3. Spread the mixture evenly on a baking sheet lined with parchment paper.
4. Bake in the preheated oven for 10-15 minutes, stirring occasionally, until lightly toasted.
5. Remove from the oven and let cool completely.
6. Store in a ziploc bag or mason jar.
7. Will keep for up to 1 month.

Optional: If you really need the extra sweetness, you can coat the mix with 30 ml (2 tablespoons) maple syrup, spread it out on a baking sheet, and allow it to dry before bagging.

Garlic and Lemon Salad Dressing

Ingredients:

- 1 small clove garlic
- 15 ml (1 tablespoon) fresh lemon juice
- 2.5 ml (1/2 teaspoon) finely grated lemon zest, optional
- 2.5 ml (1/2 teaspoon) sea salt, more to taste
- 1.25 ml (1/4 teaspoon) freshly ground black pepper, more to taste
- 1.25 ml (1/4 teaspoon) ground mustard
- 30 to 45 ml (2 to 3 tablespoons) extra-virgin olive oil, or lemon-infused olive oil
- 85 grams (3 ounces) salad greens

Directions:

1. Peel and mince the garlic (you can use a garlic press if you like; presses tend to bring out the bitterness in garlic, but some people don't seem to notice it).
2. If you're making a salad in the next few hours, put the garlic in a large salad bowl. (If you're making the dressing ahead of time, put the garlic in a sealable jar.)
3. Add the lemon juice, lemon zest, salt, pepper, and mustard.
4. Whisk to combine everything (or seal and shake the jar).
5. Whisk in the olive oil (or, again, seal the jar and shake it vigorously).
6. Taste and adjust salt and pepper to taste.
7. If the dressing is too zingy for you, feel free to add more olive oil to soften the flavor.
8. A bit more salt will help temper the acid kick, too.
9. Use the vinaigrette-style dressing immediately.
10. If you've made the dressing in the salad bowl, just add the greens to that big bowl and toss.

Kale and Quinoa Salad with Garlic and Lemon Salad Dressing

Ingredients:

- 1 cup quinoa, rinsed and drained
- 2 cups vegetable broth
- Pinch of salt
- 1/4 cup tahini
- 3 tablespoons olive oil
- 2 tablespoons apple cider vinegar
- 1 teaspoon sugar
- 1 teaspoon hot sauce (optional)

- 2 cloves garlic, minced
- 2 lemons, zested and juiced
- Salt and pepper, to taste
- 1 bunch kale, tough stems removed and leaves cut into ribbons
- 1/2 red onion, finely chopped
- 1/2 cup sunflower seeds
- 1/4 cup chopped fresh parsley

Directions:

1. Combine quinoa, broth, and a pinch of salt in a saucepan.
2. Bring to a boil, cover, and reduce the heat to a simmer.
3. Cook, without stirring, until all liquid is absorbed, about 15 minutes.
4. Remove from the heat and allow to sit, covered, for 10 additional minutes.
5. Fluff grains with a fork.
6. Combine tahini, olive oil, vinegar, sugar, hot sauce, garlic, lemon zest, lemon juice, salt, and pepper in a large bowl.
7. Stir in kale; gently mix with a wooden spoon or massage with your hands so that the kale breaks down.
8. Add onions, sunflower seeds, parsley, and reserved quinoa; mix to combine.

Mushroom and Veggie Stir Fry

Ingredients:

- 2 cloves garlic (minced // 2 cloves yield ~1 tablespoon)
- 2 teaspoons minced ginger
- 3-4 tablespoons maple syrup (or agave nectar or coconut sugar)
- 1/2 teaspoon red pepper flake (more or less to taste)
- 3-4 tablespoons tamari (or soy sauce if not gluten-free // more or less to taste)
- 1 tablespoon sesame oil (toasted or untoasted)
  Optional:
- 4 cups cooked brown rice or cauliflower rice

- 3 tablespoons lime juice
- 1 tablespoon water
- 2 portobello mushrooms (~20 grams each)
- 1 medium red bell pepper (thinly sliced)
- 1 cup chopped broccolini
- 1 cup chopped green onion (optional)

- 1 teaspoon sesame seeds

Directions:

1. Cook rice (or cauliflower rice) if serving with stir-fry.
2. Next, wipe portobello mushrooms clean with a slightly damp towel (do not immerse in water or they will get soggy) and slice into thin strips.
3. Prepare marinade by adding all ingredients to a small mixing bowl and whisking to combine.
4. Taste and adjust flavor as needed.
5. Add portobello mushrooms to a large shallow dish and top with marinade.
6. Gently stir/toss to combine.
7. Set aside to marinate for 10-12 minutes.
8. Chop vegetables and set aside.
9. Once portobellos have marinated, heat a large skillet over medium heat and add a bit of sesame oil.
10. Then add only as many portobellos as will fit comfortably in the pan and sauté for 2-4 minutes on each side or until golden brown and slightly seared.
11. Set portobellos aside and loosely cover to keep warm.
12. Then add red pepper and broccolini to the pan and increase heat to medium-high.
13. Sauté for 2-3 minutes, stirring frequently.
14. Add the green onion (optional) and any remaining portobello marinade and toss to coat.
15. Cook for 1 minute.
16. Then remove from heat and serve immediately.
17. Enjoy as is or with chili garlic sauce, sesame seeds, or a garnish of chopped green onion.
18. Best when fresh, though leftovers keep in the refrigerator up to 2-3 days.

Balsamic Sauteed Spinach

Ingredients:

- 1 pound fresh baby spinach
- 3 cloves fresh garlic
- 2 tablespoons extra virgin olive oil
- 2 tablespoons balsamic vinegar

Directions:

1. Start by cleaning the spinach in a salad spinner. Set aside.
2. Add the olive oil to a large pot or Dutch oven; then heat over medium-high heat.
3. Thinly slice the garlic with a sharp knife; then add it to the pot. Saute for 30 seconds; just until it starts to erupt with flavor; then add the spinach.
4. Stir the spinach, patting it down until it wilts; then add the balsamic vinegar. Mix well; then add to a serving bowl. If desired, sprinkle with a little cheese and serve hot.

Chickpea and Tuna Salad

Ingredients:

- 2 tablespoons mayonnaise or plain Greek yogurt
- 2 tablespoons extra-virgin olive oil
- 1 tablespoon fresh lemon juice
- 1 teaspoon Dijon mustard
- ¼ teaspoon kosher salt and black pepper
- A few dashes of hot sauce (such as Tabasco or Cholula), optional
- 1 (15-ounce) can chickpeas
- 1 (5-ounce) can tuna (packed in water), drained
- 3 tablespoons finely chopped celery
- 2 tablespoons minced red onion
- 2 tablespoons finely chopped fresh dill
- 1 tablespoon roughly chopped capers, green olives, or relish

Directions:

1. Combine mayonnaise, olive oil, lemon juice, Dijon mustard, salt, pepper, and hot sauce (if using) in a small bowl; whisk to combine.
2. Drain and rinse chickpeas, and dry with a clean kitchen towel.
3. If desired, peel and discard loose skins, and transfer chickpeas to a medium bowl. (I like to mash some of the chickpeas with a fork to help the salad better stick together, however, this is optional.)
4. Add tuna, celery, onion, capers (or olives), fresh dill, and dressing; stir to combine.
5. Serve in a sandwich or wrap, over a bed of arugula, or with crackers.

Bone Health

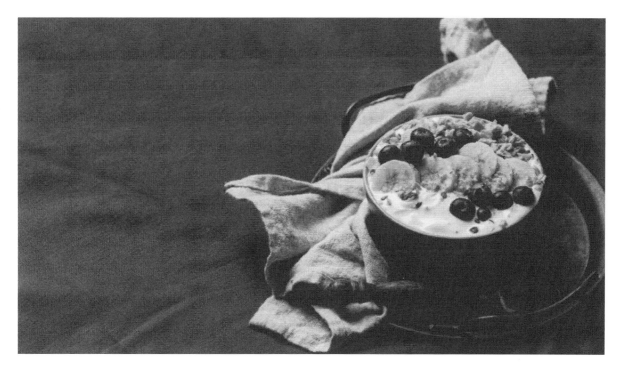

"You are a seed dropping from above. To be nurtured by the earth. And to grow into a healing herb. For the whole world to consume." –Michael Bassey Johnson

Our bones are the living, breathing architecture that shapes our physical form. They are the sturdy scaffolding that supports us through every step, every dance, every embrace in life. Calcium-rich herbs and plants are a veritable treasure trove of bone-health-friendly "medicines," designed to nourish and fortify our skeletal systems.

Topical Treatments

Epsom and Himalayan Bath Soak

Ingredients:

- 4 cups Epsom salts
- 1 cup coarse Dead Sea salt or pink Himalayan salt crystals
- 40 drops rose essential oil
- 2 tablespoons dried rose petals and 4 tablespoons dried desiccated coconut (blended)

Directions:

1. Combine all ingredients in a large bowl.
2. Be sure to break up any clumps that develop from essential oils.
3. Store in an airtight container, in a dark, cool place indefinitely.
4. For use: Add 1/2-1 cup of bath salts to your bath just before getting in.

Green Tea and Mint Facial Mist

Ingredients:

- 6 ounces (170 grams) distilled water
- 1 teaspoon loose green tea leaves or 1 green tea bag
- 3 drops lavender oil
- 3 drops aloe vera gel

Directions:

1. Make a 6-ounce cup of strong green tea and let it cool.
2. Add the 3 drops of lavender essential oil and the 3 drops of aloe vera gel, then stir well with a sterile instrument.
3. Pour into a sterilized spray bottle. Shake well every time you use it.
4. Keep it in the refrigerator.
5. If you feel you need something to help keep it fresh, add a drop of vitamin E oil to your mixture.

Calendula and Lavender Balm

Ingredients:

For the oil:

- Olive oil, preferably organic
- Dried calendula petals and lavender flowers

For the balm:

- Makes about 8 small (25ml) pots of salve, or 3 medium (60ml) pots. You can quadruple the batch for larger quantities.
- 6 fluid ounces of calendula oil (¾ cup)
- 2 fluid ounces of coconut oil (¼ cup)
- A large jar
- A large brown paper bag
- 1 ounce of beeswax (about 30g)
- Pinch of dried turmeric powder (optional, for color)
- 15-18 drops of lavender essential oil (optional, omit if you have sensitive skin)

Directions:

For the oil:

1. Dump the dried calendula and lavender petals into a large jar, filling it at least halfway.
2. Completely cover the petals with 6 fluid ounces (¾ cup) of organic olive oil.
3. Place the jar in a brown paper bag and leave it on a sunny windowsill for about a month.
4. Strain the oil from the petals using muslin or cheesecloth.
5. Place the beeswax, coconut oil, and infused calendula oil into a double boiler and heat over low heat, stirring gently, until the beeswax melts.
6. Once melted, add the essential oil (if using) and a pinch of turmeric for extra color.
7. Pour the mixture into tins or jars.
8. Allow it to set before using.

Herbal Brews and Drinks

Devils Claw and Turmeric Tea

Ingredients:

- 1 teaspoon Devil's Claw
- 1 teaspoon White Willow
- 1 teaspoon Turmeric
- 1 teaspoon St. John's Wort
- 2 cups water

Directions:

1. Boil 2 cups of water.
2. Pour the boiled water into a teapot or jug.
3. Add the remainder of the ingredients.
4. Allow to steep for 5 minutes.
5. Strain and enjoy.

Rosehip Iced Tea

Ingredients:

- 6 hibiscus tea bags
- ½ cup honey
- 1 cup fresh lime juice (from 8 to 10 limes)

Directions:

1. In a large heatproof pitcher, combine tea bags, honey, and 5 cups boiling water; let steep for 10 minutes.
2. Discard tea bags.
3. Add lime juice.
4. Pour in 3 cups of cold water.
5. Refrigerate until cold, for at least 1 hour (and up to 1 week).
6. Serve over ice.

Pain-Relieving Willowbark Iced Tea

Ingredients:

- 4 tsp white willow bark
- 2 cups filtered water
- 1 cinnamon stick (optional)
- 2 tsp honey (optional)

Directions:

1. In a saucepan, combine the water and white willow bark.
2. Bring the mixture to a boil and let it simmer for 5-10 minutes.
3. Turn off the heat and let the willow bark steep for an additional 20-30 minutes. You can optionally add a cinnamon stick for additional flavor.
4. Strain the tea into tall glasses once it has cooled.
5. Add ice cubes.
6. The tea may be bitter, so you can use honey to sweeten it according to your taste.

Spinach, Lemon, and Apple Shots

Ingredients:

- 1 medium stalk celery (about 1.6 oz or 45 g)
- 6 slices (1-inch diameter) ginger (about 0.5 oz or 14 g)
- 2/3 medium green apple (about 4 oz or 113 g)
- 4 1/2 cups spinach (about 4.6 oz or 130 g)
- 1/5 medium lemon (about 0.4 oz or 11 g)
- 2/3 cups chopped parsley (about 1.7 oz or 48 g)
- 3 cups chopped romaine lettuce (about 4.5 oz or 128 g)

Directions:

1. Wash all produce thoroughly.
2. Juice all ingredients together.

Bone Health Recipes

Kelp Berry Smoothie

Ingredients:

- 2 cups frozen mixed berries
- 1 banana, peeled & sliced into round disks
- 1 cup regular milk or almond milk
- 1/2 cup orange juice
- 3 tablespoons kelp purée or kelp powder

Directions:

1. Add all ingredients to the blender.
2. Blend for approximately one minute or until ingredients are well blended and smooth.
3. Serve immediately.

Chocolate Date Smoothie

Ingredients:

- 35g oats (about 1/3 cup)
- 240ml milk (your choice) (about 1 cup)
- 4 dates
- 1 pinch cinnamon
- 2 teaspoons cocoa powder
- 1 teaspoon peanut butter (or other nut butter)

Directions:

1. Add all ingredients to the jug of a power blender.
2. Blend until smooth.
3. Enjoy!

Cucumber and Greek Yogurt Salad

Ingredients:

- 2 English cucumbers
- Kosher salt
- ¾ cup whole milk Greek yogurt
- 2 tablespoons red wine vinegar
- Zest and juice of ½ lemon
- ¼ cup chopped fresh dill, stems removed, plus more for garnish
- ½ to ¾ teaspoon garlic powder
- Black pepper
- ½ medium red onion, thinly sliced into half-moons

Directions:

1. Partially peel the cucumbers, leaving some of the peel to create stripes. Slice them in half lengthwise.
2. Use a metal spoon to scrape out and discard the seeds, then cut crosswise into ¼-inch thick slices.
3. Place the cucumber slices into a large colander and season with a generous pinch of salt.
4. Toss well and set aside in a clean sink for about 20 to 30 minutes to drain excess liquid.
5. In a large mixing bowl, whisk together the yogurt, red wine vinegar, lemon zest and juice, chopped dill, garlic powder, and a pinch of salt and pepper.
6. Set aside in the refrigerator.
7. Once the cucumbers have drained, use a paper towel to pat them dry.
8. Add the cucumbers and onions to the bowl with the yogurt mixture and toss until they are evenly coated in the dressing.
9. Taste and adjust the seasoning as needed.
10. Serve. Garnish with additional fresh dill and serve.

Sweet Potato Black Bean Burgers

Ingredients:

- 1/2 cup mashed sweet potato from one medium sweet potato
- 1 and 1/2 cups black beans, drained and rinsed (equivalent to one 15-ounce can)
- 2 teaspoons extra virgin olive oil plus more for coating sweet potato
- 1 cup diced white onion (from one medium onion)
- 1/2 medium red bell pepper, diced
- 1/2 teaspoon salt, divided in half
- 1 small jalapeño, diced (optional)
- 3 cloves garlic, minced
- 1 teaspoon ground cumin
- 1/2 teaspoon chipotle chili powder
- 1 teaspoon dried parsley
- 1 large egg, whisked
- 1 cup plain bread crumbs
- 5 burger buns
- Lettuce and barbecue sauce for topping

Directions:

1. Preheat the oven to 400°F (200°C).
2. Lightly coat the whole sweet potato in olive oil (optional).
3. Poke several holes in the sweet potato using a knife.
4. Place on a baking sheet and roast in the oven until tender, about 45 minutes to an hour depending on the size of your sweet potato.
5. Remove the skin from the sweet potato.
6. Mash the inside until almost pureed. Measure out 1/2 cup of the mashed sweet potato.
7. Before adding black beans, pat them with a paper towel to remove excess moisture.
8. Combine the sweet potato and black beans and mash a little more. You want some whole beans to remain for texture. Set aside.
9. Heat 2 teaspoons of olive oil in a medium skillet over medium-high heat.
10. Once hot, add diced onion, diced bell pepper, and 1/4 teaspoon salt.
11. Sauté until softened, about 6 minutes.
12. Add jalapeño and garlic and sauté for a minute more, until golden and aromatic.
13. Stir the sautéed ingredients into the sweet potato mixture.
14. Add the seasonings (cumin, 1/4 teaspoon salt, chipotle chili powder, parsley), whisked egg, and bread crumbs.
15. Mix until a loose ball forms.
16. Form the mixture into patties, about the width of your palm.
17. For best results, make sure the burger is no more than 1/2 inch thick when cooking.
18. The thinner the patty, the firmer it will be.
19. Heat a skillet over medium heat (you can use the same skillet used for sautéing the onions for extra flavor).
20. Lightly spray with non-stick cooking spray.
21. Once hot, add the patties.
22. Cook until lightly browned, about 5 minutes.
23. Flip and cook the other side until browned.
24. Serve on burger buns with your favorite fixings.

Breast Health

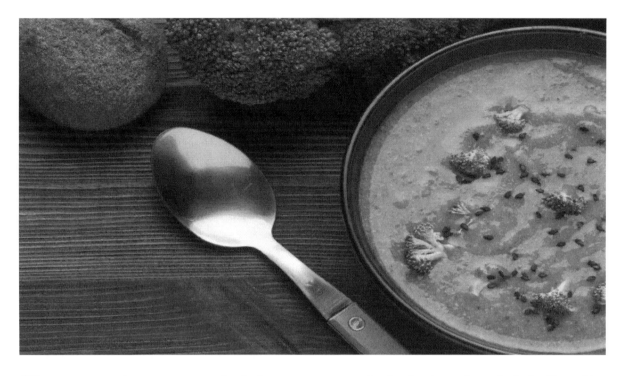

"The moment you change your perception is the moment you rewrite the chemistry of your body." —Bruce Lipton

Women's breast health is a crucial aspect of our overall well-being, yet it is often overlooked until issues arise. By proactively nourishing and supporting our breasts with targeted herbal remedies and recipes, we can harness the power of nature to maintain healthy breast tissue and promote balanced hormonal function.

Topical Treatments

One Jar Secret Breast Miracle Cream

Ingredients:

- Approximately 90 ml (3 ounces) virgin coconut oil
- 15-20 drops of Progest E* (natural progesterone in vitamin E)
- 8 drops Lavender essential oil
- (Optional) 5 drops Frankincense essential oil

Directions:

1. Preheat the oven to 350°F (175°C). Allow the oven to warm for about 5 minutes, then turn it off.

2. Place a glass jar containing the coconut oil in the warm oven for about 5-10 minutes to melt. The oven should be warm but turned off at this point.

3. Once the coconut oil is melted, carefully remove it from the oven and add the Progest E and essential oils.

4. Stir the mixture well to ensure all ingredients are thoroughly combined.

5. Transfer the jar to a cool, dark place to allow the coconut oil to solidify again.

6. Once solidified, keep the balm in your bathroom or bedside for everyday use.

7. Enjoy the benefits of this light progesterone cream as it replaces your everyday products!

Wild Yam and Chaste Tree Balm

Ingredients:

- 240 ml (1 cup) of cut and sifted wild yam root
- 120 ml (1/2 cup) of dried chaste tree berries
- 240 ml (1 cup) of coconut oil or olive oil
- 120 ml (1/2 cup) of beeswax pellets
- 15 ml (1 tablespoon) of vitamin E oil
- 10-20 drops of your favorite essential oil (optional)

Directions:

1. Place the cut and sifted wild yam root and dried chaste tree berries in a clean, dry glass jar.
2. Pour the coconut oil or olive oil over the herbs until they are completely covered.
3. Close the jar tightly and let it sit in a cool, dark place for 2-4 weeks. Shake the jar every day or so to ensure that the herbs are fully infused in the oil.
4. After the oil has been infused for the desired time, strain the mixture through a cheesecloth or fine mesh strainer to remove the solid plant material.
5. In a double boiler over low heat, melt the beeswax pellets and the infused oil together, stirring occasionally until fully combined.
6. Let the mixture simmer on low heat for about 10 minutes, stirring occasionally.
7. After 10 minutes, remove the mixture from the heat and let it cool for a few minutes.
8. Add the vitamin E oil and essential oil, if desired, and stir well.
9. Pour the mixture into a clean glass jar or container and let it cool completely.
10. Once the cream or oil has cooled and solidified, it is ready to use.
11. Apply a small amount to the desired area and massage gently into the skin. Store the cream or oil in a cool, dry place.

Hormone Balance Serum

Ingredients:

- 1 fluid ounce (30 ml) evening primrose oil
- 30 drops clary sage oil
- 30 drops thyme oil
- 30 drops ylang ylang oil

Directions:

1. Mix all ingredients together in a 2-fluid-ounce (60 ml) bottle.
2. Put the mixture into a glass vial with a dropper.
3. Rub 5 drops onto the neck 2 times daily.

Milk thistle and Dandelion Tea Bath Soak

Ingredients:

- 1 tablespoon Red Clover
- 1 tablespoon Nettle
- 1 tablespoon Dandelion
- 1 tablespoon Milk Thistle

Directions:

- Combine equal parts of red clover, nettle, dandelion, and milk thistle into a jar with an airtight lid.
- Shake to distribute the herbs together evenly.
- Add 1 tablespoon of the herbal mixture to a teapot with a mesh strainer.
- Pour boiling water over the herbs, cover, and let steep for at least 5 minutes.
- Pour the infused tea into your already-drawn bath, and enjoy!
- Optionally, you can add Epsom salts to relieve muscle pain.

Herbal Brews

Honeybush and Cinnamon Tea

Ingredients:

- 2 cups (480 ml) plant or goat's milk
- 1 pinch sea salt
- 4 bags organic honeybush tea
- 1 cup (240 ml) maple syrup
- 2 bags Rooibos Tea
- 20 ounces (591 ml) boiling water
- Garnish: chopped or shaved dark chocolate to taste

Directions:

1. In a jug, combine the tea bags and maple syrup.
2. Pour the boiling water over the tea bags and syrup, and stir

generously.

3. Allow the mixture to steep for 5-10 minutes.

4. Pour the tea into tall glasses.

5. Add milk of choice and garnish with chocolate shavings.

6. Serve and enjoy!

Iced Fenugreek and Honey Sweet Tea

Ingredients:

- 1 1/2 cups (360 ml) cold water
- Small piece of ginger, crushed, or 1/4-inch piece dried ginger*
- 1/2 teaspoon fenugreek seeds
- 1 scant teaspoon anise seeds
- 2 tablespoons honey, to taste

Directions:

1. Bring the water to a boil in a small pot.

2. Add the ginger, fenugreek, and anise seeds to the boiling water. Cover and boil for 10 minutes.

3. Strain the tea into a mug and stir in honey to taste.

4. Allow the tea to cool to room temperature, then transfer it to the refrigerator to chill.

5. Once chilled, serve the tea over ice.

6. Enjoy your refreshing Iced Fenugreek and Honey Sweet Tea!

Mint and Honey Tea

Ingredients:

- 4 cups (960 ml) water
- 4 green tea bags
- 3 sprigs fresh mint, plus more for garnish
- 1/4 cup (60 ml) honey, plus more if desired (up to 1/2 cup)
- 2 cups (480 ml) cold water
- 1-2 cups (240-480 ml) ice

Directions:

1. In a saucepan, bring 4 cups of water to a boil.

2. Remove from heat, and add in tea bags and 3 mint sprigs.

3. Cover and let steep for about 15-20 minutes. For a stronger tea flavor, steep for about 30-45 minutes.

4. Remove the tea bags and mint, and stir in honey until dissolved.

5. In a large pitcher, add green tea, about 1-2 cups of ice, and 2 cups of cold water. Mix well.

6. Serve over ice and garnish with more fresh mint.

7. Enjoy your refreshing Mint and Honey Tea!

Pomegranate and Blueberry Juice

Ingredients:

- 16 oz (approx. 454 g) pomegranate seeds
- 8 oz (approx. 227 g) blueberries
- 1/2 tbsp lemon juice
- 1 1/2 tbsp sugar (optional)
- 1/2 cup (120 ml) water
- 1 tsp rosemary

Directions:

- Place a piece of cheesecloth over a medium bowl.
- Add a handful of pomegranate seeds in the middle of the cheesecloth and fold it in half.
- Gather the corners together and twist the cloth to wring out the juice.
- Continue with the remaining pomegranate seeds.
- Put the blueberries and 1 tsp of rosemary through a juicer and collect the juice in a pitcher.
- Add 1/2 cup of water to the juicer; this helps further process the leftover blueberry flesh inside the machine.
- Add the pomegranate juice to the pitcher with the blueberry juice.
- To balance out the tartness, add no more than 1 1/2 tbsp of sugar.
- This adds more depth of flavor to the juice.
- Pour the juice into 4 glasses and serve immediately, or chill the pitcher before serving.

Breast Health Recipes

The Ultimate Pink Smoothie

Ingredients:

- 1 cup (240 ml) soy milk
- 1/2 cup (120 ml) cherries
- 1/2 cup (120 ml) raspberries
- 1 cup (240 ml) Greek yogurt
- Sprinkling of chia seeds

Directions:

1. Add all ingredients except chia seeds to the blender.
2. Blend until desired consistency is reached.
3. Pour the smoothie into a glass.
4. Sprinkle with chia seeds.
5. Enjoy your delicious pink smoothie!

Berry Spinach and Matcha Smoothie

Ingredients:

- 1 cup (250 ml) coconut-rice milk or milk of choice
- 1 teaspoon matcha tea powder
- 1 small banana, frozen
- 20-30 grams baby spinach (one handful)
- 2 teaspoons chia seeds
- 1 tablespoon coconut oil (or any nut butter)
- 1/2 cup ice cubes (optional)

Directions:

1. Place all ingredients into a blender.
2. Process until nice and smooth.
3. Serve immediately.
4. Optionally, top with something crunchy such as homemade granola, cacao nibs, or bee pollen.

Pumpkin Baked Oatmeal

Ingredients:

- 120g unsweetened pumpkin puree
- 355ml regular, almond milk, or soy milk
- 2 tablespoons raisins
- ¼ teaspoon pumpkin pie spice
- ¼ teaspoon salt
- 100g rolled oats
- 30g roughly chopped roasted pecans or walnuts
- Maple syrup

Directions:

1. In a medium saucepan, whisk together the pumpkin puree, milk, raisins, pumpkin pie spice, and salt until smooth. Bring to a boil.
2. Add the oatmeal, then turn down the heat to a simmer and cook, stirring occasionally, until the oats are tender, about 8 minutes.
3. Serve topped with pecans and a drizzle of maple syrup.

Sicilian-Style Roasted Cauliflower

Ingredients:

- 1 large head cauliflower (about 2½-3 pounds)
- 60 ml (¼ cup) extra-virgin olive oil
- Kosher salt and freshly ground black pepper
- 2 tablespoons capers, drained and roughly chopped
- 60 ml (¼ cup) golden raisins
- 1 tablespoon champagne or white wine vinegar
- ¼ cup roughly chopped fresh parsley
- 2 tablespoons toasted pine nuts
- ¼ teaspoon crushed red pepper flakes

Directions:

1. Preheat the oven to 220°C (425°F).
2. Trim the leaves from the cauliflower, remove the core, and cut the cauliflower into medium-size florets.
3. On a sheet pan, toss the cauliflower with the olive oil, 1 teaspoon salt, and ½ teaspoon pepper.
4. Roast for 25 to 35 minutes, tossing once halfway through, until tender and browned.
5. Meanwhile, in a small bowl, combine the capers, raisins, and vinegar, and set aside.
6. When the cauliflower is done, add the caper mixture, parsley,

pine nuts, and red pepper flakes to the sheet pan.

7. Toss well, sprinkle generously with salt, then transfer to a shallow dish or platter and serve.

Circulatory Health

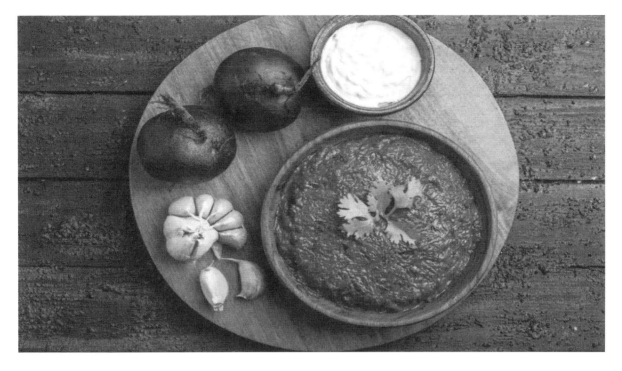

"The doctor of the future will give no medication, but will interest his patients in the care of the human frame, diet, and in the cause and prevention of disease." –Thomas A. Edison

The circulatory system is the body's superhighway, transporting vital nutrients, oxygen, and immune cells to every cell and organ. By supporting our circulatory health with targeted herbs and natural remedies, we can ensure that our bodies receive the nourishment they need to function at their best, while also promoting detoxification and overall well-being.

Topical Treatments

Healing Salve

Equipment:

- Double boiler OR glass bowl and pot
- Quart-size mason jar
- 4 oz Metal tins (or glass jars)

Ingredients:

- 475 ml olive oil (or coconut oil)
- 2 tsp echinacea root (optional)
- 1 TBSP comfrey leaf
- 2 TBSP dried plantain leaf
- 1 TBSP calendula flowers
- 2 tsp yarrow flowers
- 1 tsp rosemary
- 60 ml beeswax pellets
- 1 tsp vitamin E oil (optional)
- 20-40 drops essential oils (optional, lavender and tea tree are good options)

Directions:

Infuse the Herbs:

Combine the olive oil and herbs in a jar with an airtight lid and leave for 3-4 weeks, shaking daily. This option doesn't work well with coconut oil.

OR heat the olive oil (or other oil) and herbs over low heat in a double boiler for 3 hours (low heat!) until the oil is very green.

1. Another option is to put the herbs and oil in mason jars with lids. Place in a water bath in a crockpot set to low and let this infuse for at least 24 hours. Refill the water in the slow cooker as needed.

Make the Salve:

2. Pour the oil through a cheesecloth and strain out the herbs. Squeeze the cheesecloth to get as much oil out as possible. Compost the herbs.

3. Combine the infused oil and beeswax in a double boiler.

4. Heat over low heat, stirring occasionally, until the wax is melted.

5. Add essential oils if desired.

6. Pour into small tins, glass jars, or lip balm tubes and use as needed.

Notes:

• Store in a cool, dry place for up to 2 years.

Arnica Hand Balm

Equipment:

• 4 – 2 oz tins

Ingredients:

• 175 ml Arnica oil
• 60 g beeswax pellets
• 2.5 ml vitamin E oil
• 20 drops peppermint essential oil

Directions:

1. Using a double boiler, add a couple of cups of water into a pot. Then place a heat-proof bowl over the top of the pot.

2. Turn the burner on and allow the water to come to a boil.

3. Meanwhile, measure out the ingredients. Once the water is boiling, add arnica oil and beeswax pellets to the bowl of your double-boiler and stir consistently until the beeswax has melted (about 5 minutes).

4. Once the beeswax has melted, remove the bowl from the heat and let it sit for a few minutes on the counter to cool slightly.

5. Combine vitamin E oil and essential oils, then pour into the oil and beeswax mixture.

6. Stir to incorporate all oils then pour into a clean, dry pourable measuring cup.

7. Carefully divide the oil equally between the four 2-ounce tins. Don't forget to label your tins!

8. Let cool completely and store in a cool, temperature-controlled cupboard.

Warming Hand Balm For Winter Hands and Feet

Ingredients:

• 60 g shea butter
• 30 ml sweet almond oil
• 15 g beeswax
• 10 drops myrrh essential oil
• 10 drops cedarwood essential oil

Directions:

1. Melt the shea butter, beeswax, and sweet almond oil together in a double boiler. (You can use a Pyrex measuring cup placed in a pot of simmering water).

2. Stir the mixture as it melts.

3. Once everything is melted, remove it from the heat and allow it to cool for 5-10 minutes.

4. Stir in the essential oils, and pour the liquid hand cream into a small glass container. Allow it to harden completely (this usually takes several hours).

5. Apply this homemade hand cream recipe to your dry hands as often as needed.

6. Store in the fridge to preserve the freshness.

Homemade Hot Tiger Balm

Ingredients:

• 1 oz (60 ml) olive oil
• 1 1/2 tablespoons beeswax pastilles
• 1 tablespoon menthol crystals
• 12 drops camphor essential oil
• 11 drops peppermint essential oil
• 9 drops eucalyptus essential oil
• 7 drops clove essential oil
• 7 drops cinnamon essential oil

Equipment:

- Double boiler
- 4 oz (approx. 120 ml) glass jar for storage

Directions:

1. Using a double boiler, melt the beeswax, menthol, and olive oil until fully melted.
2. Allow the mixture to cool for 2 minutes, then add your essential oils.
3. Stir the mixture well then pour into your tin or jar.
4. Allow the mixture to set and harden completely before using.
5. Use a small amount for pain where needed.

Tips and Cautions:

- IMPORTANT: Do not rub Tiger Balm on open wounds, or irritated, sunburned, or chapped skin. The menthol can cause further irritation.
- Avoid getting this mixture in your eyes or mouth, so be sure to wash your hands after applying.
- Use the recommended amount of essential oils in this recipe as they are very potent and can cause burning sensations if used in excess.

Herbal Brews and Drinks

Pomegranate Green Tea Iced Tea

Ingredients:

- 4 green tea bags
- 1 (16 oz) bottle organic pomegranate juice or make your own juice
- 8 teaspoons honey
- Ice cubes
- 1 cup fresh or frozen berries for garnish, optional

Directions:

1. In a pot, bring 6 cups (approx. 1.4 liters) of water to a boil.
2. Dunk the tea bags several times and then let them sit in the pot.
3. Steep the tea for 10 minutes.
4. Stir in the pomegranate juice and honey, to taste.
5. Pour the cooled tea into a pitcher. Store the tea in the refrigerator.
6. To serve: Add ice to a cup. Pour in 1 cup of tea.
7. Garnish with 2 tablespoons of frozen berries, if desired.

Beetroot and Lemon Juice

Ingredients:

- 2 medium beets, scrubbed clean and tops trimmed
- 1 medium seedless cucumber, rinsed
- 1-inch length piece fresh ginger, scrubbed clean
- 1 medium lemon

Directions:

1. Chop the beets, cucumber, and ginger into thin pieces small enough to easily go through the juicer.
2. Cut away the yellow peel from the lemon, leaving most of the white pith and lemon flesh. Cut into slices and remove any seeds.
3. Reserve about half of the lemon.
4. Turn the juicer on and push everything through, alternating between the beets and the softer cucumber and lemon.
5. When everything but the reserved lemon has been juiced, stir the juice and taste for tartness.
6. Add the remaining lemon if you feel it can take it. Or if the juice is too tart, consider adding a couple scrubbed unpeeled carrots or a small cored apple.

Homemade Fire Cider

Ingredients:

- A clean 1-liter or 1-quart jar with a lid
- A selection of pungent roots, bulbs, and rhizomes: onion, ginger, horseradish, garlic, and turmeric
- A selection of fresh seasonal herbs: oregano, rosemary, thyme, tulsi, calendula flowers
- Spice: fresh or dried chili, black pepper, long pepper
- Raw unpasteurized apple cider vinegar
- Raw honey
- Lemon
- Fresh hot chili or cayenne powder

Directions:

Preparation:

1. Fill one-quarter of the jar with loosely packed chopped or grated pungent roots, bulbs, and rhizomes. Ensure they are in small pieces to increase the surface area for the vinegar to draw out the medicinal compounds.

2. Fill the other two-quarters of the jar with chopped fresh herbs such as oregano, rosemary, thyme, tulsi, and calendula flowers.

3. Add three slices of fresh lemon and 1 – 2 fresh hot chili (or ¼ – ½ tsp of powdered cayenne).

4. Pour in ¼ cup raw local honey.

5. Top the jar with raw/unpasteurized organic apple cider vinegar.

6. Cap the jar and place it out of direct sunlight. Remember to shake the jar once a day.

After 4 - 6 Weeks:

7. Place a colander over a heavy pot or jug. Line the colander with cheesecloth (use three to four layers).

8. Pour the fire cider into the lined colander and allow it to drain until most of the liquid has collected in the pot, leaving wet organic matter.

9. Gather the corners of the cheesecloth and squeeze the remaining liquid through into the pot.

10. Add honey to taste and pour the strained liquid into sterilized jars or bottles for storage.

Empty Stomach Garlic Water

Ingredients:

- 12 garlic cloves
- 1 cup raw honey

Directions:

Preparation:

1. To make fermented garlic honey, you will need a clean 1-quart (liter) heatproof glass jar with a wide mouth for easier access to the garlic cloves.

2. Prepare the garlic cloves according to your preference. You can choose to peel them fully or keep the thin papery layer on. You can also decide whether to use the whole garlic clove, lightly crush it, or mince it.

3. Place the garlic cloves in the jar and pour the honey over them. Stir to ensure all the garlic cloves are coated with honey.

4. Close the lid of the jar and let it sit for 3 days.

Fermentation:

5. After 3 days, remove the lid of the jar to release any gases that may have built up. You may notice tiny bubbles at this stage.

6. Let the jar sit for another week, opening the lid every other day to stir the mixture slightly.

To Use:

7. Place 1 teaspoon of fermented garlic honey in 1/3 cup boiling water.

8. Stir and drink as soon as it has cooled enough to consume it on an empty stomach.

Note: You can store fermented garlic honey at room temperature for up to a month.

Circulatory Health Recipes

Lentil and Barley Casserole

Ingredients:

- 2 tablespoons canola oil, divided
- 1 onion, chopped
- 1 stalk celery, chopped
- 1 carrot, chopped
- 3 cloves garlic, minced
- 1 teaspoon dried thyme leaves
- 1/4 teaspoon hot pepper flakes
- 1/2 cup pearl barley
- 1/2 cup green lentils
- 3 cups hot low-sodium vegetable broth (710 ml)
- 1 can (19 oz) petite-cut stewed tomatoes
- 2 tablespoons tomato paste
- 1/2 cup whole wheat fresh breadcrumbs
- 1/4 cup crumbled feta (optional) (60 g)
- 2 tablespoons chopped fresh parsley

Directions:

Preparation:

1. Lightly spray a deep 10-cup (2.5 L) casserole dish and set it aside.

2. Preheat the oven to 400°F (200°C).

Cooking:

3. In a large nonstick skillet, heat 1 tablespoon of the oil over medium heat. Add onion, celery, carrot, garlic, thyme, and hot pepper flakes. Cook, stirring for about 6 minutes or until softened.

4. Stir in barley and lentils to coat. Scrape the mixture into the prepared casserole dish. Pour in the broth and stir to combine. Cover and bake for 45 minutes.

5. Uncover and stir in tomatoes and tomato paste. Cover and return to the oven for about 15 minutes or until barley and lentils are tender and most of the liquid has been absorbed. Stir gently.

6. Meanwhile, in a small bowl, stir together breadcrumbs, feta (if using), parsley, and the remaining oil. Sprinkle over the casserole, leaving it uncovered, and broil for 2 minutes or until golden brown.

7. Let cool slightly before serving.

Beetroot Hummus

Ingredients:

- 1 can chickpeas (15 oz / 430 g), drained and rinsed
- 2 medium cooked beetroots, cut into quarters
- 2 cloves garlic
- Zest and juice from 1 medium lemon
- 2-3 tablespoons tahini
- 2-3 tablespoons olive oil
- 1/4 teaspoon salt
- 1/2 teaspoon ground cumin

Directions:

Preparation:

1. Cook the beetroots according to your preferred method until they are tender. Let them cool down before using.

Cooking:

2. Place the beetroots, chickpeas, and garlic into a food processor and process for 1 minute until ground.

3. Add all the remaining ingredients: lemon zest, lemon juice, tahini, olive oil, salt, and ground cumin.

4. Process until creamy. It should have some grainy texture, which is okay. If it's dry or you want to thin it out and make it more creamy, add more tahini or water until you reach the desired consistency.

5. Adjust seasonings, adding more salt, cumin, olive oil, or lemon juice if needed.

6. Scrape into a serving bowl to use immediately. Serve at room temperature. Refrigerate in an airtight container if you aren't serving right away.

7. Beetroot hummus will keep in the fridge, covered well, for 4-5 days.

Jeweled Couscous Salad

Ingredients:

- 1 cup (200g) couscous
- 1 1/4 cups (300ml) boiling water
- 1/4 cup (60ml) olive oil
- 2 tablespoons lemon juice
- 1 teaspoon honey
- Salt and pepper to taste
- 1/2 cup (75g) dried cranberries
- 1/2 cup (75g) golden raisins
- 1/4 cup (30g) chopped pistachios
- 1/4 cup (30g) chopped almonds

- 1/4 cup (30g) chopped dried apricots
- 2 tablespoons chopped fresh mint
- 2 tablespoons chopped fresh parsley
- 2 tablespoons chopped fresh coriander (cilantro)
- 1/4 cup (30g) crumbled feta cheese (optional)

Directions:

1. Place the couscous in a large heatproof bowl. Pour the boiling water over the couscous, cover the bowl with a plate or lid, and let it sit for about 5-10 minutes until the water is absorbed and the couscous is tender.

2. In a small bowl, whisk together the olive oil, lemon juice, honey, salt, and pepper to make the dressing.

3. Fluff the couscous with a fork to separate the grains. Pour the dressing over the couscous and toss to coat evenly.

4. Add the dried cranberries, golden raisins, chopped pistachios, chopped almonds, chopped dried apricots, chopped fresh mint, chopped fresh parsley, and chopped fresh coriander (cilantro) to the couscous. Toss gently to combine.

5. If desired, sprinkle crumbled feta cheese over the top of the salad.

6. Serve the jeweled couscous salad immediately, or cover and refrigerate until ready to serve. Enjoy!

Spiced Okra

Ingredients:

- 1 pound (450g) fresh okra pods, washed and dried
- 2 tablespoons (30ml) olive oil
- 1 teaspoon (5g) ground cumin
- 1 teaspoon (5g) ground coriander
- 1/2 teaspoon (2.5g) ground turmeric
- 1/4 teaspoon (1.25g) cayenne pepper (adjust to taste)
- Salt to taste
- Freshly ground black pepper to taste
- Lemon wedges, for serving (optional)

Directions:

1. Preheat your oven to 400°F (200°C).

2. Trim the stems off the okra pods and slice them into 1/2-inch (1.25cm) rounds.

3. In a large bowl, toss the sliced okra with olive oil, ground cumin, ground coriander, ground turmeric, cayenne pepper, salt, and black pepper until evenly coated.

4. Spread the seasoned okra in a single layer on a baking sheet lined with parchment paper or aluminum foil.

5. Roast the okra in the preheated oven for 15-20 minutes, or until tender and slightly crispy, stirring halfway through cooking.

6. Once done, remove the spiced okra from the oven and transfer it to a serving dish.

7. Serve the spiced okra hot as a side dish or appetizer, garnished with lemon wedges if desired. Enjoy!

Red Plum Compote

Ingredients:

- 1 pound (450g) red plums, pitted and quartered
- 1 tsps (10 ml) corn starch
- 1/4 cup (60ml) water
- 1 cinnamon stick
- 1 teaspoon (5ml) vanilla extract
- Zest of 1 lemon
- Juice of 1/2 lemon

Directions:

1. In a saucepan, combine the red plums, cornstarch, water, cinnamon stick, vanilla extract, and lemon zest.

2. Place the saucepan over medium heat and bring the mixture to a simmer, stirring occasionally to prevent the cornstarch from clumping.

3. Once simmering, reduce the heat to low and let the mixture cook gently for about 15-20 minutes, or until the plums are soft and the liquid has thickened slightly, stirring occasionally.

4. Remove the saucepan from the heat and stir in the lemon juice.

5. Allow the compote to cool slightly before serving. It can be served warm or cold.

6. Once cooled, transfer the compote to a jar or container and store it in the refrigerator.

7. It will keep for about a week.

8. Serve the red plum compote as a topping for yogurt, ice cream, pancakes, or toast. Enjoy!

Cognitive Function

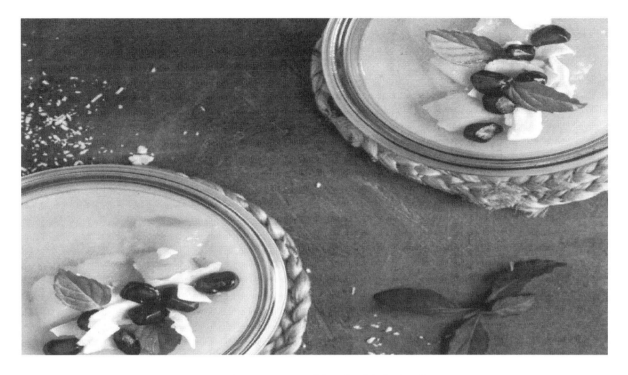

"The greatest wealth is health." –Virgil

In today's fast-paced, information-driven world, maintaining optimal cognitive function is more important than ever. By nourishing our brains with targeted herbs and natural remedies, we can support mental clarity, focus, and memory, while also promoting overall brain health and resilience in the face of daily stressors.

Topical Treatments

Aloe Vera Salve

Ingredients:

- 1/2 cup (120ml) coconut oil
- 2 tablespoons (30ml) beeswax pellets
- 1/4 cup (60ml) aloe vera gel
- 10 drops lavender essential oil (optional)
- 5 drops tea tree essential oil (optional)

Directions:

1. In a double boiler or a heatproof bowl set over a pot of simmering water, melt the coconut oil and beeswax pellets together, stirring occasionally until fully melted.
2. Once melted, remove from heat and let it cool slightly.
3. Stir in the aloe vera gel until well combined. If desired, add the lavender and tea tree essential oils for additional benefits.
4. Pour the mixture into clean, dry containers or jars. Allow it to cool and solidify completely before sealing the jars.
5. Store the aloe vera salve in a cool, dry place. It can be kept at room temperature for several months.
6. Apply the salve to dry or irritated skin as needed. Enjoy the soothing and moisturizing benefits of this homemade aloe vera salve!

Whipped Tallow Butter

Ingredients:

- 1 cup (240 ml) beef tallow
- 1/4 cup (60 ml) coconut oil
- 1/4 cup (60 ml) shea butter
- Optional: Essential oils for fragrance (e.g., lavender, peppermint, or citrus)

Directions:

- In a heatproof bowl, combine the beef tallow, coconut oil, and shea butter.
- Place the bowl over a pot of simmering water to create a double boiler. Alternatively, you can melt the ingredients in the microwave using short bursts of heat, stirring in between, until fully melted.
- Once melted, remove the bowl from the heat and let the mixture cool to room temperature. You can speed up this process by placing the bowl in the refrigerator for a short while, but be careful not to let it solidify completely.
- Once the mixture has cooled but is still soft, add any desired essential oils for fragrance. Start with a few drops and adjust according to your preference.
- Using a hand mixer or stand mixer, whip the mixture on high speed until it becomes light and fluffy, resembling the texture of whipped cream.
- Transfer the whipped tallow body butter to clean, airtight jars or containers for storage.
- Store the body butter in a cool, dry place away from direct sunlight. It should keep well for several months.
- To use, simply scoop out a small amount of the whipped body butter and massage it into your skin. Enjoy the nourishing and moisturizing benefits!

Herbal Brews and Drinks

Ginseng Tea

Ingredients:

- 1 teaspoon dried ginseng root (or 1 ginseng tea bag)
- 1 cup (240 ml) water
- Honey or lemon, to taste (optional)

Directions:

1. Heat 1 cup (240 ml) of water in a kettle or saucepan until it reaches a gentle boil. You can adjust the amount of water and ginseng according to your preference.
2. Place the dried ginseng root or ginseng tea bag in a teapot or mug. Pour the hot water over the ginseng.
3. Let the ginseng steep in the hot water for about 5 to 10 minutes. This allows the beneficial compounds in the ginseng to be released into the water.
4. If you used loose ginseng root, strain the tea to remove the root particles before drinking. You can use a fine mesh strainer or a tea infuser for this purpose.
5. If desired, add honey or lemon to taste for sweetness and flavor. Ginseng has a slightly bitter taste on its own, so sweetening can help balance the flavor.
6. Pour the ginseng tea into a cup and enjoy it while it's still warm. You can also chill it in the refrigerator and serve it over ice for a refreshing iced ginseng tea.
7. If you have leftover tea, you can store it in a sealed container in the refrigerator for up to 24 hours. Reheat it gently before serving if desired.

Lion's Mane Mushroom Brew

Ingredients:

- 1 teaspoon dried Lion's Mane mushroom powder (or 1 Lion's Mane mushroom tea bag)
- 1 cup (240 ml) water
- Optional: honey or other sweetener, to taste

Directions:

1. Heat 1 cup (240 ml) of water in a kettle or saucepan until it reaches a gentle boil.
2. Place the dried Lion's Mane mushroom powder or tea bag in a teapot or mug.
3. Pour the hot water over the Lion's Mane mushroom powder or tea bag.
4. Let the mushroom steep in the hot water for about 5 to 10 minutes. This allows the beneficial compounds in the Lion's Mane mushroom to be released into the water.
5. If you used loose Lion's Mane mushroom powder, strain the brew to remove any remaining particles before drinking. You can use a fine mesh strainer or a tea infuser for this purpose.
6. If desired, add honey or your preferred sweetener to taste. Lion's Mane mushroom brew has a mild flavor, so sweetening is optional but can enhance the taste.
7. Pour the brewed Lion's Mane mushroom tea into a cup and enjoy it while it's still warm.
8. If you have leftover brew, you can store it in a sealed container in the refrigerator for up to 24 hours. Reheat it gently before serving, if desired.

Rosemary and Nutmeg Iced Tea

Ingredients:

- 4 cups (960 ml) water
- 2 tablespoons fresh rosemary leaves
- 1/2 teaspoon ground nutmeg
- 4 black tea bags
- Ice cubes
- Honey or sweetener (optional)
- Lemon slices for garnish (optional)

Directions:

1. In a medium saucepan, bring 4 cups (960 ml) of water to a boil.
2. Once the water is boiling, reduce the heat to low and add the fresh rosemary leaves and ground nutmeg to the saucepan. Let it simmer for about 5 minutes to infuse the water with the flavors.
3. Remove the saucepan from the heat and add the black tea bags to the infused water. Let the tea bags steep for 3-5 minutes, depending on how strong you prefer your tea.
4. After steeping, remove the tea bags and allow the tea to cool to room temperature.
5. Once cooled, transfer the tea to a pitcher and refrigerate for at least 1 hour to chill.
6. When ready to serve, fill glasses with ice cubes and pour the chilled rosemary and nutmeg tea into each glass.
7. If desired, add honey or your preferred sweetener to taste, stirring until dissolved.
8. Garnish each glass with a slice of lemon for added freshness and visual appeal.
9. Serve immediately and enjoy!

Brain Booster Morning Juice

Ingredients:

- 1 bunch coriander leaves & roots
- 2 green apples
- 2 stalks celery
- 400 grams (about 2 cups) grapes

Directions:

Prepare **Ingredients:**

1. Roughly chop coriander leaves, stems, and roots.
2. Remove stems from celery and chop into small pieces.

   Juicing:
3. Wash grapes thoroughly.
4. Juice the coriander, celery, and grapes in handfuls at a time, feeding them into the juicer chute.
5. If the grapes have seeds, juice them whole with the skin on.
6. For the apples, juice them whole with the skin and seeds, or cut them into halves or quarters if they are too large to fit into the chute.
7. Assembly:
8. Start by juicing the coriander, then add the grapes in handfuls to help push the coriander down onto the press.
9. Follow with the celery pieces, juicing them in handfuls at a time.
10. Finish with the apples, allowing the juicer to press each one before adding the next.

Tip: Select fresh and fragrant coriander bunches with brightly colored leaves for maximum juice and nutrition. Juice the ingredients on the same day as purchased for the best results.

Watermelon, Ginger, and Lemon Shots

Ingredients:

- 2 cups watermelon cubes
- 1 tablespoon fresh ginger, peeled and grated
- Juice of 1 lemon
- Optional: Honey or agave syrup for sweetness

Directions:

1. Cut the watermelon into cubes, removing any seeds if necessary.
2. Peel and grate the fresh ginger.
3. Juice the lemon to extract the lemon juice.
4. In a blender, combine the watermelon cubes, grated ginger, and lemon juice.
5. If desired, add a drizzle of honey or agave syrup for sweetness.
6. Blend the ingredients until smooth and well combined.
7. If you prefer a smoother consistency, strain the mixture through a fine mesh sieve to remove any pulp or fibers.
8. Pour the health shot into small glasses or shot glasses.
9. Serve immediately for a refreshing and invigorating health boost.
10. Enjoy

Cognitive Function Recipes

Turmeric Smoothie Bowl

Ingredients:

- 1 ripe banana, frozen
- 1/2 cup frozen pineapple chunks
- 1/2 cup frozen mango chunks
- 1/2 teaspoon ground turmeric
- 1/4 teaspoon ground ginger
- 1/2 cup coconut milk (or any milk of choice)
- 1 tablespoon chia seeds (optional, for topping)
- Fresh fruit, nuts, seeds, or granola, for topping (optional)

Directions:

1. In a blender, combine the frozen banana, pineapple chunks, mango chunks, ground turmeric, ground ginger, and coconut milk.
2. Blend until smooth and creamy, adding more coconut milk if needed to reach your desired consistency.
3. Pour the smoothie into a bowl.
4. Top with chia seeds and any additional toppings you like, such as fresh fruit, nuts, seeds, or granola.
5. Serve immediately and enjoy your vibrant turmeric smoothie bowl!

Brain Boosting Lemon Balm

Ingredients:

- 2 cups (480ml) water
- 1/2 cup (about 15g) fresh lemon balm leaves
- Honey or sweetener of choice, to taste (optional)
- Lemon slices for garnish (optional)

Directions:

- In a small saucepan, bring the water to a boil over medium-high heat.
- Once boiling, remove the saucepan from the heat and add the fresh lemon balm leaves to the hot water.
- Cover the saucepan and let the lemon balm leaves steep in the hot water for about 10-15 minutes to infuse the water with their flavor and beneficial properties.
- After steeping, strain the lemon balm leaves from the infused water using a fine mesh strainer or cheesecloth, and discard the leaves.
- If desired, sweeten the infused lemon balm water with honey or your preferred sweetener to taste, stirring until dissolved.
- Pour the infused lemon balm water into cups or mugs for serving.
- Optionally, garnish each cup with a slice of lemon for extra flavor and visual appeal.
- Serve the brain-boosting lemon balm tea hot and enjoy its refreshing and revitalizing effects!

One Pan Salmon

Ingredients:

- 4 salmon filets (about 6 ounces each) 170 grams each
- 1 pound baby potatoes, halved
- 1 bunch asparagus, trimmed
- 2 tablespoons olive oil
- 2 cloves garlic, minced
- 1 teaspoon dried dill (or 1 tablespoon fresh dill, chopped)
- 1 teaspoon paprika
- Salt and pepper, to taste
- Lemon wedges, for serving

Directions:

1. Preheat your oven to 400°F (200°C).
2. Place the salmon filets, baby potatoes, and asparagus on a large baking sheet.
3. Drizzle the olive oil over the salmon, potatoes, and asparagus. Sprinkle with minced garlic, dried dill, paprika, salt, and pepper.
4. Toss everything together on the baking sheet until evenly coated with the seasonings.
5. Arrange the ingredients in a single layer, ensuring the salmon filets are skin-side down.
6. Roast in the preheated oven for 15-20 minutes, or until the salmon is cooked through and flakes easily with a fork, and the potatoes are tender.
7. Remove from the oven and serve immediately with lemon wedges.
8. Enjoy your delicious one-pan salmon dish!

Chickpea, Tomato, and Spinach Stew

Ingredients:

- 1 tablespoon olive oil
- 1 onion, diced
- 2 cloves garlic, minced
- 1 teaspoon ground cumin
- 1 teaspoon ground coriander
- 1/2 teaspoon smoked paprika
- 1 can (400g/14 oz) chickpeas, drained and rinsed
- 1 can (400g/14 oz) chopped tomatoes
- 2 cups fresh spinach leaves
- Salt and pepper to taste
- Fresh parsley, chopped (for garnish, optional)

Directions:

1. Heat the olive oil in a large saucepan over medium heat.

2. Add the diced onion and cook until softened, about 5 minutes.

3. Add the minced garlic, ground cumin, ground coriander, and smoked paprika. Cook for another 1-2 minutes until fragrant.

4. Stir in the drained chickpeas and chopped tomatoes. Bring the mixture to a simmer.

5. Reduce the heat to low and let the stew simmer for 15-20 minutes, stirring occasionally, until the flavors meld together and the sauce thickens slightly.

6. Add the fresh spinach leaves to the stew and cook for an additional 2-3 minutes, until wilted.

7. Season with salt and pepper to taste.

8. Serve the stew hot, garnished with chopped fresh parsley if desired. Enjoy your delicious and nutritious chickpea, tomato, and spinach stew!

Discover Time-Honored Herbal Wisdom with Exclusive Access to Video Recipes

Are you looking for a natural way to support your health and well-being? Are you sick and tired of being sick and tired?

The Barbara O'Neill Herbal Remedies & Medicine Encyclopedia is your comprehensive guide to harnessing the power of medicinal herbs, and now, you have access to this timeless wisdom through a never-been-seen-before transformative video course.

By gaining exclusive access, you will be introduced to:

- Detailed profiles of common healing herbs, including their traditional uses and modern applications.
- Step-by-step instructions for preparing some of the herbal teas, tinctures, salves, and other natural remedies featured in The Babara O'Neill Herbal Remedies & Natural Medicine Encyclopedia.
- Guidance on using herbs safely and effectively to address common health concerns including dosages.
- Fascinating insights into what herbs can do for you and your well-being.
- In-depth video tutorials demonstrating advanced herbal preparation techniques.
- Simply scan the QR code below to unlock your access to a time-honored wisdom and tradition.

Whether you're a beginner exploring herbal remedies for the first time or a seasoned herbalist seeking to deepen your knowledge, The Barbara O'Neill Herbal Remedies & Natural Medicine Encyclopedia and bonus video course will empower you to take control of your health naturally now and in the future.

Don't miss this opportunity to tap into the profound wisdom of medicinal herbs.

Colds and Flu

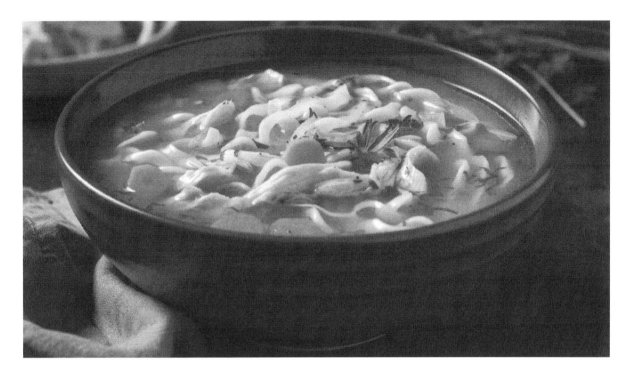

"Nature itself is the best physician." –Hippocrates

As seasons change and our bodies adapt to new environmental challenges, our immune systems can become compromised, leaving us vulnerable to colds and flu. By fortifying our natural defenses with targeted herbal remedies and nourishing recipes, we can help to prevent illness, reduce the severity of symptoms, and promote a swift recovery while our bodies build immunity.

Topical Treatments

Ingredients:

- 1 cup (286 g) baking soda
- 1/2 cup (118 g) citric acid
- 3/4 - 1 tsp peppermint essential oil
- 3/4 - 1 tsp eucalyptus essential oil
- 1 Tbsp dried mint leaves, crushed
- Witch hazel (in a spray bottle)

Directions:

1. In a bowl, mix together the baking soda and citric acid. Crush any clumps with your hands.

2. Add the peppermint and eucalyptus essential oils to the dry mixture, stirring with a spatula. Avoid direct contact with the oils.

3. Once combined, pour witch hazel into a small spray bottle. Spritz the dry mixture 3 to 4 times, stirring to incorporate.

4. If the mixture is still crumbly, lightly spray it with more witch hazel.

5. Sprinkle the crushed dried mint leaves into the bottom of a 1/4 measuring cup.

6. Pack the shower bomb mixture into the measuring cup, pressing firmly as you fill.

7. Invert the measuring cup onto a flat surface, like a plate or cutting board, to release the shower steamer.

8. Allow it to dry for approximately 3 hours.

9. Once dry, store the shower steamers in an airtight container in a cool, dark place.

10. Place the shower steamer at the back of your shower, away from direct water contact.

11. As you shower, the splashes of water will dissolve the steamer, releasing the invigorating scents of eucalyptus and mint.

12. Use as needed.

Thyme and Honey Homemade Cough Syrup

Ingredients:

- 1/2 lemon, sliced
- Handful of fresh thyme (or dried thyme)
- 1/2 cup honey
- 1 pint water (2 cups)

Directions:

- Place the lemon slices in a pint jar.
- Pour the honey over the lemon slices, ensuring they are completely covered. The honey will macerate the lemons and draw out their liquids.
- In a saucepan, combine the fresh thyme with the water.
- Bring the water to a gentle simmer, then reduce the heat to maintain a simmer for about 20 minutes.
- If using dried thyme, you can skip this step and simply add the dried thyme directly to the jar.
- Allow the thyme-infused water to cool slightly, then strain it to remove the thyme leaves.
- Add the infused water to the jar containing the lemon and honey mixture.
- Stir the contents of the jar well to combine all the ingredients.
- Cover the jar tightly and shake it to ensure everything is well-mixed.
- Store the homemade cough syrup in the refrigerator for up to 1 month.
- Take a spoonful of the syrup as needed to soothe coughs and sore throats.

Nasal Congestion Massage Oil

Ingredients:

- 1 ounce (30ml) Jojoba oil
- 10 drops peppermint essential oil
- 5 drops tea tree oil
- 5 drops lavender oil

Directions:

1. Begin by selecting a clean, empty glass bottle or container to mix and store your massage oil.
2. Pour the jojoba oil into the bottle, filling it almost to the top.
3. Add the essential oils to the jojoba oil base.
4. Close the bottle tightly and shake it well to thoroughly blend the oils together.
5. Your nasal congestion massage oil is now ready to use.
6. Before each use, shake the bottle gently to ensure the oils are mixed evenly.
7. To use, apply a small amount of the oil to your fingertips and gently massage it onto the chest, neck, and sinus areas, avoiding contact with the eyes.

Chest Congestion Massage Oil

Ingredients:

- 1 ounce (30ml) carrier oil like coconut, jojoba, sweet almond, or olive oil
- 5 drops eucalyptus essential oil
- 5 drops peppermint essential oil
- 3 drops tea tree essential oil
- 3 drops lavender essential oil

Directions:

1. In a clean glass bottle or container, pour in the carrier oil.
2. Add the drops of eucalyptus, peppermint, tea tree, and lavender essential oils to the carrier oil.
3. Close the bottle tightly and shake well to mix the oils together thoroughly.
4. Massage a small amount of the chest congestion oil onto the chest area in a circular motion, focusing on the upper chest and throat.
5. You can also apply it to the back between the shoulder blades.

Herbal Brews and Drinks

Echinacea and Elderberry Warm Tea

Ingredients:

- 6 cups (1.40 L) water
- 2 tablespoons dried elderberries
- 2 tablespoons honey
- 2 lemons

Directions:

1. Pour the water into a heavy saucepan.
2. Add the dried elderberries to the water.
3. Bring the water to a boil over medium-high heat.
4. Once boiling, reduce the heat to low and let the mixture simmer for 20 minutes.
5. After simmering, strain the mixture to remove the elderberries.
6. Stir in the honey until it dissolves completely.
7. Juice one lemon and add the juice to the tea.
8. Cut the remaining lemon into slices for garnish.
9. Serve the tea in cups or mugs, garnished with lemon slices.
10. Enjoy the warm and soothing Echinacea and Elderberry tea!

Ginger and Lemon Throat Soother

Ingredients:

- ¼ cup (60 ml) honey, or to taste
- 1 lemon, juiced
- 1 tablespoon finely grated ginger root
- ¼ teaspoon ground cinnamon
- 3 ½ cups (830 ml) boiling water

Directions:

1. Gather all ingredients. Boil water.
2. Place honey, lemon juice, ginger, and cinnamon in a teapot or 4-cup (946 ml) glass measuring beaker with spout.
3. Pour boiling water over the mixture; stir until honey is dissolved.
4. Cover the teapot and let steep for 5 minutes. The ginger should sink to the bottom but may be strained while pouring into a mug.

Peppermint, Honey, and Ginger Tea

Ingredients:

- 2 cups (480 ml) water
- 10 Mint leaves
- 2 tsp (10 ml) Honey
- 1 tsp (5 ml) Ginger, grated

Directions:

1. Place water in a saucepan, and add in mint leaves and ginger.
2. Bring this to a boil and simmer for 5 minutes or so.
3. Now place honey in a serving mug.
4. Pour the tea over a strainer into the cup.
5. Mix well and enjoy.

Basic Body Healing Bone Broth

Ingredients:

- 1 whole chicken carcass, meat removed but some scraps are OK
- 1-2 bay leaves
- 1 sprig fresh herbs like thyme (optional)
- 128 ounces (1 gallon or approximately 3.78 liters) filtered water
- 1 yellow onion, chopped
- 1 carrot, chopped
- 2-3 garlic cloves, smashed
- 2 tbsp (30 ml) apple cider vinegar
- A good amount of salt, about 1 tbsp (15 ml)
- Black pepper or whole black peppercorns

Directions:

- Add the chicken carcass, vegetables, and herbs to a large pot.
- Add 1 gallon (128 ounces or approximately 3.78 liters) of filtered water, making sure to fully submerge the chicken bones.
- Add the apple cider vinegar, salt, and black pepper.
- Cover with a lid and place the pot over low heat.
- Allow the chicken bone broth to simmer on low for 6-8 hours.
- Once the bone broth has simmered for at least 6 hours, it's time to strain it.
- Place a large bowl or pot in the kitchen sink with a colander or other strainer on top.
- Slowly pour the bone broth through the strainer.
- Don't worry about any herbs or large bits getting in the broth. If you would like to really filter the bone broth and remove any herb leaves or larger bits, strain one more time with cheesecloth covering the strainer.
- Once the broth has been strained, it can be poured into glass containers and the lids screwed on tight.
- Allow to sit on the counter to cool before placing in the refrigerator or freezer.

Colds and Flu Recipes

Coconut and Chili Poached Chicken

Ingredients:

- 4 skinless, boneless chicken breasts
- 1 can (14 ounces / 400ml) coconut milk
- 2 red chili peppers, sliced (adjust to taste)
- 2 cloves garlic, minced
- 1 tablespoon ginger, minced
- 2 tablespoons soy sauce
- 1 tablespoon fish sauce
- 1 tablespoon brown sugar
- Juice of 1 lime
- Salt and pepper to taste
- Fresh cilantro leaves for garnish
- Cooked rice or noodles, for serving (optional)

Directions:

1. In a large skillet or saucepan, combine the coconut milk, red chili peppers, garlic, ginger, soy sauce, fish sauce, brown sugar, and lime juice. Stir to combine.
2. Place the skillet over medium heat and bring the coconut milk mixture to a simmer.
3. Once the mixture is simmering, add the chicken breasts to the skillet. Ensure the chicken is submerged in the liquid.
4. Reduce the heat to low and let the chicken poach gently for about 15-20 minutes, or until cooked through. Cooking time may vary depending on the thickness of the chicken breasts.
5. Once the chicken is cooked, remove it from the skillet and set aside to rest for a few minutes.
6. Meanwhile, increase the heat to medium-high and simmer the coconut milk mixture until it thickens slightly, about 5-7 minutes.
7. Season with salt and pepper to taste.
8. Slice the chicken breasts and serve them over cooked rice or noodles, if desired.
9. Spoon the coconut chili sauce over the chicken and garnish with fresh cilantro leaves.
10. Serve hot and enjoy your delicious Coconut and Chili Poached Chicken!

Chicken Noodle Soup

Ingredients:

- 1 tablespoon olive oil
- 1 onion, chopped
- 2 carrots, sliced
- 2 celery stalks, sliced
- 2 cloves garlic, minced
- 6 cups (1.4 liters) chicken broth
- 2 boneless, skinless chicken breasts, cooked and shredded
- 2 cups (150g) egg noodles
- 1 teaspoon dried thyme
- Salt and pepper to taste
- Fresh parsley, chopped (for garnish)
- Optional: lemon wedges for serving

Directions:

1. In a large pot, heat the olive oil over medium heat.
2. Add the chopped onion, carrots, and celery. Cook, stirring occasionally, until the vegetables are softened, about 5-7 minutes.
3. Add the minced garlic and cook for an additional 1-2 minutes until fragrant.
4. Pour in the chicken broth and bring the mixture to a simmer.
5. Add the shredded chicken, egg noodles, and dried thyme to the pot. Season with salt and pepper to taste.
6. Simmer the soup for about 10-12 minutes, or until the noodles are cooked and tender.
7. Taste and adjust seasoning if needed.
8. Serve hot, garnished with chopped fresh parsley. Optionally serve with lemon wedges on the side for squeezing over the soup

Cambodian Seafood Broth

Ingredients:

- 1 tablespoon coconut oil
- 1 onion, finely chopped
- 2 cloves garlic, minced
- 1 stalk lemongrass, bruised and finely chopped
- 2 teaspoons grated fresh ginger
- 2 red chilies, thinly sliced (adjust to taste)
- 4 cups (950 ml) fish or seafood stock
- 1 can (14 ounces / 400 ml) coconut milk

- 1 tablespoon fish sauce
- 1 tablespoon low-sodium soy sauce
- Juice of 1 lime
- Salt and pepper to taste
- 500g mixed seafood, cleaned and deveined
- Fresh cilantro leaves for garnish
- Cooked rice or noodles, for serving (optional)

Directions:

1. In a large pot, heat the coconut oil over medium heat.
2. Add the chopped onion and cook until softened, about 3-4 minutes.
3. Add the minced garlic, lemongrass, grated ginger, and sliced red chilies to the pot. Cook for another 2 minutes until fragrant.
4. Pour in the fish or seafood stock and bring the mixture to a simmer.
5. Stir in the coconut milk, fish sauce, soy sauce, and lime juice.

Season with salt and pepper to taste.

6. Add the mixed seafood to the pot and simmer gently until cooked through, about 5-7 minutes depending on the type of seafood used.
7. Taste and adjust seasoning if needed.
8. Serve hot, garnished with fresh cilantro leaves. Optionally, serve with cooked rice or noodles on the side.

Flu-Busting Super Greens Soup

Ingredients:

- 1 tablespoon olive oil
- 1 onion, chopped
- 2 cloves garlic, minced
- 1-inch piece of ginger, grated
- 2 celery stalks, chopped
- 2 carrots, chopped
- 6 cups (1.4 liters) vegetable broth (low sodium or homemade)

- 4 cups (120g) mixed greens (such as spinach, kale, Swiss chard), chopped
- 1 cup (150g) frozen green peas
- 1 tablespoon lemon juice
- Salt and pepper to taste
- Optional toppings: sliced green onions, fresh herbs, or a dollop of Greek yogurt

Directions:

1. In a large pot, heat the olive oil over medium heat.
2. Add the chopped onion and cook until softened, about 3-4 minutes.
3. Add the minced garlic and grated ginger to the pot. Cook for another 1-2 minutes until fragrant.
4. Add the chopped celery and carrots to the pot and cook for 5 minutes, stirring occasionally.
5. Pour in the vegetable broth and bring the mixture to a simmer.
6. Once simmering, add the mixed greens and frozen green peas to the pot. Cook for another 5-7 minutes until the greens are wilted and the peas are heated through.
7. Remove the pot from the heat and stir in the lemon juice. Season with salt and pepper to taste.
8. Using an immersion blender or regular blender, blend the soup until smooth and creamy. Be careful when blending hot liquids.
9. Taste and adjust seasoning if needed.
10. Serve hot, garnished with sliced green onions, fresh herbs, or a dollop of Greek yogurt or sour cream if desired.

Detox and Cleanse

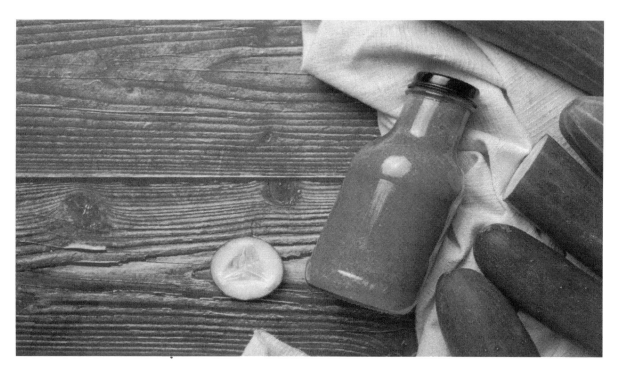

"The body is a self-healing organism, so it's really about clearing things out of the way and letting the body heal itself." –Barbara Brennan

We are constantly exposed to toxins and pollutants in the air we breathe, the water we drink, and the food we eat. Over time, these substances can accumulate in our bodies, leading to a range of health issues, from fatigue and digestive problems to chronic diseases. By periodically cleansing and detoxifying our systems, we can support our body's natural ability to eliminate harmful toxins, restore balance and promote optimal health.

Topical Treatments

Cleansing Cucumber and Mint Facial Mist

Ingredients:

- 1 cucumber
- Handful of fresh mint leaves
- 2 cups (480 ml) filtered water
- Optional: a few drops of essential oil (such as lavender or tea tree oil) for added fragrance and benefits

Directions:

1. Wash the cucumber thoroughly and cut it into slices.
2. Rinse the fresh mint leaves under cold water.
3. In a blender or food processor, combine the cucumber slices, fresh mint leaves, and filtered water.
4. Blend the ingredients until they form a smooth liquid.
5. If desired, strain the mixture through a fine mesh strainer or cheesecloth to remove any solids and achieve a finer mist.
6. Pour the cucumber and mint liquid into a clean spray bottle.
7. Optional: add a few drops of your favorite essential oil for added fragrance and benefits. Shake the bottle well to combine.
8. Store the facial mist in the refrigerator for a cooling effect.
9. To use, close your eyes and spritz the mist onto your face, holding the bottle about 6-8 inches away.
10. You can also apply it to a cotton pad and gently wipe your face with it.
11. Use the facial mist as part of your skincare routine to refresh and cleanse your skin, especially on hot days or after exercising.

Kelp Herbal Soak

Ingredients:

- 1 cup dried kelp seaweed
- 1/2 cup Epsom salt
- 1/4 cup sea salt
- 1/4 cup dried lavender flowers
- 1/4 cup dried chamomile flowers
- 1/4 cup dried calendula flowers
- Optional: a few drops of your favorite essential oil (such as lavender or eucalyptus) for added fragrance and benefits

Directions:

1. In a large mixing bowl, combine the dried kelp seaweed, Epsom salt, sea salt, dried lavender flowers, dried chamomile flowers, and dried calendula flowers.
2. Mix well to evenly distribute the ingredients.
3. If desired, add a few drops of your favorite essential oil to the mixture for added fragrance and therapeutic benefits.
4. Stir well to incorporate the essential oil.
5. Transfer the herbal bath soak mixture to a clean, airtight container or jar for storage.
6. To use, draw a warm bath and add 1/2 to 1 cup of the kelp herbal bath soak mixture to the running water.
7. Allow the salts to dissolve completely.
8. Soak in the bath for at least 20-30 minutes to fully experience the relaxing and rejuvenating benefits of the kelp and herbal blend.
9. After your bath, rinse off with warm water and pat your skin dry with a soft towel.
10. Store any remaining herbal bath soak mixture in a cool, dry place for future use.

ACV and Epsom Salt Foot Soak

Ingredients:

- 1 cup Epsom salt
- 1/2 cup apple cider vinegar (ACV)
- Warm water (enough to cover your feet in a basin or foot tub)
- Optional: a few drops of your favorite essential oil (such as lavender or peppermint) for added fragrance and benefits

Directions:

1. Fill a basin or foot tub with warm water. Make sure there's enough water to comfortably cover your feet.
2. Add 1 cup of Epsom salt to the warm water in the basin or foot tub.
3. Pour in 1/2 cup of apple cider vinegar (ACV) into the water.
4. If desired, add a few drops of your favorite essential oil to the foot soak mixture for added fragrance and therapeutic benefits.
5. Stir the ingredients in the foot soak mixture until the Epsom salt and ACV are dissolved.
6. Sit back and relax as you soak your feet in the mixture for 15-20 minutes. You can gently massage your feet while soaking to help relieve tension and improve circulation.
7. After soaking, rinse your feet with warm water and pat them dry with a soft towel.
8. Follow up with your favorite moisturizer to keep your feet soft and hydrated.

Herbal Brews and Drinks

Dandelion Tea

Ingredients:

- 1-2 tablespoons dried dandelion roots or leaves (or 2-3 fresh dandelion flowers)
- 1 cup (240 ml) water
- Optional: honey or lemon for flavor

Directions:

1. If using fresh dandelion flowers, rinse them thoroughly under cold water to remove any dirt or debris. If using dried dandelion roots or leaves, skip this step.
2. Bring 1 cup of water to a boil in a small saucepan.
3. Add the dried dandelion roots, leaves, or flowers to the boiling water.
4. Reduce the heat to low and let the mixture simmer for 5-10 minutes. Cover the saucepan to retain the volatile oils in the tea.
5. Remove the saucepan from the heat and let the tea steep for an additional 5-10 minutes.
6. Strain the tea using a fine mesh strainer or cheesecloth to remove the dandelion roots, leaves, or flowers.
7. If desired, sweeten the tea with honey or add a squeeze of lemon for extra flavor.
8. Serve the dandelion tea hot and enjoy!

Note: Dandelion tea has a slightly bitter taste, so you may want to adjust the brewing time or add sweeteners to suit your taste preferences.

Black Lemonade

Ingredients:

- 2-3 activated charcoal capsules (about 1/2 to 1 teaspoon of activated charcoal powder)
- 4 cups (about 950 ml) water
- 1/2 cup (about 120 ml) freshly squeezed lemon juice (about 3-4 lemons)
- 1/4 cup (about 60 ml) maple syrup or honey, adjust to taste
- Ice cubes
- Lemon slices or mint leaves for garnish (optional)

Directions:

1. In a pitcher or large mixing bowl, combine the activated charcoal powder and water. Stir well until the charcoal is evenly distributed and the water turns black.
2. Add the freshly squeezed lemon juice to the black water. Stir to combine.
3. Sweeten the black lemonade with maple syrup or honey according to your taste preferences. Start with 1/4 cup and adjust as needed.
4. Stir the lemonade until the sweetener is completely dissolved.
5. Place ice cubes in serving glasses and pour the black lemonade over the ice.
6. Garnish each glass with a lemon slice or mint leaves, if desired.
7. Serve immediately and enjoy your refreshing and visually striking Black Lemonade!

Note: Activated charcoal may interact with certain medications and supplements, so it's always best to consult with a healthcare professional before consuming it, especially if you're taking any medications or have any health concerns.

Super Green Detox Juice

Ingredients:

- 2 cups spinach
- 1 cucumber
- 2 celery stalks
- 1 green apple
- 1 inch piece of ginger
- 1 lemon, peeled
- Handful of parsley or cilantro
- Optional: a small knob of turmeric root

Directions:

1. Wash all the vegetables and fruits thoroughly.
2. Cut the cucumber, celery, and green apple into chunks that will fit into your juicer chute.
3. Peel the ginger and cut it into smaller pieces.
4. Cut the lemon into quarters or eighths, removing any seeds.
5. Rinse the parsley or cilantro and remove any tough stems.
6. If using turmeric, peel it and cut it into smaller pieces.
7. Feed all the ingredients through a juicer, alternating between the leafy greens and the harder vegetables and fruits.
8. Once all the ingredients have been juiced, stir the juice well to combine the flavors.
9. Pour the juice into glasses and serve immediately, over ice desired.

Early Morning ACV

Ingredients:

- 1 tablespoon of raw, unfiltered apple cider vinegar (with the "mother")
- 1/2 cup (120 ml) of warm water
- Optional: 1 teaspoon of honey or maple syrup (for sweetness)

Directions:

1. Measure out 1 tablespoon of raw, unfiltered apple cider vinegar and pour it into a small glass.
2. Heat 1/2 cup of water until it's warm but not boiling.
3. Pour the warm water into the glass with the apple cider vinegar.
4. If desired, add 1 teaspoon of honey or maple syrup to sweeten the shot.
5. Stir the mixture well until the apple cider vinegar and sweetener are fully dissolved.
6. Drink the ACV shot first thing in the morning on an empty stomach, before consuming any food or beverages.

Note: It's important to dilute apple cider vinegar with water before consuming it as a shot, as undiluted ACV can be harsh on the throat and stomach lining. Additionally, be sure to rinse your mouth with plain water after drinking the ACV shot to protect tooth enamel.

Detox Carrot Shot

Ingredients:

- 1 medium-sized carrot, washed and peeled
- 1/2 inch piece of fresh ginger, peeled
- 1/2 lemon, juiced
- Pinch of ground turmeric
- Pinch of cayenne pepper
- 1/4 cup (60 ml) filtered water

Directions:

1. Cut the carrot into smaller pieces that will fit into your juicer chute.
2. Cut the ginger into smaller pieces as well.
3. Juice the carrot and ginger using a juicer.
4. Pour the freshly squeezed carrot and ginger juice into a small glass.
5. Add the freshly squeezed lemon juice to the glass.
6. Add a pinch of ground turmeric and cayenne pepper for extra detoxifying and anti-inflammatory benefits.
7. Stir the mixture well to combine all the ingredients.
8. Dilute the mixture with 1/4 cup of filtered water.
9. Drink the detox carrot shot immediately after preparing it, before consuming any food or beverages.

Liver Cleansing Beetroot Juice

Ingredients:

- 1 medium-sized beetroot, washed and peeled
- 2 carrots, washed and peeled
- 1 apple, cored and sliced
- 1/2 lemon, juiced
- 1-inch piece of ginger, peeled
- Handful of fresh parsley or cilantro

Directions:

- Cut the beetroot, carrots, and apple into smaller pieces that will fit into your juicer chute.
- Cut the ginger into smaller pieces as well.
- Juice the beetroot, carrots, apple, and ginger using a juicer.
- Pour the freshly squeezed juice into a pitcher or large glass.
- Add the freshly squeezed lemon juice to the juice mixture.
- Add a handful of fresh parsley or cilantro for added detoxifying benefits.
- Optional: add a pinch of ground turmeric for its anti-inflammatory properties.
- Stir the mixture well to combine all the ingredients.
- Serve the liver-cleansing beetroot juice immediately after preparing it, over ice if desired.

Detox and Cleanse Recipes

Crunchy Detox Salad

Ingredients:

For the salad:

- 4 cups mixed greens like kale, spinach, arugula, or romaine lettuce, chopped
- 1 cup red cabbage, thinly sliced
- 1 cup carrots, julienned or grated
- 1 cucumber, thinly sliced

For the dressing:

- 1/4 cup extra virgin olive oil
- 2 tablespoons apple cider vinegar
- 1 tablespoon lemon juice
- 1 teaspoon Dijon mustard

- 1 bell pepper (any color), thinly sliced
- 1 cup broccoli florets, chopped
- 1/4 cup fresh parsley, chopped
- 1/4 cup sunflower seeds or pumpkin seeds for extra crunch

- 1 clove garlic, minced
- 1 teaspoon honey or maple syrup (optional)
- Salt and pepper to taste

Directions:

1. In a large mixing bowl, combine the chopped mixed greens, red cabbage, carrots, cucumber, bell pepper, broccoli florets, and fresh parsley. If using, add the sunflower seeds or pumpkin seeds for extra crunch.

2. In a small bowl or jar, whisk together the extra virgin olive oil, apple cider vinegar, lemon juice, Dijon mustard, minced garlic, honey or maple syrup (if using), and salt and pepper to taste. Alternatively, you can shake the ingredients together in a sealed jar to emulsify the dressing.

3. Pour the dressing over the salad and toss well to coat all the ingredients evenly.

4. Allow the salad to sit for a few minutes to allow the flavors to meld together.

5. Serve.

Glowing Body Summer Salad

Ingredients:

For the Grill:

- 3 ears fresh sweet corn, husked (about 375g)
- 4 hearts Romaine lettuce
- 1 lb. jumbo tail-on shrimp (about 450g) (use more for a higher

Other Salad Stuff:

- 2 cups chopped tomatoes (about 300g)
- 2 cups chopped cucumbers (about 300g)

shrimp-to-veg ratio)

- Lime juice, olive oil, and salt

- 2 cups chopped yellow bell pepper (about 300g)
- Cilantro avocado dressing

Directions:

1. Salad Prep:
- Make the avocado cilantro dressing.
- Chop the tomatoes, cucumbers, and bell peppers. Set aside about

2. Grilling:
- Heat the grill to medium-high heat.
- Brush the corn with olive oil and sprinkle with salt. Wrap in foil.
- Wash and dry the Romaine lettuce, cut in half lengthwise keeping the stem intact, and brush with olive oil and salt.
- Thread the shrimp on skewers for easy grilling. Brush with olive

3. Assembly:
- Cut the stem off the romaine and loosely chop it up.
- Cut the corn off the cob.
- Toss everything together with the remaining dressing.

80ml (1/3 cup) of dressing to brush on the shrimp while grilling.

oil, lime juice, and salt.

- Grill the corn (wrapped in foil) for 20-25 minutes, turning every 5 minutes. Grill the lettuce (directly on the grill) for about 5 minutes. Grill the shrimp (directly on the grill) for about 5 minutes. Brush the reserved dressing onto the shrimp as it grills for extra flavor.

Turmeric-Spiced Bone Broth

Ingredients:

- 2-3 lbs (about 1-1.5 kg) beef, chicken, or turkey bones (you can also use a combination)
- 2 carrots, chopped
- 2 celery stalks, chopped
- 1 onion, peeled and quartered
- 4 cloves garlic, smashed
- 1-inch piece of ginger, sliced
- 1 tablespoon ground turmeric
- 1 teaspoon whole black peppercorns
- 2 bay leaves
- 2 tablespoons apple cider vinegar
- Water, enough to cover the bones (about 10-12 cups)
- Salt, to taste

Directions:

1. Preheat your oven to 400°F (200°C). Place the bones on a baking sheet and roast them in the oven for about 30-40 minutes, or until they are browned and caramelized.
2. Transfer the roasted bones to a large stockpot or slow cooker. Add the chopped carrots, celery, onion, garlic, ginger, ground turmeric, black peppercorns, bay leaves, and apple cider vinegar.
3. Pour enough water into the pot to cover the bones by about 1-2 inches (about 10-12 cups).
4. If using a stockpot, bring the mixture to a boil over high heat. Once boiling, reduce the heat to low and let the broth simmer, partially covered, for at least 6-8 hours. Skim off any foam or impurities that rise to the surface during cooking. If using a slow cooker, set it to low and let the broth cook for 8-10 hours, or overnight.
5. Once the broth is done cooking, remove the bones and vegetables with a slotted spoon or mesh strainer. Discard the solids.
6. Strain the broth through a fine mesh sieve or cheesecloth to remove any remaining solids and achieve a clear broth.
7. Season the broth with salt, to taste.
8. Allow the broth to cool before transferring it to containers for storage. Store the broth in the refrigerator for up to 5 days, or freeze it for longer storage.
9. Enjoy your homemade Turmeric-Spiced Bone Broth as a nutritious base for soups, and stews, or simply sipped on its own for a comforting and healing beverage!

Roasted Carrot Hummus Dip

Ingredients:

- 3 large carrots, peeled and cut into 1-inch pieces
- 1 can (15 ounces) chickpeas, drained and rinsed
- 2 cloves garlic, minced
- 3 tablespoons tahini
- 3 tablespoons lemon juice
- 2 tablespoons olive oil
- 1 teaspoon ground cumin
- 1/2 teaspoon ground coriander
- Salt and pepper, to taste
- Water (as needed for consistency)
- Optional garnish: olive oil, chopped parsley, paprika

Directions:

1. Preheat your oven to 400°F (200°C). Place the chopped carrots on a baking sheet lined with parchment paper. Drizzle with olive oil and season with salt and pepper. Toss to coat.
2. Roast the carrots in the preheated oven for 20-25 minutes, or until they are tender and slightly caramelized.
3. In a food processor, combine the roasted carrots, chickpeas, minced garlic, tahini, lemon juice, olive oil, ground cumin, and ground coriander.
4. Pulse the mixture until smooth, scraping down the sides of the bowl as needed. If the mixture is too thick, add water, 1 tablespoon at a time, until you reach your desired consistency.
5. Taste the hummus and adjust the seasoning with salt, pepper, and additional lemon juice, if needed.
6. Transfer the hummus to a serving bowl. Drizzle with olive oil and sprinkle with chopped parsley and paprika, if desired, for garnish.
7. Serve the Roasted Carrot Hummus Dip with pita bread, crackers, or vegetable sticks for dipping.
8. Enjoy your flavorful and nutritious homemade hummus dip!

Protein Balls

Ingredients:

5 dates, pitted
¼ cup raw cashews (about 30g)
½ scoop clean chocolate protein powder (we like Truvani protein powder)
2 tablespoons shredded unsweetened coconut
1 tablespoon cashew butter (make sure it's all-natural, with no sugar)
1 tablespoon dark chocolate pieces

Directions:

. Place everything in a food processor and mix until you have a crumbly mixture that will stick together if pressed.

2. Remove the mixture from the food processor, rolling it between your hands into 6 evenly sized balls. If you have any extra coconut, roll the power bites in the coconut to prevent them from sticking together.

3. Transfer the protein bites to an airtight container and store them in the fridge for a firmer texture or at room temperature if you like them super soft. These will keep for up to 5 days.

Coconut Matcha Pudding

Ingredients:

- 1 cup (240ml) coconut milk
- 2 tablespoons chia seeds
- 1 teaspoon matcha powder
- 1-2 tablespoons honey or maple syrup, to taste
- Optional toppings: shredded coconut, sliced almonds, fresh berries

Directions:

1. In a mixing bowl, whisk together the coconut milk, matcha powder, and honey or maple syrup until well combined.

2. Add the chia seeds to the mixture and stir until they are evenly distributed.

3. Let the mixture sit for about 5 minutes, then give it another stir to prevent clumping.

4. Cover the bowl and refrigerate for at least 2 hours, or preferably overnight, to allow the chia seeds to absorb the liquid and thicken.

5. Once the pudding has thickened to your desired consistency, give it a final stir.

6. Divide the pudding into serving bowls or jars.

7. If desired, top each serving with shredded coconut, sliced almonds, or fresh berries for added flavor and texture.

8. Serve chilled and enjoy your delicious Coconut Matcha

ChiazPudding!

Digestive Health

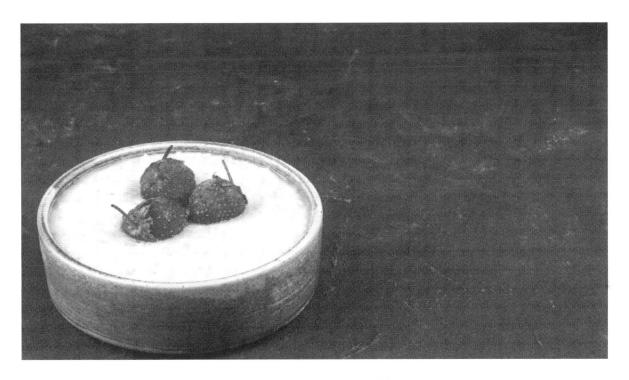

"All disease begins in the gut." –Hippocrates

Digestive health is the foundation of overall well-being, as it is through the gut that we absorb the nutrients necessary to fuel our bodies and minds. When our digestive system is out of balance, we may experience a range of symptoms, from bloating and discomfort to more serious health issues. By supporting our gut health with targeted herbs and nourishing recipes, we can promote optimal digestion, nutrient absorption, and overall vitality.

Topical Treatments

Digestion Tincture

Equipment:

- Quart-size mason jar
- Dropper bottles

Ingredients:

- 60g (1/2 cup) dried peppermint leaf
- 30g (1/4 cup) dried ginger root pieces (or 115g (1/2 cup) fresh, finely chopped)
- 30g (1/4 cup) dried fennel (or chamomile)
- 475ml (2 cups) 95-proof alcohol (like Everclear)
- 240ml (1 cup) distilled water

Directions:

1. Crush the fennel. Put peppermint, ginger, and fennel (or chamomile) in the glass jar.
2. Fill the rest of the jar with alcohol and water. If you don't have enough liquid to cover your herbs fully, add a little more alcohol and water in a 2:1 ratio until you do.
3. Cap the jar and keep in a cool dark place for at least two weeks, but up to six. Shake occasionally.
4. After 2-6 weeks, strain the herbs out with a fine mesh strainer or cheesecloth. Compost the herbs.
5. Store your tincture in glass dropper bottles in a cool, dark place.

Notes:

- Start small with the dose and increase as needed.
- Dosage: 10 to 20 drops

Herbal Brews and Drinks

After Meal Tea

Ingredients:

- 2 cups (500ml) filtered water
- 1 teaspoon anise seed, lightly crushed using a mortar and pestle
- 1 teaspoon fennel seeds, lightly crushed using a mortar and pestle
- ½ a cinnamon stick
- Strips of zest from ½ a small orange
- 1-inch (2.5 cm) piece of ginger, peeled and finely grated
- Sweetener of choice to taste
- Orange slices and cinnamon stick for serving if desired

Directions:

1. Combine all the ingredients in a small saucepan.
2. Bring to a gentle simmer over medium heat, then lower the heat and keep warm (just a couple of bubbles around the sides of the pan) for 10 minutes.
3. Strain the tea through a fine mesh strainer into cups or mugs.
4. Sweeten to taste with your preferred sweetener.
5. Serve hot with orange slices and a cinnamon stick if desired.

Peppermint and Fennel Tea

Ingredients:

- 2 cups (500ml) filtered water
- 1 teaspoon dried peppermint leaves
- 1 teaspoon fennel seeds
- Sweetener of choice, such as honey or sugar, to taste (optional)
- Lemon slices or fresh mint leaves for garnish (optional)

Directions:

1. In a small saucepan, bring the filtered water to a boil over medium-high heat (100°C / 212°F).
2. Once the water reaches a boil, remove it from the heat.
3. Add the dried peppermint leaves and fennel seeds to the hot water.
4. Cover the saucepan with a lid and let the herbs steep for 5-7 minutes.
5. After steeping, strain the tea through a fine mesh strainer to remove the peppermint leaves and fennel seeds.
6. If desired, sweeten the tea with honey or sugar to taste.
7. Pour the tea into cups or mugs.
8. Garnish with lemon slices or fresh mint leaves, if desired.
9. Serve hot and enjoy your soothing Peppermint and Fennel Tea!

Cumin Seed Tea

Ingredients:

- 2 cups (500ml) filtered water
- 1 tablespoon cumin seeds
- Sweetener of choice, such as honey or sugar, to taste (optional)
- Lemon slices or fresh mint leaves for garnish (optional)

Directions:

1. In a small saucepan, bring the filtered water to a boil over medium-high heat (100°C / 212°F).
2. Add the cumin seeds to the boiling water.
3. Reduce the heat to low and let the cumin seeds simmer in the water for 5-10 minutes.
4. After simmering, remove the saucepan from the heat and let the tea cool slightly.
5. Strain the tea through a fine mesh strainer to remove the cumin seeds.
6. If desired, sweeten the tea with honey or sugar to taste.
7. Pour the tea into cups or mugs.
8. Garnish with lemon slices or fresh mint leaves, if desired.

Cardamom Iced Tea

Ingredients:

- 4 cups (1 liter) water
- 4-5 black tea bags or 2 tablespoons loose black tea leaves
- 4-5 green cardamom pods, lightly crushed
- Sweetener of choice, such as honey or sugar, to taste
- Ice cubes
- Lemon slices and fresh mint leaves for garnish (optional)

Directions:

1. In a medium saucepan, bring the water to a boil over medium-high heat.
2. Once the water boils, remove it from the heat and add the black tea bags or loose black tea leaves to the hot water.
3. Add the lightly crushed green cardamom pods to the tea.
4. Cover the saucepan and let the tea steep for 5-7 minutes to infuse the flavors.
5. After steeping, remove the tea bags or strain the tea leaves and cardamom pods from the liquid.
6. If desired, sweeten the tea with honey or sugar while it's still warm, stirring until dissolved.
7. Let the tea cool to room temperature, then transfer it to a pitcher and refrigerate until chilled, for about 1-2 hours.
8. To serve, fill glasses with ice cubes and pour the chilled cardamom-infused tea over the ice.
9. Garnish with lemon slices and fresh mint leaves, if desired.

Ginger Pepper Shot

Ingredients:

- 1 small piece of ginger (about 1 inch / 2.5 cm), peeled
- 1/4 teaspoon ground black pepper
- 1/4 cup (60 ml) water
- Optional: a squeeze of lemon juice or a pinch of cayenne pepper for extra kick

Directions:

- Peel the ginger and chop it into smaller pieces to make it easier to blend.
- In a blender or food processor, combine the chopped ginger, ground black pepper, and water.
- Blend on high speed until the mixture is smooth and well combined.
- If desired, add a squeeze of lemon juice or a pinch of cayenne pepper for extra flavor and kick.
- Once blended, strain the mixture through a fine mesh strainer or cheesecloth to remove any fibrous bits.
- Pour the strained juice into a shot glass or small glass.
- Serve immediately and enjoy your invigorating Ginger Pepper Juice Shot!

Digestive Health Recipes

Gut-Friendly Oatmeal

Ingredients:

- 1/2 cup rolled oats (gluten-free if needed)
- 1 cup water or milk of choice (such as almond milk, oat milk, or dairy milk)
- 1 tablespoon ground flaxseed
- 1 tablespoon chia seeds
- 1/2 ripe banana, mashed
- 1/2 teaspoon ground cinnamon
- 1/4 teaspoon ground ginger
- Pinch of salt
- Optional toppings: sliced banana, berries, nuts, seeds, honey, or maple syrup

Directions:

1. In a small saucepan, combine the rolled oats and water or milk. Bring to a boil over medium-high heat.
2. Once boiling, reduce the heat to low and simmer, stirring occasionally, for about 5 minutes, or until the oats are cooked and the mixture has thickened to your desired consistency.
3. Stir in the ground flaxseed, chia seeds, mashed banana, ground cinnamon, ground ginger, and a pinch of salt. Cook for an additional 1-2 minutes, stirring occasionally, until the mixture is well combined and heated through.
4. Remove the oatmeal from the heat and transfer it to a serving bowl.
5. Serve the Gut-Friendly Oatmeal hot, topped with your favorite toppings such as sliced banana, berries, nuts, seeds, honey, or maple syrup.

Mango and Aloe Smoothie

Ingredients:

- 1 ripe mango, peeled, pitted, and chopped (about 1 cup)
- 1/2 cup aloe vera juice (unsweetened)
- 1/2 cup plain Greek yogurt (or coconut yogurt for a dairy-free option)
- 1/2 cup coconut water
- 1 tablespoon honey or maple syrup (optional, depending on sweetness of mango)
- Ice cubes (optional)

Directions:

1. Place the chopped mango, aloe vera juice, Greek yogurt, coconut water, and honey or maple syrup (if using) in a blender.
2. Blend on high speed until smooth and creamy. If the smoothie is too thick, you can add more coconut water or aloe vera juice to reach your desired consistency.
3. If desired, add a handful of ice cubes to the blender and blend again until the smoothie is chilled and frothy.
4. Pour the Mango and Aloe Smoothie into glasses and serve immediately.
5. Optionally, garnish with a slice of mango or a sprig of mint for a decorative touch.
6. Enjoy your refreshing and hydrating Mango and Aloe Smoothie!

Sweet ACV Salad Dressing

Ingredients:

- 60ml (1/4 cup) apple cider vinegar
- 30ml (2 tablespoons) honey or maple syrup
- 60ml (1/4 cup) extra virgin olive oil
- Salt and pepper to taste

Directions:

1. In a small bowl or jar, combine the apple cider vinegar, and honey or maple syrup until well combined.
2. Slowly drizzle in the extra virgin olive oil while continuing to whisk or shake, until the dressing is emulsified and smooth.
3. Season the dressing with salt and pepper to taste, and adjust the sweetness or acidity as desired by adding more honey or vinegar.
4. Serve the Sweet Apple Cider Vinegar Salad Dressing immediately over your favorite salad greens, or store it in an airtight container in the refrigerator for up to one week.
5. Shake or whisk the dressing again before using, as the ingredients may separate over time.

Quick Kimchi

Ingredients:

- 1 small head Napa cabbage (about 1 pound), thinly sliced
- 1 medium carrot, julienned or grated
- 4 green onions, thinly sliced
- 2 cloves garlic, minced
- 1 tablespoon grated fresh ginger
- 2 tablespoons gochugaru (Korean red pepper flakes)
- 2 tablespoons fish sauce or soy sauce
- 1 tablespoon rice vinegar or apple cider vinegar
- 1 tablespoon sugar
- 1 teaspoon salt
- Optional: 1 tablespoon sesame seeds

Directions:

1. In a large mixing bowl, combine the sliced Napa cabbage, julienned or grated carrot, thinly sliced green onions, minced garlic, grated ginger, gochugaru, fish sauce or soy sauce, rice vinegar or apple cider vinegar, sugar, and salt.
2. Using clean hands, massage the mixture thoroughly, squeezing and pressing the vegetables to help them release their juices and soften. Continue massaging for about 5-7 minutes, or until the vegetables have reduced in volume and are well coated in the seasoning mixture.
3. Once the vegetables are well combined and softened, transfer the quick kimchi to a clean glass jar or airtight container, pressing it down firmly to remove any air bubbles and ensuring that the vegetables are submerged in their own juices.
4. If desired, sprinkle sesame seeds over the top of the kimchi for added flavor and texture.
5. Seal the jar or container tightly and let the quick kimchi ferment at room temperature for at least 1-2 hours before transferring it to the refrigerator.
6. Allow the kimchi to ferment in the refrigerator for at least 24 hours before serving. The longer it ferments, the more flavorful it will become.

Creamy Yogurt Pudding

Ingredients:

- 3 tablespoons (25g) porridge oats
- 150g pot 0% fat probiotic yogurt

Directions:

1. Tip 200 ml water into a small non-stick pan and stir in porridge oats.
2. Cook over a low heat until bubbling and thickened. (To make in a microwave, use a deep container to prevent spillage as the mixture will rise up as it cooks, and cook for 3 minutes on High.)
3. Stir in the probiotic yogurt – or swirl in half and top with the rest.

Apricot Seed Bars

Ingredients:

- 1 cup dried apricots
- 1 cup pitted dates
- 1 cup raw almonds
- 1/2 cup raw sunflower seeds
- 1/4 cup raw pumpkin seeds
- 1/4 cup unsweetened shredded coconut
- 1/4 cup honey or maple syrup
- 1 teaspoon vanilla extract
- Pinch of salt

Directions:

1. Preheat your oven to 180°C (350°F) and line a baking dish with parchment paper.
2. In a food processor, combine the dried apricots, pitted dates, raw almonds, sunflower seeds, pumpkin seeds, shredded coconut, honey or maple syrup, vanilla extract, and a pinch of salt.
3. Pulse the mixture until it forms a sticky dough-like consistency. You may need to stop and scrape down the sides of the food processor occasionally to ensure that all the ingredients are well combined.
4. Transfer the mixture to the prepared baking dish and press it down firmly into an even layer using the back of a spoon or your hands.
5. Bake in the preheated oven for 15-20 minutes, or until the edges are golden brown and the bars are set.
6. Remove the baking dish from the oven and let the bars cool completely before slicing them into bars or squares.
7. Once cooled, store the Apricot Seed Bars in an airtight container at room temperature for up to one week, or in the refrigerator for a longer shelf life.

Electrolyte Balancing

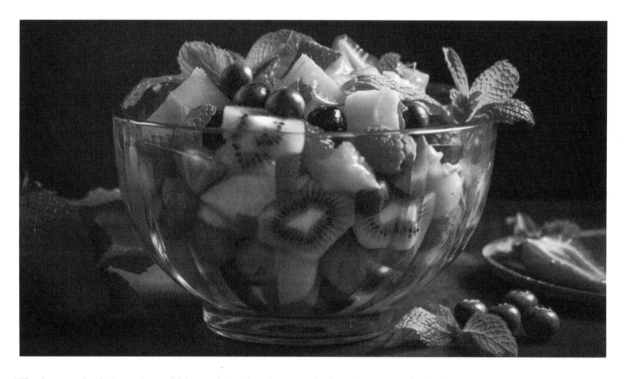

"The human body is an incredible machine, but it can only function properly if it's given the right fuel." —Dr. Mark Hyman

Electrolytes are essential minerals that play a crucial role in maintaining fluid balance, muscle function, and overall health. When our electrolyte levels become imbalanced, whether due to illness, intense exercise, or poor diet, we may experience symptoms such as fatigue, muscle cramps, and dizziness. By supporting our body's natural electrolyte balance with targeted herbs and nourishing recipes, we can help to restore optimal hydration, energy levels, and vitality.

Topical Treatments

Pink Himalayan Soak

- 1 cup Natural Epsom Salt
- 1 cup Pink Himalayan Salt, Extra-Fine Grain

Directions:

1. Combine all ingredients in a large bowl.
2. Be sure to break up any clumps that develop from essential oils.

   For use:

- Add 1/2 to 1 cup of bath salts to your bath just before getting in.

- 1/4 cup Arm & Hammer Pure Baking Soda
- 6 drops Grapefruit 100% Essential Oil, Therapeutic Grade

3. Store the mixture in an airtight container, in a dark, cool place indefinitely.

Herbal Brews and Drinks

Salt Lemonade

Ingredients:

- 4 cups (960ml) water
- 1 cup (240ml) freshly squeezed lemon juice (about 4-6 lemons)
- 1/4 teaspoon salt
- Natural sweetener of choice, to taste (such as stevia or monk fruit sweetener)
- Ice cubes
- Lemon slices and mint leaves, for garnish (optional)

Directions:

1. In a large pitcher, combine the water and freshly squeezed lemon juice.
2. Add the salt to the pitcher and stir until dissolved.
3. Taste the lemonade and adjust the saltiness or tartness by adding more salt or lemon juice, if desired.
4. Add your natural sweetener of choice to the pitcher, starting with a small amount, and adjust to taste. Remember that natural sweeteners are much sweeter than sugar, so you'll need less.
5. Stir until the sweetener is dissolved.
6. Refrigerate the lemonade for at least 1-2 hours to chill.
7. Once chilled, fill glasses with ice cubes and pour the salted lemonade over the ice.
8. Garnish with lemon slices and mint leaves, if desired.
9. Serve immediately and enjoy your refreshing Natural Sweetener Salted Lemonade!

Note: Stevia and monk fruit sweetener are both natural, zero-calorie sweeteners that can be used as alternatives to sugar. They provide sweetness without the calories or blood sugar spike associated with sugar, making them ideal choices for those looking to reduce their sugar intake.

Pineapple, Lemon, Salt Electrolyte Drink

Ingredients:

- 2 cups (480ml) coconut water
- 1 cup (240ml) pineapple juice (freshly squeezed or store-bought, without added sugar)
- Juice of 1 lemon
- 1/4 teaspoon salt (preferably sea salt or Himalayan salt)
- Optional: Honey or natural sweetener of choice, to taste
- Ice cubes
- Lemon slices and pineapple wedges, for garnish (optional)

Directions:

1. In a large pitcher, combine the coconut water, pineapple juice, lemon juice, and salt.
2. If desired, add honey or a natural sweetener of choice to taste. Keep in mind that pineapple juice is naturally sweet, so you may not need much, if any, additional sweetener.
3. Stir until all the ingredients are well combined and the salt is dissolved.
4. Taste the electrolyte drink and adjust the sweetness or saltiness as needed.
5. Refrigerate the drink for at least 1-2 hours to chill.
6. Once chilled, fill glasses with ice cubes and pour the electrolyte drink over the ice.
7. Garnish each glass with a slice of lemon and a pineapple wedge, if desired.

Lemon, Lime, and Coconut Water

Ingredients:

- 2 cups (480ml) coconut water
- Juice of 1 lemon
- Juice of 1 lime
- Ice cubes
- Lemon and lime slices, for garnish (optional)
- Mint leaves, for garnish (optional)

Directions:

1. In a pitcher or large jug, combine the coconut water, freshly squeezed lemon juice, and freshly squeezed lime juice.
2. Stir well to mix the juices with the coconut water.
3. Taste the drink and adjust the tartness by adding more lemon or lime juice if desired.
4. If desired, add ice cubes to the pitcher to chill the drink, or add ice cubes directly to individual glasses.
5. Garnish each glass with slices of lemon and lime, and a sprig of mint if desired.

Basil and Watermelon Shot

Ingredients:

- 1 cup diced watermelon, seeds removed
- 4-5 fresh basil leaves
- Juice of 1/2 lime
- Optional: A pinch of salt or a dash of honey, to taste
- Ice cubes (optional)

Directions:

1. In a blender, combine the diced watermelon, fresh basil leaves, and lime juice.
2. If desired, add a pinch of salt for flavor enhancement or a dash of honey for sweetness. Adjust according to your taste preferences.
3. Blend the ingredients until smooth and well combined.
4. Strain the juice through a fine mesh sieve or cheesecloth to remove any pulp or seeds, if desired. This step is optional depending on your preference for texture.
5. Pour the juice into shot glasses or small cups.
6. If desired, add ice cubes to chill the juice before serving.
7. Garnish each shot with a small basil leaf or a slice of watermelon, if desired.

Cucumber and Mint Shot

Ingredients:

- 1 cucumber
- Handful of fresh mint leaves
- Juice of 1 lemon
- Optional: A pinch of salt or a dash of honey, to taste
- Ice cubes (optional)

Directions:

- Wash the cucumber and mint leaves thoroughly under cold running water.
- Cut the cucumber into smaller pieces, removing the ends.
- In a blender or food processor, combine the cucumber pieces, fresh mint leaves, and lemon juice.
- If desired, add a pinch of salt for flavor enhancement or a dash of honey for sweetness. Adjust according to your taste preferences.
- Blend the ingredients until smooth and well combined. If the mixture is too thick, you can add a splash of water to thin it out.
- Strain the mixture through a fine mesh sieve or cheesecloth to remove any pulp or fibers, if desired. This step is optional depending on your preference for texture.
- Pour the juice into shot glasses or small cups.
- If desired, add ice cubes to chill the juice before serving.
- Garnish each shot with a small mint leaf or a slice of cucumber, if desired.

Electrolyte Balancing Recipes

Banana, Coconut Milk, and Avocado Smoothie

Ingredients:

- 1 ripe banana, peeled and sliced
- 1/2 ripe avocado, peeled and pitted
- 1 cup (240ml) coconut milk (you can use canned or homemade)
- 1/2 cup (120ml) water or coconut water
- 1 tablespoon honey or maple syrup (optional, for sweetness)
- Ice cubes (optional)
- Toasted coconut flakes, for garnish (optional)

Directions:

1. In a blender, combine the sliced banana, ripe avocado, coconut milk, and water or coconut water.
2. If you prefer a sweeter smoothie, add honey or maple syrup to taste. You can adjust the amount based on your preference for sweetness.
3. If desired, add a handful of ice cubes to the blender to make the smoothie colder and more refreshing.
4. Blend the ingredients on high speed until smooth and creamy. If the smoothie is too thick, you can add more water or coconut milk to reach your desired consistency.
5. Once blended, taste the smoothie and adjust the sweetness or creaminess as needed.
6. Pour the smoothie into glasses and garnish with toasted coconut flakes, if desired.
7. Serve immediately and enjoy!

Cucumber, Lime, and Pomegranate Salad

Ingredients:

- 2 large cucumbers, peeled and thinly sliced
- Seeds from 1 large pomegranate
- Juice of 2 limes
- Zest of 1 lime
- 2 tablespoons extra virgin olive oil
- 1 tablespoon honey or maple syrup (optional, for sweetness)
- Salt and pepper, to taste
- Fresh mint leaves, chopped, for garnish (optional)

Directions:

1. In a large mixing bowl, combine the thinly sliced cucumbers and pomegranate seeds.
2. In a separate small bowl, whisk together the lime juice, lime zest, extra virgin olive oil, and honey or maple syrup (if using). Season with salt and pepper to taste.
3. Pour the dressing over the cucumber and pomegranate mixture and toss until well combined.
4. Taste the salad and adjust the seasoning or sweetness as needed.
5. Transfer the salad to a serving dish or individual plates.
6. Garnish the salad with chopped fresh mint leaves, if desired, for an extra burst of freshness.

Not Just One Fruit Salad

Ingredients:

- 1 mango (a bit ripe), cut into cubes
- 8 strawberries, cut in half
- 2 kiwis, peeled and cut into cubes
- 2 teaspoons honey
- 3 tablespoons fresh lime juice
- 1 teaspoon chia seeds

Directions:

1. In a large mixing bowl, combine the cubed mango, halved strawberries, and cubed kiwis.
2. In a small bowl, warm the honey slightly using a hot water bath or microwave, so it is easier to stir.
3. Stir in the fresh lime juice and chia seeds into the warmed honey until well combined.
4. Drizzle the dressing over the fruit salad in the mixing bowl.
5. Gently toss the fruit salad until all the fruits are evenly coated with the dressing.
6. Transfer the fruit salad to a serving dish or individual plates.
7. Serve immediately as a refreshing and colorful dessert or snack.

Cool as Cucumber Salad

Ingredients:

- 2 large cucumbers, thinly sliced
- 1/4 cup red onion, thinly sliced
- 2 tablespoons fresh dill, chopped
- 2 tablespoons fresh parsley, chopped
- 2 tablespoons extra virgin olive oil
- 1 tablespoon white wine vinegar or apple cider vinegar
- Salt and black pepper, to taste
- Optional: Feta cheese, crumbled, for garnish

Directions:

1. In a large mixing bowl, combine the thinly sliced cucumbers, sliced red onion, chopped fresh dill, and chopped fresh parsley.
2. In a small bowl, whisk together the extra virgin olive oil and white wine vinegar (or apple cider vinegar) to make the dressing.
3. Pour the dressing over the cucumber mixture in the large mixing bowl.
4. Season the salad with salt and black pepper to taste.
5. Toss the salad gently until all the ingredients are evenly coated with the dressing.
6. If desired, sprinkle crumbled feta cheese over the top of the salad for extra flavor and creaminess.
7. Transfer the Cool as Cucumber Salad to a serving dish or individual plates.
8. Serve immediately.

Energy Boosters

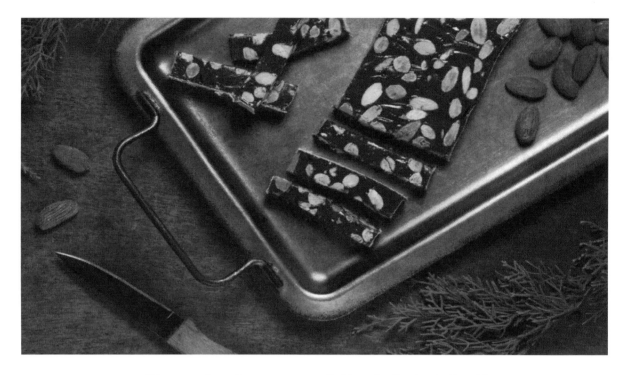

"Energy and persistence conquer all things." —Benjamin Franklin

The pace of modern living is frenetic at best and many of us find ourselves struggling to maintain the energy levels needed to power through our daily responsibilities and pursue our passions. Turning to natural energy boosters, like invigorating herbs and nutrient-dense recipes can help to combat fatigue, enhance mental clarity, and support our body's natural vitality.

Topical Treatments

Witch Hazel Toning Water

Ingredients:

- 1/2 cup witch hazel extract
- 1/2 cup distilled water
- 5-10 drops essential oil of choice (optional, for fragrance and additional benefits)
  - Examples: lavender, tea tree, rosemary, or chamomile

Directions:

1. In a clean glass bottle or container, combine the witch hazel extract and distilled water.
2. If using essential oils for added fragrance and benefits, add 5-10 drops of your chosen essential oil to the mixture. You can use a single essential oil or a combination of oils, depending on your preference.
3. Secure the lid tightly on the bottle or container and shake well to thoroughly mix all the ingredients together.
4. Store the Witch Hazel Face Toning Water in a cool, dark place away from direct sunlight.

Usage:

- After cleansing your face, apply the Witch Hazel Face Toning Water to a cotton pad or ball.
- Gently swipe the soaked cotton pad or ball across your face and neck, avoiding the delicate eye area.
- Allow the toning water to air dry on your skin or lightly pat it into your skin with clean hands.

- Follow up with your favorite moisturizer or serum.

Herbal Brews and Drinks

Green Tea and Mint Cold Drink

Ingredients:

- 2 green tea bags
- 4 cups (960ml) water
- 1/4 cup (60ml) fresh mint leaves, loosely packed
- 2 tablespoons honey or maple syrup (optional, for sweetness)
- Ice cubes
- Fresh mint sprigs, for garnish (optional)
- Lemon slices, for garnish (optional)

Directions:

1. Bring the water to a boil in a medium saucepan. Once boiling, remove from heat.
2. Add the green tea bags and fresh mint leaves to the hot water.
3. Allow the tea bags and mint leaves to steep in the hot water for about 5-7 minutes, or until the desired strength is reached.
4. Once steeped, remove the tea bags and mint leaves from the saucepan. Discard the tea bags and strain out the mint leaves.
5. If using honey or maple syrup for sweetness, stir it into the hot tea until dissolved. Adjust the sweetness according to your taste preferences.
6. Allow the tea to cool to room temperature, then transfer it to a pitcher or large glass jar.
7. Refrigerate the tea until chilled, about 1-2 hours.
8. Once chilled, fill glasses with ice cubes.
9. Pour the chilled Green Tea and Mint Cold Drink into the glasses over the ice cubes.
10. Garnish each glass with a fresh mint sprig and a slice of lemon, if desired.

Berry Coconut Water

Ingredients:

- 1 cup mixed berries (such as strawberries, blueberries, raspberries, or blackberries), fresh or frozen
- 2 cups (480ml) coconut water
- Ice cubes (optional)
- Fresh mint leaves, for garnish (optional)

Directions:

1. If using fresh berries, rinse them under cold water and remove any stems or leaves. If using frozen berries, thaw them slightly at room temperature or microwave them for a few seconds until they are partially thawed.
2. In a blender, combine the mixed berries and coconut water.
3. Blend on high speed until the berries are completely pureed and the mixture is smooth.
4. If desired, strain the mixture through a fine mesh sieve or cheesecloth to remove any seeds or pulp. This step is optional depending on your preference for texture.
5. Pour the berry coconut water into glasses filled with ice cubes, if using.
6. Garnish each glass with fresh mint leaves for a pop of color and additional freshness, if desired.
7. Serve immediately

Ginseng Green Tea

Ingredients:

- 1 green tea bag or 1 teaspoon loose green tea leaves
- 1 cup (240ml) water
- 1 teaspoon ginseng powder or 1 ginseng tea bag (optional)
- Honey or sweetener of choice (optional)

Directions:

1. Bring the water to a boil in a small saucepan or kettle.
2. Place the green tea bag or loose green tea leaves in a mug.
3. If using ginseng powder, add it to the mug with the green tea. If using a ginseng tea bag, you can steep it separately or add it to the mug with the green tea.
4. Once the water reaches a boil, pour it over the green tea and ginseng in the mug.
5. Allow the tea to steep for 3-5 minutes, depending on your preference for strength.
6. If desired, add honey or sweetener of choice to taste for a touch of sweetness. Stir until the sweetener is fully dissolved.
7. Remove the tea bag or strain out the loose tea leaves, if necessary.

Energy Boosting Recipes

Avocado and Green Tea Smoothie

Ingredients:

- 1 ripe avocado, peeled and pitted
- 1 cup (240ml) brewed green tea, cooled
- 1/2 cup (120ml) unsweetened almond milk or coconut milk
- 1 tablespoon honey or maple syrup (optional, for sweetness)
- Juice of 1/2 lime
- Handful of ice cubes

Directions:

- Brew green tea and allow it to cool to room temperature.
- In a blender, combine the ripe avocado, brewed green tea, almond milk or coconut milk, honey or maple syrup (if using), lime juice, and ice cubes.
- Blend on high speed until smooth and creamy, scraping down the sides of the blender as needed.
- Taste the smoothie and adjust sweetness or tartness by adding more honey, lime juice, or green tea as desired.
- Once blended to your desired consistency, pour the Avocado and Green Tea Smoothie into glasses.

Energy Smoothie with Maca Root

Ingredients:

- 1 ripe banana, peeled
- 1 tablespoon maca root powder
- 1 cup (240ml) unsweetened almond milk or coconut milk
- 1 tablespoon almond butter or peanut butter
- 1 tablespoon honey or maple syrup (optional, for sweetness)
- 1/2 teaspoon ground cinnamon
- Handful of ice cubes

Directions:

- In a blender, combine the ripe banana, maca root powder, almond milk or coconut milk, almond butter or peanut butter, honey or maple syrup (if using), ground cinnamon, and ice cubes.
- Blend on high speed until smooth and creamy, scraping down the sides of the blender as needed.
- Taste the smoothie and adjust sweetness or flavorings as desired.

You can add more honey for sweetness or more cinnamon for a spicier flavor.
- Once blended to your desired consistency, pour the Energy Smoothie with Maca Root into glasses.
- Serve immediately and enjoy

Quinoa and Almond Salad Bowl

Ingredients:

- 1 cup quinoa, rinsed
- 2 cups water or vegetable broth
- 1/4 cup sliced almonds, toasted
- 1 cup cherry tomatoes, halved
- 1/2 cucumber, diced
- 1/4 red onion, thinly sliced
- 2 tablespoons chopped fresh parsley or cilantro
- Juice of 1 lemon
- 2 tablespoons extra virgin olive oil
- Salt and pepper, to taste
- Optional toppings: avocado slices, crumbled feta cheese, grilled chicken or tofu

Directions:

- In a medium saucepan, combine the rinsed quinoa and water or vegetable broth.
- Bring to a boil over medium-high heat.
- Reduce the heat to low, cover, and simmer for 15-20 minutes, or until the quinoa is cooked and the liquid is absorbed.
- Remove from heat and let it sit, covered, for 5 minutes. Fluff the quinoa with a fork and let it cool slightly.
- In a large mixing bowl, combine the cooked quinoa, toasted sliced almonds, cherry tomatoes, diced cucumber, thinly sliced red onion, and chopped fresh parsley or cilantro.
- In a small bowl, whisk together the lemon juice, extra virgin olive oil, salt, and pepper to make the dressing.
- Pour the dressing over the quinoa salad in the mixing bowl and toss until all the ingredients are evenly coated.
- Taste the salad and adjust the seasoning or add more lemon juice, olive oil, salt, or pepper as needed.
- Divide the Quinoa and Almond Salad among serving bowls.
- If desired, top each salad bowl with avocado slices, crumbled feta cheese, or grilled chicken or tofu for added flavor and protein.
- Serve immediately.

Walnut Avocado and Rocket Salad

Ingredients:

- 2 cups fresh rocket (arugula) leaves
- 1 ripe avocado, sliced
- 1/2 cup walnuts, toasted
- 1/4 cup crumbled feta cheese (optional)
- 1 tablespoon lemon juice
- 2 tablespoons extra virgin olive oil
- Salt and pepper, to taste

Directions:

- In a large mixing bowl, combine the fresh rocket leaves, sliced avocado, and toasted walnuts.
- If using, sprinkle the crumbled feta cheese over the salad ingredients in the mixing bowl.
- In a small bowl, whisk together the lemon juice, extra virgin olive oil, salt, and pepper to make the dressing.
- Pour the dressing over the salad ingredients in the mixing bowl.
- Gently toss the salad until all the ingredients are evenly coated with the dressing.
- Taste the salad and adjust the seasoning or add more lemon juice, olive oil, salt, or pepper as needed.
- Transfer the Walnut, Avocado, and Rocket Salad to serving plates or a large serving platter.
- Serve immediately as a delicious and nutritious side dish or light meal.

Chia Energy Bars

Ingredients:

- 1 cup (240ml) rolled oats
- 1/2 cup (120ml) almond butter or peanut butter
- 1/4 cup (60ml) honey or maple syrup
- 1/4 cup (60ml) chia seeds
- 1/4 cup (60ml) chopped nuts (such as almonds, walnuts, or ca-shews)
- 1/4 cup (60ml) dried fruit (such as raisins, cranberries, or chopped apricots)
- 1/4 teaspoon salt
- 1/2 teaspoon vanilla extract

Directions:

1. Preheat your oven to 350°F (180°C) and line an 8x8 inch (20x20cm) baking dish with parchment paper, leaving some overhang on the sides for easy removal later.

2. In a large mixing bowl, combine the rolled oats, almond butter or peanut butter, honey or maple syrup, chia seeds, chopped nuts, dried fruit, salt, and vanilla extract.

3. Mix all the ingredients together until well combined and the mixture starts to come together. You may need to use your hands to fully incorporate the ingredients.

4. Transfer the mixture to the prepared baking dish and press it down firmly and evenly into the bottom of the dish.

5. Bake in the preheated oven for 15-20 minutes, or until the edges are golden brown.

6. Remove from the oven and let it cool completely in the baking dish.

7. Once cooled, use the parchment paper overhang to lift the Chia Energy Bars out of the dish. Place them on a cutting board and cut into bars or squares of your desired size.

8. Store the bars in an airtight container at room temperature for up to one week, or in the refrigerator for longer freshness.

Enzyme Support

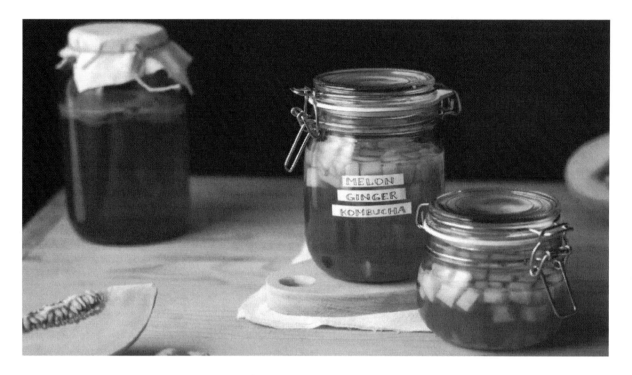

"The road to health is paved with good intestines!" —Sherry A. Rogers

Enzymes are the unsung heroes of our digestive system, working tirelessly to break down the foods we eat into the nutrients our bodies need to thrive. When our enzyme levels are low, we may experience digestive discomfort, nutrient deficiencies, and a range of other health issues. Supporting our body's natural enzyme production with targeted herbs and nourishing recipes ensure we can optimize digestion, enhance nutrient absorption, and promote overall well-being.

Topical Treatments

Aloe Digestive Aid

Ingredients:

- 1 cup (240ml) pure aloe vera juice
- 1 tablespoon freshly squeezed lemon juice
- 1 tablespoon raw honey or maple syrup (optional)
- 1/2 teaspoon ground ginger
- 1/4 teaspoon ground turmeric
- Pinch of ground black pepper
- Pinch of ground cinnamon
- 1-2 cups (240-480ml) cold water or coconut water
- Ice cubes (optional)
- Fresh mint leaves, for garnish (optional)

Directions:

- In a pitcher or large mixing bowl, combine the pure aloe vera juice, freshly squeezed lemon juice, raw honey or maple syrup (if using), ground ginger, ground turmeric, ground black pepper, and ground cinnamon.
- Stir all the ingredients together until well combined and the honey or maple syrup is fully dissolved.
- Gradually add 1-2 cups of cold water or coconut water to the mixture, depending on your desired strength and taste preferences. Stir well to dilute the tonic to your liking.
- If desired, add ice cubes to the pitcher or individual serving glasses to chill the tonic further.
- Garnish each glass with fresh mint leaves for a refreshing touch.

and added aroma, if desired.

• Serve the Aloe Digestive Aid Tonic immediately and enjoy!

Herbal Brews and Drinks

Barley Tea

Ingredients:

- 56 grams (2 ounces) barley seeds
- Clean water for soaking
- 5 gallons (about 18.9 liters) water for brewing

Directions:

1. Place the barley seeds in a large bowl or container and cover them with clean water.
2. Allow the barley seeds to soak for 8 hours. After soaking, the seeds should weigh a minimum of 84 grams. If not, continue soaking until they reach this weight.
3. Once the barley seeds have been soaked and have reached the desired weight, drain and rinse them thoroughly.
4. Sprout the barley seeds by placing them in a sprouting tray or container. Allow them to sprout until the tail is as long as the seed or for about 1-2 days. Rinse the seeds with water once or twice a day during the sprouting process.
5. After the barley seeds have sprouted, transfer them to a food blender or food processor. Add a little water to help them blend, and blend until smooth.
6. In a large pot or container, add 5 gallons of water.
7. Pour the blended barley mixture into the water and stir to combine.
8. Allow the barley tea to steep for several hours or overnight to extract the nutrients from the barley.
9. Once steeped, strain the barley tea to remove any solids.
10. Serve the barley tea chilled or over ice, if desired.

Kombucha

Ingredients:

- 1 SCOBY (Symbiotic Culture Of Bacteria and Yeast)
- 1 cup starter tea (previously brewed Kombucha)
- 3 1/2 quarts (approximately 14 cups or 3.3 liters) filtered water
- 1 cup white sugar
- 8 bags black tea (or 2 tablespoons loose leaf tea)

Equipment:

- Large pot
- Glass jar or brewing vessel (at least 1-gallon capacity)
- Breathable cloth cover (cheesecloth, coffee filter, or paper towel)
- Rubber band or string
- pH strips or pH meter (optional)

Directions:

1. Boil 3 1/2 quarts of filtered water in a large pot.
2. Once the water reaches a boil, remove it from heat and stir in 1 cup of white sugar until dissolved.
3. Add 8 bags of black tea (or 2 tablespoons loose leaf tea) to the hot water and allow it to steep for about 10-15 minutes.
4. After steeping, remove the tea bags or strain out the loose tea leaves and allow the sweet tea to cool to room temperature.
5. Once the sweet tea has cooled, transfer it to a clean glass jar or brewing vessel.
6. Carefully add the SCOBY and 1 cup of starter tea (previously brewed Kombucha) to the sweet tea mixture.
7. Cover the jar with a breathable cloth cover (cheesecloth, coffee filter, or paper towel) and secure it with a rubber band or string. This allows air to flow in and out while preventing dust and insects from getting into the brew.
8. Place the jar in a warm, dark area away from direct sunlight and let it ferment for 7-10 days. The ideal temperature for fermentation is around 70-75°F (21-24°C).
9. After 7-10 days, taste the Kombucha using a clean straw or spoon. It should be slightly tangy and fizzy. If it's too sweet, let it ferment for a few more days.
10. Once the Kombucha reaches your desired flavor, carefully remove the SCOBY and 1-2 cups of the brewed Kombucha to use as starter tea for your next batch.
11. Bottle the remaining Kombucha in glass bottles with a tight-fitting lid. You can also add fruit juice, herbs, or spices for flavoring at this stage if desired.
12. Let the bottled Kombucha sit at room temperature for 1-3 days for a second fermentation to create carbonation.
13. After the second fermentation, transfer the bottled Kombucha to the refrigerator to chill before serving.

Chia ACV Shot

Ingredients:

- 1 tablespoon chia seeds
- 1 tablespoon raw, unfiltered apple cider vinegar (ACV)
- 1/2 cup water
- 1 teaspoon honey
- Squeeze of fresh lemon juice (optional)

Directions:

- In a small glass or jar, combine the chia seeds, raw apple cider vinegar, and water.
- Stir well to mix the ingredients together.
- Let the mixture sit for about 5-10 minutes to allow the chia seeds to absorb some of the liquid and become gel-like.
- If desired, add a teaspoon of honey for sweetness, and a squeeze of fresh lemon juice for added flavor.
- Stir the mixture again to incorporate any additional ingredients.
- Once mixed, drink the Chia ACV Shot immediately.

Enzyme Support Recipes

Pineapple and Melon Smoothie

Ingredients:

- 1 cup fresh pineapple chunks
- 1 cup fresh melon chunks (such as honeydew, cantaloupe, or watermelon)
- 1 ripe banana, peeled
- 1/2 cup Greek yogurt (or dairy-free alternative)
- 1/2 cup coconut water or water
- Optional: a handful of ice cubes for a colder smoothie

Directions:

1. Place all the ingredients in a blender.
2. Blend on high speed until smooth and creamy. If the smoothie is too thick, you can add more coconut water or water to reach your desired consistency.
3. Taste the smoothie and adjust sweetness by adding a bit of honey, maple syrup, or more banana if desired.
4. Pour the Pineapple and Melon Smoothie into glasses.
5. If desired, garnish with additional pineapple chunks or melon balls.

Fermented Ginger Side Salad

Ingredients:

- 4 medium carrots
- 1 tablespoon (approx 25g) fresh ginger, grated
- 2 tablespoons chopped chives
- 1/2 tablespoon dried chili flakes
- 1 tablespoon coriander seeds
- 1 tablespoon Celtic Sea or Himalayan salt

Directions:

1. Grate the carrots using a food processor or a grater. Place them in a bowl.
2. Add the grated ginger, chopped chives, dried chili flakes, coriander seeds, and Celtic Sea or Himalayan salt to the bowl with the grated carrots. Stir well to incorporate all the ingredients.
3. Transfer the mixture to a glass jar. Kilner jars are ideal for this purpose. Do not use plastic jars as they may react with the fermentation process.
4. Use the end of a rolling pin or your fist to press the mixture down firmly into the jar. Continue pressing until the brine, which leaks out from the shredded carrots, covers the mixture. The carrots will reduce in size significantly during this process.
5. Seal the jar and allow it to ferment at a cool room temperature for anywhere between 3-7 days, or until it reaches your desired level of tanginess. This batch was fermented for 4 days.
6. Once fermented to your liking, transfer the jar to the refrigerator. The fermented carrots will keep for a few weeks when stored in the fridge.
7. Enjoy your tangy and flavorful Fermented Carrots as a tasty and nutritious condiment or snack!

Note: Fermented carrots are not only delicious but also rich in probiotics, which can promote gut health. Experiment with different spices and herbs to customize the flavor to your liking.

Miso Soup

Ingredients:

- 4 cups (946 ml) water
- 2 tablespoons (30 ml) miso paste
- 1 sheet nori (dried seaweed), torn into small pieces
- 1/2 cup (100 g) tofu, diced
- 2 green onions, thinly sliced
- 1 tablespoon (15 ml) soy sauce (or tamari for gluten-free option)
- 1 tablespoon (15 ml) rice vinegar
- 1 teaspoon (5 ml) sesame oil
- 1 teaspoon (5 ml) grated fresh ginger
- 1 clove garlic, minced
- Optional: cooked soba noodles or rice, for serving
- Optional: sliced mushrooms, spinach, or other vegetables of choice

Directions:

1. In a large saucepan, bring the water to a gentle boil over medium heat.
2. In a small bowl, whisk together the miso paste and a small amount of hot water until smooth.
3. Add the miso paste mixture to the saucepan of hot water and stir until well combined.
4. Add the torn nori pieces, diced tofu, sliced green onions, soy sauce (or tamari), rice vinegar, sesame oil, grated ginger, and minced garlic to the saucepan.
5. If desired, add any optional ingredients such as cooked soba noodles or rice, sliced mushrooms, spinach, or other vegetables of choice.
6. Simmer the soup gently for about 5-7 minutes, stirring occasionally, until the tofu is heated through and the vegetables are tender.
7. Taste the soup and adjust seasoning if needed, adding more miso paste, soy sauce, or rice vinegar to taste.
8. Once ready, ladle the Miso Soup into bowls and serve immediately.

Thai Green Papaya Salad

Ingredients:

Dressing:

- 2 tablespoons garlic, roughly chopped (about 10 normal or 4 large garlic cloves)
- 6 bird eye chillies, roughly chopped with seeds (use fewer for less spiciness)
- 6 tablespoons dried shrimp

Green Papaya Salad:

- 1 cup roasted peanuts, unsalted
- 20 snake beans, cut into 5 cm/2⊠ pieces (raw)
- 3 cups grape tomatoes, cut in half (about 400g / 14oz)
- 1 cup palm sugar, grated using standard box grater, loosely packed
- 1/2 cup lime juice
- 1/2 cup fish sauce
- 500g / 4 cups green papaya, shredded, tightly packed cups (about 1 medium or 2/3 large)
- 1/2 cup Thai basil leaves

Directions:

1. Place peanuts in a mortar and pestle. Pound lightly to break them up into large pieces, not into powder. Transfer to a bowl.
2. Place garlic and chili in the mortar. Pound into a paste. Add shrimp and pound to crush them – no need to grind them to a paste.
3. Stir in palm sugar, lime juice, and fish sauce until the sugar dissolves. Pour Dressing into a large bowl.
4. Add snake beans to the mortar (in batches if needed). Pound to bruise, split, and soften (they are raw, so they need to be bashed to soften). Add to Dressing.
5. Grab handfuls of tomato, crush with your hands, then add into the bowl.
6. Add papaya: Add papaya and 3/4 of the peanuts. Toss well with 2 wooden spoons or tongs.
7. Once everything is coated in Dressing, immediately pile up onto plates. Spoon over some dressing (there will be a bit of dressing still left in the bowl, that's normal).
8. Garnish with Thai basil leaves, sprinkle with remaining peanuts. Serve immediately.

Eye Health

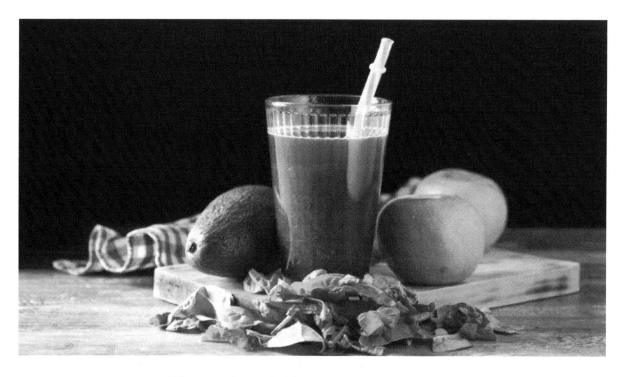

"The eye is the jewel of the body." –Henry David Thoreau

Our eyes are precious organs that allow us to experience the world in all its vibrant colors, shapes, and forms. However, in today's digital age, our eyes are increasingly subjected to strain and stress from prolonged screen time, artificial lighting, and environmental factors. Neglecting eye health can lead to a range of issues, from minor discomforts like dry eyes and headaches to more severe conditions such as cataracts and macular degeneration.

Topical Treatments

Chamomile and Cornflower Soothing Soak

Ingredients:

- 2 chamomile tea bags
- 2 cornflower tea bags
- 2 cups (475 ml) hot water
- Ice cubes (optional)

Directions:

- Place the chamomile and cornflower tea bags in a heatproof bowl or container.
- Heat 2 cups of water until just boiling, then pour it over the tea bags.
- Allow the tea bags to steep in the hot water for 5-10 minutes, or until the water has cooled to a comfortable temperature.
- Once the tea has cooled slightly, remove the tea bags and discard them.
- To use the eye soak, tilt your head back and close your eyes. Place a clean washcloth soaked in the warm tea over your closed eyelids.
- Relax and allow the soothing herbal infusion to soak into your eyes for 5-10 minutes.
- If desired, you can chill the tea beforehand or add ice cubes to the eye soak for a cooling effect.
- After the allotted time, gently remove the washcloth and discard it.
- Pat your eyelids dry with a clean towel, being careful not to rub or irritate the delicate skin around your eyes.

Note: Never put anything in your eyes without first consulting a medical professional.

Chamomile and Castor Oil Gentle Massage Oil

Ingredients:

- 1/4 cup (60 ml) castor oil
- 2 chamomile tea bags
- 1/2 teaspoon (2.5 ml) vitamin E oil (optional)

Directions:

1. Heat the castor oil in a small saucepan over low heat until warm, but not hot. You can also warm it by placing the container in a bowl of hot water.
2. Place the chamomile tea bags in a heatproof bowl or container.
3. Pour the warm castor oil over the chamomile tea bags, ensuring they are fully submerged.
4. Allow the chamomile tea bags to steep in the warm castor oil for at least 30 minutes to infuse the oil with the soothing properties of chamomile.
5. After steeping, remove the chamomile tea bags from the oil and discard them.
6. If desired, you can add vitamin E oil to the infused castor oil for its additional nourishing benefits.
7. Transfer the infused castor oil to a clean, airtight container for storage.

How to Use:

- Before using the Chamomile and Castor Oil Gentle Eye Massage Oil, ensure your face is clean and free of makeup.
- Using clean fingertips, gently apply a small amount of the oil to the skin around your eyes.
- Using light, circular motions, massage the oil into the skin around your eyes, starting from the inner corners and working outwards.
- Be gentle and avoid applying too much pressure to prevent pulling or stretching the delicate skin around your eyes.
- Leave the oil on overnight for maximum benefits, or you can use it as a daytime treatment if preferred.
- Repeat this process daily or as needed to soothe and nourish the delicate skin around your eyes.

Herbal Brews and Drinks

Tumeric and Carrot Health Shot

Ingredients:

- 1 pound (450g) carrots, very coarsely chopped
- 1 (2-inch) piece fresh turmeric, peeled and coarsely chopped
- 1 (2-inch) piece fresh ginger, peeled and coarsely chopped
- 3/4 cup (180ml) unsweetened coconut water, divided
- Pinch of salt

Directions:

1. Process carrots, turmeric, ginger, and 1/2 cup (120ml) coconut water in a blender on high speed until completely smooth, about 2 minutes.
2. Pour the mixture through a fine-mesh strainer into a clean jar or container, pressing lightly with a rubber spatula to extract juice; discard solids.
3. Stir in salt and the remaining 1/4 cup (60ml) coconut water.
4. Serve the ginger and turmeric shot immediately or refrigerate until ready to use.

Citrus Zest Green Tea

Ingredients:

- 4 cups (950 ml) water
- 4 green tea bags
- Zest of 1 lemon (about 1 tablespoon)
- Zest of 1 lime (about 1 tablespoon)
- Zest of 1 orange (about 1 tablespoon)
- Honey or sweetener of choice, to taste (optional)
- Ice cubes (optional)

Directions:

1. In a medium saucepan, bring the water to a boil over medium-high heat.
2. Once boiling, remove the saucepan from the heat and add the green tea bags.
3. Allow the tea bags to steep in the hot water for 3-5 minutes, depending on your desired strength of tea.
4. While the tea is steeping, use a fine grater or zester to zest the lemon, lime, and orange. Make sure to only zest the outer colored part of the citrus fruits, avoiding the bitter white pith underneath.
5. After steeping, remove the tea bags from the saucepan and discard them.
6. Stir the citrus zest into the hot tea and let it steep for an additional 2-3 minutes to infuse the flavors.

7. If desired, sweeten the tea with honey or your preferred sweetener to taste, stirring until dissolved.

8. Allow the tea to cool slightly before serving. You can serve it hot or chilled over ice cubes for a refreshing iced tea.

9. Garnish with additional citrus slices or mint leaves, if desired.

Bilberry Iced Tea

Ingredients:

- 4 cups (950 ml) water
- 4 bilberry tea bags
- 1 tablespoon (15 ml) honey or sweetener of choice (optional)
- Ice cubes
- Fresh bilberries or lemon slices for garnish (optional)

Directions:

1. In a medium saucepan, bring the water to a boil over medium-high heat.

2. Once boiling, remove the saucepan from the heat and add the bilberry tea bags.

3. Allow the tea bags to steep in the hot water for 5-7 minutes, depending on your desired strength of tea.

4. After steeping, remove the tea bags from the saucepan and discard them.

5. If desired, sweeten the tea with honey or your preferred sweetener, stirring until dissolved.

6. Allow the tea to cool to room temperature, then transfer it to a pitcher and refrigerate until chilled.

7. Once chilled, fill glasses with ice cubes and pour the bilberry tea over the ice.

8. Garnish with fresh bilberries or lemon slices, if desired.

9. Stir the tea gently before serving.

Eye Health Recipes

Blueberry and Spinach Smoothie

Ingredients:

- 1 cup (240 ml) unsweetened almond milk or any milk of your choice
- 1 ripe banana, peeled and sliced
- 1 cup (150g) frozen blueberries
- 1 cup (30g) fresh spinach leaves
- 1 tablespoon (15 ml) honey
- 1/2 cup (120g) Greek yogurt or dairy-free yogurt
- Ice cubes (optional)

Directions:

1. In a blender, combine the unsweetened almond milk, sliced banana, frozen blueberries, fresh spinach leaves, honey (if using), and Greek yogurt.

2. Blend on high speed until the mixture is smooth and creamy, about 1-2 minutes. If the smoothie is too thick, you can add more almond milk to reach your desired consistency.

3. Taste the smoothie and adjust the sweetness if needed by adding more honey or maple syrup.

4. If you prefer a colder smoothie, you can add a handful of ice cubes to the blender and blend until smooth.

5. Once blended to your liking, pour the blueberry and spinach smoothie into glasses and serve immediately.

Sweet Potato Ginger Soup

Ingredients:

- 2 medium sweet potatoes, peeled and cubed (about 500g)
- 1 tablespoon (15 ml) olive oil
- 1 onion, chopped
- 2 cloves garlic, minced
- 1 tablespoon (15g) fresh ginger, grated
- 4 cups (950 ml) vegetable broth
- 1 can (400 ml) coconut milk
- Salt and pepper to taste
- Fresh cilantro or parsley for garnish (optional)

Directions:

1. In a large pot, heat the olive oil over medium heat. Add the chopped onion and cook until softened, about 5 minutes.

2. Add the minced garlic and grated ginger to the pot, and cook for another 1-2 minutes until fragrant.

3. Add the cubed sweet potatoes to the pot, along with the vegetable broth. Bring the mixture to a boil, then reduce the heat to low and let it simmer for about 15-20 minutes, or until the sweet potatoes are tender and cooked through.

4. Once the sweet potatoes are cooked, use an immersion blender to blend the soup until smooth. Alternatively, you can transfer

the soup to a blender in batches and blend until smooth, then return it to the pot.

5. Stir in the coconut milk until well combined. Season the soup with salt and pepper to taste.

6. Continue to simmer the soup for another 5 minutes to heat through and allow the flavors to meld together.

7. Serve the sweet potato ginger soup hot, garnished with fresh cilantro or parsley if desired.

Roasted Mediterranean Salad with Super Green Sauce

Ingredients:

Roasted Vegetables:
- 1 large sweet potato, chopped (about 500g)
- 6-7 baby yellow or red potatoes, quartered
- 2 whole carrots, halved and chopped
- 2 tablespoons melted coconut oil (divided) // or sub water
- 2 teaspoons curry powder (divided)

Magic Green Sauce:
- 5 cloves garlic, peeled and crushed
- 1 medium serrano or jalapeño pepper, seeds and stems removed (omit if not into spicy food)
- 1 cup packed cilantro, thick bottom stems cut off
- 1 cup packed flat-leaf parsley
- 3 tablespoons ripe avocado

Salad:
- 4 cups hearty greens (spinach, kale, or mustard greens), chopped
- 1 medium ripe avocado, chopped
- 3 tablespoons hemp seeds

- 1/2 teaspoon sea salt (divided)
- 1 cup chopped broccolini
- 2 cups chopped red cabbage
- 1 medium red bell pepper, sliced

- 1/4 teaspoon salt (plus more to taste)
- 3 tablespoons lime juice
- 1 tablespoon maple syrup (or other sweetener of choice)
- Water to thin (about 3 tablespoons or 45 ml)

- Fresh herbs (cilantro, parsley, thyme, etc.), optional
- 5-7 medium sliced radishes, optional
- 1/4 cup Macadamia Nut Cheese, optional

Directions:

1. Preheat the oven to 375°F (190°C) and line 2 baking sheets with parchment paper.

2. Add the sweet potato, potato, and carrots to one baking sheet and toss with half of the oil (or water), half of the curry powder, and half of the sea salt (1 tablespoon (15 ml) oil (or water), 1 teaspoon curry powder, and 1/4 teaspoon sea salt).

3. Bake for 25 minutes or until golden brown and tender.

4. To a separate baking sheet, add broccolini, cabbage, and bell pepper and toss with the remaining half of the oil (or water), half of the curry powder, and half of the sea salt (1 tablespoon (15 ml) oil (or water), 1 teaspoon curry powder, and 1/4 teaspoon sea salt).

5. Bake for 15-20 minutes or until golden brown and tender (place in the oven once the potatoes have been cooking for 5-10 minutes).

6. Meanwhile, make the magic green sauce. Place garlic and pepper in a food processor along with the cilantro, parsley, avocado, salt, lime juice, and maple syrup.

7. Process until smooth, scraping down sides as needed. Thin with water until a semi-thick but pourable sauce is formed. Adjust flavor as needed.

8. Plate the salad by adding mixed greens to a serving platter and topping with roasted vegetables. Arrange avocado along the edges, along with radishes and macadamia nut cheese (optional). Sprinkle the top with hemp seeds and serve with dressing on the side. Garnish with herbs if desired.

9. Leftover salad will keep covered in the refrigerator for up to 3 days. Eat cold or at room temperature, or reheat on the stovetop

Pumpkin Seed and Goji Trail Mix

Ingredients:

1 cup (140g) pumpkin seeds (pepitas)

1/2 cup (75g) goji berries

1/2 cup (60g) almonds, chopped

1/2 cup (60g) cashews

1/2 cup (75g) dried cranberries

- 1/4 cup (35g) sunflower seeds
- 1/4 cup (40g) dark chocolate chips or chunks (optional)
- 1/2 teaspoon ground cinnamon (optional)
- Pinch of sea salt

Directions:

. Preheat your oven to 325°F (160°C) and line a baking sheet with parchment paper.

. In a large mixing bowl, combine the pumpkin seeds, goji berries, almonds, cashews, dried cranberries, sunflower seeds, and dark

chocolate chips or chunks (if using).

3. If desired, sprinkle the mixture with ground cinnamon and a pinch of sea salt, and toss to combine.

4. Spread the trail mix out evenly on the prepared baking sheet.

5. Bake in the preheated oven for 10-15 minutes, stirring occasionally, until the pumpkin seeds are toasted and golden brown.

6. Remove the baking sheet from the oven and allow the trail mix to cool completely before transferring it to an airtight container for storage.

Gut Healing, Nausea, Vomiting, and Diarrhea

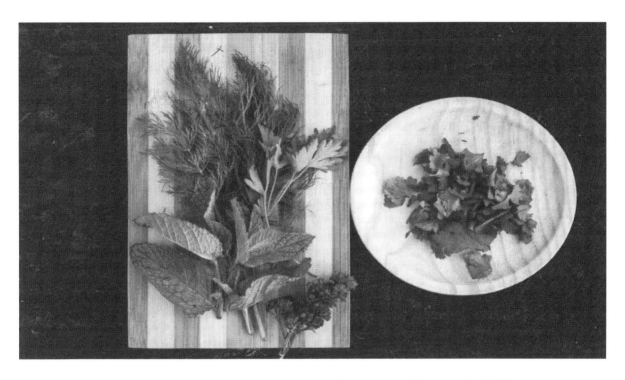

"Healing is a matter of time, but it is sometimes also a matter of opportunity." –Hippocrates

The gut is the foundation of our health, playing a crucial role in digestion, nutrient absorption, immune function, and overall well-being. When our gut is out of balance, we may experience a range of symptoms, from digestive discomfort and inflammation to mood imbalances and chronic illness. By nurturing our gut with healing herbs and nourishing recipes, we can help restore balance, soothe inflammation, and promote optimal gut health.

Topical Treatments

Ease the Quease Tincture

Ingredients:

- 6 fl oz (175 ml) OAC Organic Cane 190-proof Alcohol
- 3 fl oz (90 ml) Distilled Water
- Organic Ginger Root, approximately 4-6 oz (115-170 g) (enough to fill a Mason jar 1/3-1/2 full)
- 12 fl oz (350 ml) Mason Jar
- Cheesecloth

Directions:

1. Mix the OAC Organic Cane alcohol and distilled water in a clean container.
2. Wash and slice the ginger root lengthwise.
3. Add the sliced ginger to the Mason jar.
4. Pour the diluted Organic Alcohol mixture into the Mason jar, filling it to the top.
5. Close the Mason jar tightly and shake well to combine the ingredients.
6. Place the Mason jar in a dark, cool place for at least 6 weeks, shaking it weekly to ensure thorough infusion.
7. After 6 weeks, strain out the ginger pieces using a cheesecloth, pressing to extract as much liquid as possible.

8. Pour the tincture into dark bottles and label them with the name and date.
   Dose:
- Take 5 to 10 drops of the Ease the Quease Tincture twice daily, or as needed for relief from nausea or digestive discomfort.

Mugwort Bitters

Equipment:
- 32 oz. (946 ml) glass jar
- Glass dropper bottles (optional)

Ingredients:
- ½ cup dried hawthorn berries (Crataegus spp.) or 100g fresh berries
- 2 tablespoons cacao nibs (Theobroma cacao)
- 2 tablespoons dried orange peel (Citrus x sinensis)
- 1 tablespoon hulled cardamom seeds (Elettaria cardamomum)
- 2 teaspoons cut and sifted dried mugwort leaves (Artemisia vulgaris) or 4 teaspoons chopped fresh leaves
- 2 cinnamon sticks (Cinnamomum verum)
- 2 cups (473 ml) brandy or vodka

Directions:
- In a 32 oz. (946 ml) glass jar, combine all herbs and spices.
- Cover with alcohol of choice. Brandy makes for a smooth and drinkable blend, while vodka provides a stronger and more medicinal extraction.
   Dosage: 5 to 10 drops.
- Store in a cool, dark place for six weeks, shaking often.
- After six weeks, strain out the herbs and store your bitters in a glass jar in a dark cabinet. Best used within one year.

Herbal Brews and Drinks

Electrolyte Coconut Sip

Ingredients:
- 2 cups (480 ml) coconut water
- 1/4 cup (60 ml) freshly squeezed lime juice
- 2 tablespoons (30 ml) honey or maple syrup
- 1/4 teaspoon sea salt

Directions:
1. In a pitcher, combine the coconut water, freshly squeezed lime juice, honey or maple syrup, and sea salt.
2. Stir the mixture until the honey or maple syrup is fully dissolved and the ingredients are well combined.
3. Taste the drink and adjust the sweetness or tartness by adding more honey or lime juice as desired.
4. Refrigerate the electrolyte coconut drink until chilled or serve over ice for immediate enjoyment.
5. Stir the drink before serving to ensure the ingredients are evenly distributed.
6. Sip slowly to replenish lost electrolytes.

Peppermint Ginger Tea

Ingredients:
- 2 cups (480 ml) water
- 1 tablespoon (15 ml) fresh ginger root, thinly sliced or grated
- 2 tablespoons (30 ml) dried peppermint leaves or 10-12 fresh peppermint leaves
- Honey or maple syrup, to taste (optional)
- Lemon slices, for garnish (optional)

Directions:
1. In a saucepan, bring the water to a gentle boil over medium heat.
2. Add the fresh ginger root slices or grated ginger to the boiling water.
3. Reduce the heat to low and simmer the ginger in the water for 5-7 minutes to infuse its flavor.
4. Remove the saucepan from the heat and add the dried peppermint leaves or fresh peppermint leaves to the ginger-infused water.
5. Cover the saucepan with a lid and let the peppermint steep in the hot water for 5-10 minutes.
6. After steeping, strain the tea through a fine mesh sieve or tea strainer to remove the ginger root and peppermint leaves.
7. If desired, sweeten the tea with honey or maple syrup to taste, stirring until dissolved.
8. Pour the peppermint ginger tea into cups or mugs and garnish with lemon slices if desired.

Licorice and Chamomile Tea

Ingredients:

- 2 cups (480 ml) water
- 2 teaspoons (10 ml) dried chamomile flowers
- 1 teaspoon (5 ml) dried licorice root
- Honey or maple syrup, to taste (optional)

Directions:

- In a small saucepan, bring the water to a boil over medium heat.
- Once the water reaches a boil, remove the saucepan from the heat.
- Add the dried chamomile flowers and licorice root to the hot water.
- Cover the saucepan with a lid and let the herbs steep in the hot water for 5-7 minutes to infuse their flavors.
- After steeping, strain the tea through a fine mesh sieve or tea strainer to remove the chamomile flowers and licorice root.
- If desired, sweeten the tea with honey or maple syrup to taste, stirring until dissolved.
- Pour the licorice and chamomile tea into cups or mugs and serve immediately.

Gut Healing, Nausea, Vomiting, and Diarrhea

Pink Kefir Smoothie

Ingredients:

- 1 cup (240 ml) kefir
- 1/2 cup (75 g) frozen mixed berries (such as strawberries, raspberries, and blueberries)
- 1/2 cup (75 g) frozen chopped mango
- 1 small banana, frozen
- 1 tablespoon (15 ml) honey or maple syrup (optional, to taste)
- 1/2 teaspoon (2.5 ml) vanilla extract
- 1/2 cup (120 ml) water or coconut water (for desired consistency)
- Ice cubes (optional, for extra chill)

Directions:

1. In a blender, combine the kefir, frozen mixed berries, frozen mango, frozen banana, honey or maple syrup (if using), and vanilla extract.
2. Add water or coconut water to help with blending and achieve the desired consistency. If you prefer a thicker smoothie, use less liquid; for a thinner smoothie, add more liquid.
3. Optionally, add ice cubes to the blender for an extra-chilled smoothie.
4. Blend all the ingredients on high speed until smooth and creamy, scraping down the sides of the blender if necessary.
5. Taste the smoothie and adjust the sweetness if needed by adding more honey or maple syrup.
6. Once the smoothie reaches your desired consistency and taste, pour it into glasses and serve immediately.

BRAT Chicken Casserole

Ingredients:

- 4 boneless, skinless chicken breasts (about 500g / 1 lb)
- 2 medium potatoes, peeled and diced (about 300g / 10 oz)
- 1 large carrot, peeled and sliced (about 150g / 5 oz)
- 1 medium onion, diced (about 150g / 5 oz)
- 2 cloves garlic, minced
- 1 cup (240ml) chicken broth
- 1 cup (240ml) tomato passata (or tomato sauce)
- 1 tablespoon (15ml) olive oil
- 1 teaspoon (5ml) dried thyme
- 1 teaspoon (5ml) dried rosemary
- Salt and pepper, to taste
- Chopped fresh parsley, for garnish

Directions:

1. Preheat your oven to 375°F (190°C). Grease a baking dish and set aside.
2. In a large skillet, heat the olive oil over medium heat. Add the diced onion and minced garlic, and cook until softened and fragrant, about 2-3 minutes.
3. Add the chicken breasts to the skillet and cook until lightly browned on both sides, about 3-4 minutes per side.
4. Remove the chicken breasts from the skillet and set aside. In the same skillet, add the diced potatoes and sliced carrots. Cook for about 5 minutes, until slightly softened.
5. Pour in the chicken broth and tomato passata (or tomato sauce), and stir to combine. Season with dried thyme, dried rosemary, salt, and pepper.
6. Transfer the cooked vegetables and sauce to the greased baking dish. Arrange the browned chicken breasts on top.
7. Cover the baking dish with foil and bake in the preheated oven for 25-30 minutes, or until the chicken is cooked through and the vegetables are tender.
8. Once cooked, remove the foil and sprinkle chopped fresh parsley

over the casserole for garnish.

Shredded Apple Salad

Ingredients:

- 4 medium apples, cored and shredded (about 600g / 20 oz)
- 2 cups (480ml) shredded carrots (about 200g / 7 oz)
- 1 cup (240ml) raisins
- 1 cup (240ml) chopped walnuts
- 1/2 cup (120ml) plain Greek yogurt
- 4 tablespoons (60ml) honey
- 2 tablespoons (30ml) lemon juice
- 1 teaspoon (5ml) ground cinnamon
- Salt, to taste

Directions:

1. In a large mixing bowl, combine the shredded apples, shredded carrots, raisins, and chopped walnuts.

2. In a separate small bowl, whisk together the plain Greek yogurt, honey, lemon juice, ground cinnamon, and a pinch of salt until well combined.

3. Pour the yogurt dressing over the shredded apple mixture and toss gently until everything is evenly coated.

4. Taste the salad and adjust seasoning if needed, adding more honey or lemon juice according to your taste preference.

5. Chill the shredded apple salad in the refrigerator for at least 30 minutes before serving to allow the flavors to meld together.

6. Serve chilled.

Baked Sweet Potato

Ingredients:

- 4 medium sweet potatoes (about 800g / 28 oz)
- 2 tablespoons (30ml) olive oil
- 1 teaspoon (5ml) paprika
- 1 teaspoon (5ml) garlic powder
- 1 teaspoon (5ml) onion powder
- Salt and pepper, to taste
- Chopped fresh parsley or chives, for garnish (optional)

Directions:

1. Preheat the oven to 400°F (200°C). Line a baking sheet with parchment paper.

2. Wash and scrub the sweet potatoes under cold water to remove any dirt or debris. Pat them dry with a paper towel.

3. Cut the sweet potatoes into evenly sized wedges or rounds, about 1/2 inch (1.25cm) thick.

4. In a large mixing bowl, toss the sweet potato wedges with olive oil, paprika, garlic powder, onion powder, salt, and pepper until evenly coated.

5. Arrange the seasoned sweet potato wedges in a single layer on the prepared baking sheet.

6. Bake in the preheated oven for 25-30 minutes, flipping halfway through, or until the sweet potatoes are tender and lightly browned.

7. Once baked, remove from the oven and sprinkle with chopped fresh parsley or chives for garnish, if desired.

Hair and Nail Health

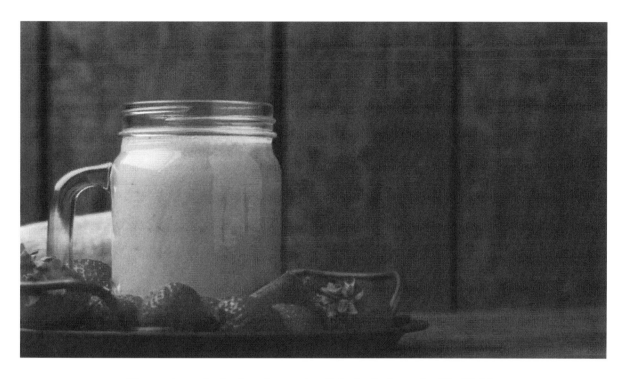

"Beauty is not in the face; beauty is a light in the heart." —Khalil Gibran

Our hair and nails are often a reflection of our inner health, with lustrous locks and strong, healthy nails signifying a well-nourished body. When our hair and nails are brittle, weak, or lackluster, it may be a sign that we need to support our body with targeted nutrients and healing herbs. Incorporating hair and nail-strengthening ingredients into our daily routines can help promote healthy growth, reduce breakage, and restore the natural beauty of our hair and nails.

Topical Treatments

ACV Anti Dandruff Rinse

Ingredients:

- 1/2 cup (120ml) apple cider vinegar (ACV)
- 1/2 cup (120ml) water
- 5 drops tea tree essential oil
- 5 drops lavender essential oil

Directions:

1. In a mixing bowl or a clean bottle, combine the apple cider vinegar and water.
2. Add the tea tree essential oil and lavender essential oil to the mixture.
3. Stir or shake well to ensure that all ingredients are thoroughly combined.
4. After shampooing your hair, pour the ACV hair rinse over your scalp and hair.
5. Gently massage the mixture into your scalp for a few minutes to ensure even distribution.
6. Let the ACV hair rinse sit on your hair for about 1-2 minutes.
7. Rinse your hair thoroughly with lukewarm water.
8. Optionally, follow with a conditioner if desired, although it's not usually necessary.
9. Use this ACV hair rinse once or twice a week as needed to help control dandruff and promote a healthy scalp.

Rice Water Rinse

Ingredients:

- 1/2 cup (120ml) uncooked rice
- 2 cups (480ml) water
- Optional: 5 drops of your favorite essential oil (such as lavender or rosemary)

Directions:

1. Rinse the uncooked rice thoroughly under cold water to remove any impurities.
2. Place the rinsed rice in a clean bowl and cover it with 2 cups of water.
3. Let the rice soak in the water for about 30 minutes to 1 hour. This allows the nutrients from the rice to seep into the water.
4. After soaking, stir the rice and water mixture to release more of the rice's nutrients into the water.
5. Strain the rice water into a clean container to remove the rice grains. You should be left with a milky liquid.
6. If desired, add 5 drops of your favorite essential oil to the rice water for added fragrance and benefits.
7. After shampooing your hair, pour the rice water over your scalp and hair, making sure to massage it into your scalp.
8. Allow the rice water to sit on your hair for 5-10 minutes to allow the nutrients to penetrate the hair shaft.
9. Rinse your hair thoroughly with lukewarm water to remove the rice water.
10. Optionally, follow with a conditioner if desired.
11. Use this rice water hair rinse once or twice a week as needed to promote stronger, shinier hair.

Rosemary Scalp Oil

Ingredients:

- 1/4 cup (60ml) carrier oil (such as jojoba oil, coconut oil, or olive oil)
- 2 tablespoons (30ml) dried rosemary leaves
- 5 drops rosemary essential oil
- Optional: 5 drops peppermint essential oil for added scalp stimulation

Directions:

1. In a small saucepan, heat the carrier oil over low heat until warm. Be careful not to overheat or boil the oil.
2. Once warm, add the dried rosemary leaves to the carrier oil.
3. Allow the rosemary leaves to infuse into the oil over low heat for about 30 minutes, stirring occasionally.
4. After 30 minutes, remove the saucepan from the heat and let the oil cool to room temperature.
5. Once cooled, strain the infused oil into a clean container to remove the rosemary leaves, ensuring you extract all the oil.
6. Add the rosemary essential oil (and peppermint essential oil, if using) to the infused oil and stir well to combine.
7. Your rosemary scalp oil is now ready to use.

Usage:

8. Before using the rosemary scalp oil, ensure your hair is dry or slightly damp.
9. Using your fingertips or a dropper, apply the oil directly to your scalp.
10. Gently massage the oil into your scalp using circular motions for 5-10 minutes to stimulate circulation and promote absorption.
11. Once applied, leave the oil on your scalp and hair for at least 30 minutes, or overnight for a more intensive treatment.
12. After the desired time, shampoo your hair as usual to remove the oil.

Clove Nail Oil

Ingredients:

- 1/4 cup (60ml) carrier oil (such as jojoba oil, sweet almond oil, or olive oil)
- 10-15 whole cloves

Directions:

1. In a clean, dry glass jar or bottle, combine the carrier oil and whole cloves.
2. Seal the jar or bottle tightly.
3. Place the jar or bottle in a cool, dark place to infuse for at least 1-2 weeks. Shake the jar gently every day to help release the clove's essential oils into the carrier oil.

Usage:

4. After 1-2 weeks, strain the infused oil through a fine-mesh sieve or cheesecloth to remove the cloves, ensuring that only the oil remains.
5. Transfer the strained clove-infused oil into a clean, airtight container for storage.
6. Before using the clove nail oil, ensure your nails and surrounding skin are clean and dry.
7. Using a clean dropper or your fingertips, apply a small amount of the clove nail oil to each nail and massage it into the nail bed and cuticles.
8. Allow the oil to absorb into the nails and cuticles for at least 10-15 minutes.

9. For best results, use the clove nail oil treatment daily, preferably before bedtime, to nourish and strengthen the nails and promote healthy cuticles.

Herbal Brews and Drinks

Berry and Lemon Shot

Ingredients:

- 1 cup (240ml) mixed berries (such as strawberries, blueberries, raspberries)
- 1 lemon, juiced
- Optional: Honey or agave syrup, to taste
- Optional: Fresh mint leaves, for garnish

Directions:

1. Wash the mixed berries thoroughly under cold water and pat them dry with a paper towel.
2. In a blender or food processor, combine the mixed berries and freshly squeezed lemon juice.
3. Blend the mixture until smooth and well combined.
4. Taste the berry and lemon mixture and adjust the sweetness if desired by adding well-mixed agave syrup to taste.
5. Once sweetened to your liking, blend the mixture again briefly to incorporate the sweetener.
6. Strain the berry and lemon mixture through a fine-mesh sieve or cheesecloth to remove any seeds or pulp, if desired. This step is optional depending on your preference for texture.
7. Pour the strained berry and lemon mixture into shot glasses or small serving glasses.

Homemade Biotin Powder Drink

Ingredients:

- 2 tablespoons (30ml) water
- 1 tablespoon (15ml) honey or agave syrup
- 1 tablespoon (15ml) powdered biotin
- 1/2 lemon, juiced
- Optional: A pinch of ground cinnamon or ginger for flavor

Directions:

1. In a glass, combine the water and honey or agave syrup. Stir until the sweetener is dissolved.
2. Add the powdered biotin to the sweetened water. Stir well to ensure the biotin is evenly distributed and dissolved.
3. Squeeze the juice from half a lemon into the glass. Stir to combine with the biotin mixture.
4. If desired, add a pinch of ground cinnamon or ginger to the drink for added flavor.
5. Stir the drink once more to ensure all ingredients are well-mixed.
6. Serve the homemade biotin powder drink immediately.

Carrot, Cucumber Hair and Nail Drink

Ingredients:

- 1 large carrot, peeled and chopped
- 1/2 cucumber, peeled and chopped
- 1 cup (240ml) water
- Juice of 1 lemon
- Optional: Honey or agave syrup, to taste

Directions:

1. In a blender, combine the chopped carrot, chopped cucumber, water, and lemon juice.
2. Blend the ingredients until smooth and well combined.
3. Taste the mixture and adjust sweetness if desired by adding honey or agave syrup to taste. Blend again briefly to incorporate.
4. Once sweetened to your liking, strain the mixture through a fine-mesh sieve or cheesecloth to remove any pulp or solids. This step is optional depending on your preference for texture.
5. Pour the strained carrot and cucumber drink into glasses.

Hair and Nail Health Recipes

Biotin Smoothie

Ingredients:

- 1 tablespoon sesame seeds
- 1 tablespoon flax seeds
- 1 tablespoon sunflower seeds
- 1 tablespoon pistachios
- 5-6 almonds
- 2 figs
- 1 apple
- 1 beetroot

Directions:

1. Place sesame seeds, flax seeds, sunflower seeds, and figs in a bowl. Cover them with water and let them soak overnight.
2. In the morning, drain the soaked seeds and figs.
3. In a blender, add the soaked seeds and figs along with the chopped apple and beetroot.
4. Blend the ingredients until smooth and well combined. Add a little water if needed to achieve the desired consistency.
5. Pour the blended mixture into a glass.
6. Garnish the shake with chopped pistachios.

Spicy Peanut Noodles

Ingredients:

- 8 oz (225g) noodles (such as spaghetti or linguine)
- 1/3 cup (80ml) smooth peanut butter
- 3 tablespoons (45ml) soy sauce
- 2 tablespoons (30ml) rice vinegar
- 1 tablespoon (15ml) sesame oil
- 1 tablespoon (15ml) honey or maple syrup
- 1 clove garlic, minced
- 1 teaspoon (5ml) grated ginger
- 1/2 teaspoon (2.5ml) red pepper flakes (adjust to taste)
- 1/4 cup (60ml) warm water, or more as needed
- Optional toppings: chopped green onions, chopped cilantro chopped peanuts, lime wedges

Directions:

1. Cook the noodles according to the package Directions until al dente. Drain and rinse under cold water to stop the cooking process. Set aside.
2. In a medium bowl, whisk together the peanut butter, soy sauce, rice vinegar, sesame oil, honey or maple syrup, minced garlic, grated ginger, and red pepper flakes until smooth.
3. Gradually whisk in the warm water, adding a little at a time until you reach your desired consistency for the sauce. You may need more or less water depending on the thickness of your peanut butter.
4. In a large mixing bowl, toss the cooked noodles with the spicy peanut sauce until well coated.
5. Serve the spicy peanut noodles immediately, garnished with chopped green onions, cilantro, chopped peanuts, and lime wedges if desired.

Chicken Liver Pate

Ingredients:

- 1 lb (450g) chicken livers, trimmed and cleaned
- 1 medium onion, finely chopped
- 2 cloves garlic, minced
- 4 tablespoons (60g) unsalted butter
- 2 tablespoons (30ml) brandy or cognac
- 2 tablespoons (30ml) heavy cream
- 1/2 teaspoon (2.5ml) dried thyme
- 1/4 teaspoon (1.25ml) ground nutmeg
- Salt and pepper, to taste
- Optional garnish: melted butter, chopped fresh parsley

Directions:

1. In a large skillet, melt 2 tablespoons of butter over medium heat. Add the chopped onion and minced garlic, and sauté until softened and fragrant, about 5 minutes.
2. Add the cleaned chicken livers to the skillet and cook until browned on all sides, but still slightly pink in the center, about 3-4 minutes per side.
3. Pour in the brandy or cognac and cook for an additional 1-2 minutes, allowing the alcohol to evaporate.
4. Remove the skillet from the heat and let the mixture cool slightly.
5. Transfer the cooked onion, garlic, and chicken livers to a food processor or blender. Add the remaining 2 tablespoons of butter heavy cream, dried thyme, ground nutmeg, salt, and pepper.
6. Blend the mixture until smooth and creamy, scraping down the sides of the bowl as needed to ensure everything is well incorporated.
7. Taste the chicken liver pate and adjust seasoning if needed, adding more salt, pepper, or spices according to your taste preference.
8. Transfer the pate to a serving dish or small ramekins. Smooth the

top with a spatula.

9. Optional: Melt additional butter and pour a thin layer over the top of the pate to seal it and preserve freshness. Garnish with

chopped fresh parsley if desired.

10. Cover the pate with plastic wrap and refrigerate for at least 1-2 hours, or until firm.

Hair Nourishing Smoothie Bowl

Ingredients:

- 1/2 cup cooked sweet potato, chilled or frozen
- 1/2 cup almond milk
- 2 tablespoons maple syrup
- 1 tablespoon almond butter or cashew butter
- 1 scoop Biotin Marine Collagen Peptides
  Toppings:
- Pumpkin seeds
- Berries

- 1 teaspoon turmeric powder
- 1 teaspoon ground cinnamon
- 1/4 teaspoon ground ginger
- Pinch of sea salt

- Coconut flakes

Directions:

1. In a blender or food processor, combine all the ingredients until completely smooth.
2. Add more almond milk if a thinner texture is desired.

3. Pour the mixture into a bowl.
4. Top the smoothie bowl with pumpkin seeds, berries, and coconut flakes.

Headaches and Migraines

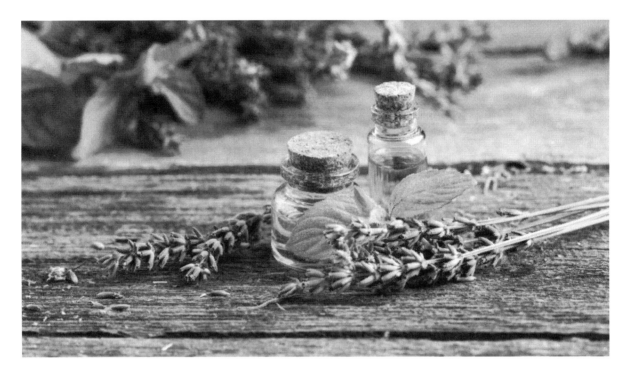

"Your body is a temple, but only if you treat it as one." —Astrid Alauda

Headaches and migraines can be debilitating, affecting our ability to work, enjoy life, and even carry out simple daily tasks. While over-the-counter medications may provide temporary relief, they often come with unwanted side effects and fail to address the underlying causes of our pain. By turning to natural remedies and lifestyle changes, we can help prevent headaches and migraines, reduce their frequency and severity, and promote overall well-being.

Topical Treatments

Lavender and Peppermint Oil Temple Rub

Ingredients:

- 2 tablespoons (30ml) carrier oil (such as jojoba oil, sweet almond oil, or coconut oil)
- 3 drops lavender essential oil
- 2 drops peppermint essential oil

Directions:

1. In a small bowl or container, combine the carrier oil with the lavender and peppermint essential oils.

2. Stir the mixture well to ensure the essential oils are evenly distributed throughout the carrier oil.

3. To use, dip your fingertips into the oil blend and gently massage it onto your temples using circular motions.

4. Continue massaging for 1-2 minutes, focusing on the temples and forehead area.

5. Take slow, deep breaths as you massage to enhance the relaxation and calming effects of the essential oils.

6. Use as needed whenever you feel tension or discomfort in your temples or head.

7. Store any leftover oil blend in a sealed container in a cool, dark place for future use.

Headache Essential Oil Vapor

Ingredients:

- 3 cups (720ml) hot water
- 3 drops peppermint essential oil
- 3 drops lavender essential oil
- 2 drops eucalyptus essential oil

Directions:

1. Boil 3 cups of water in a pot or kettle.
2. Once the water is boiling, carefully pour it into a heat-safe bowl or basin.
3. Add the drops of peppermint, lavender, and eucalyptus essential oils to the hot water.
4. Lean over the bowl, ensuring a safe distance to avoid burns, and cover your head with a towel to create a tent-like effect that traps the steam.
5. Close your eyes and breathe deeply, inhaling the aromatic steam for 5-10 minutes.
6. Take slow, deep breaths to fully experience the therapeutic benefits of the essential oils.
7. After inhaling the steam, remove the towel and allow the vapor to dissipate naturally.
8. Repeat this process as needed to help alleviate headache symptoms and promote relaxation.
9. Store any leftover essential oil blend in a dark, cool place for future use.

Cayenne Pepper Balm

Ingredients:

- 2 tablespoons (30ml) carrier oil (such as coconut oil, almond oil, or olive oil)
- 1/2 teaspoon (2.5ml) cayenne pepper powder

Directions:

- In a small bowl or container, mix the carrier oil and cayenne pepper powder until well combined.
- Stir the mixture thoroughly to ensure the cayenne pepper is evenly distributed throughout the carrier oil.
- To use, dip your fingertips into the cayenne pepper oil blend and gently massage it onto your temples using circular motions.
- Be cautious to avoid getting the mixture near your eyes, nose, or mouth, as cayenne pepper can cause irritation.
- Massage the temples for 1-2 minutes, applying gentle pressure as desired.
- Wash your hands thoroughly after applying the cayenne pepper temple rub to prevent accidental contact with sensitive areas.
- Use as needed to help alleviate tension headaches or discomfort in the temples.

Herbal Brews and Drinks

Feverfew Tea

Ingredients:

- 1 teaspoon dried feverfew leaves or 1 tablespoon fresh feverfew leaves
- 1 cup (240ml) water
- Optional: Honey or lemon for flavor

Directions:

1. Boil one cup of water in a small saucepan or kettle.
2. Once the water reaches a boil, remove it from the heat.
3. Place the dried or fresh feverfew leaves in a teapot or heatproof mug.
4. Pour the hot water over the feverfew leaves.
5. Cover the teapot or mug and let the feverfew leaves steep in the hot water for about 10-15 minutes. Steep longer if you prefer a stronger tea.
6. After steeping, strain the tea to remove the feverfew leaves.
7. If desired, add honey or lemon to sweeten or flavor the tea.
8. Serve the feverfew tea hot and enjoy its potential benefits for relieving headaches or migraines.
9. Store any leftover tea in a sealed container in the refrigerator for up to 24 hours.

Migraine Herbal Brew

Ingredients:

- 5 tablespoons peppermint
- 3 tablespoons feverfew
- 2 tablespoons chamomile
- 2 tablespoons lemon balm

Directions:

1. Mix all the herbs together in a bowl or jar.
2. For each cup of tea, measure out 2 tablespoons of the herbal mixture.
3. Bring 1.5 cups of water to a boil in a small saucepan or tea kettle.
4. Add the herbal mixture to your tea infuser or reusable tea bag.
5. Place the tea infuser or bag in your mug.
6. Pour hot water over your herbal blend in the cup and cover. Let steep for 5-7 minutes.
7. After steeping, remove the infuser from the mug and discard or compost the spent herbs.
8. Optionally, add honey or lemon to taste.
9. Enjoy your soothing herbal tea!
10. Store any remaining herbal mixture in an airtight container in a cool, dark place for future use.

Willowbark and Ginger Tea

Ingredients:

- 1 tablespoon dried willow bark
- 1 teaspoon grated fresh ginger root or 1/2 teaspoon dried ginger
- 1.5 cups (360ml) water
- Optional: Honey or lemon for flavor

Directions:

- In a small saucepan, combine the dried willow bark and grated fresh ginger root (or dried ginger) with 1.5 cups of water.
- Bring the water to a gentle boil over medium heat.
- Once boiling, reduce the heat to low and let the mixture simmer for 10-15 minutes.
- After simmering, remove the saucepan from the heat.
- Strain the tea into a cup using a fine-mesh sieve or tea strainer to remove the willow bark and ginger particles.
- If desired, add honey or lemon to sweeten or flavor the tea.
- Stir the tea well and enjoy it while it's warm.
- Store any leftover tea in a sealed container in the refrigerator for up to 24 hours.

Headache and Migraine Recipes

Boursin Pasta

Ingredients:

- 8 oz fettuccine pasta
- 2 tablespoons butter
- 2 cloves garlic, minced
- 3/4 cup heavy cream
- 4 ounces Boursin Garlic & Fine Herbs Cheese
- Kosher salt and fresh pepper to taste
- Fresh Italian parsley for garnish

Directions:

1. Cook the pasta according to package directions and drain. Reserve about a cup of pasta water just in case you need to thin out the sauce later.
2. Meanwhile, melt the butter in a large saucepan over medium heat.
3. Add the minced garlic and cook for about a minute or two until fragrant, but not browned.
4. Pour in the heavy cream and bring the sauce to a simmer, which should take about 5-7 minutes, until it thickens. You'll know it's ready when the sauce coats the back of a spoon and leaves a line or trail as you run it through the sauce.
5. Reduce the heat to low and add the Boursin cheese to the saucepan, stirring continuously until the cheese is fully melted and incorporated into the sauce.
6. Taste the sauce and adjust the seasoning with kosher salt and freshly ground black pepper as needed.
7. Add the drained pasta to the saucepan and toss everything together until the pasta is well coated with the creamy sauce.
8. Serve the fettuccine immediately, garnished with fresh Italian parsley.

Chicken Zucchini Poppers

Ingredients:

- 1 lb (450g) ground chicken
- 1 medium zucchini, grated and excess moisture squeezed out
- 1/4 cup grated Parmesan cheese
- 1/4 cup breadcrumbs
- 2 cloves garlic, minced
- 1 teaspoon Italian seasoning
- 1/2 teaspoon onion powder
- 1/2 teaspoon paprika
- Salt and pepper, to taste
- Cooking spray or olive oil for greasing

Directions:

1. Preheat your oven to 400°F (200°C). Line a baking sheet with parchment paper or grease it lightly with cooking spray or olive oil.

2. In a large mixing bowl, combine the ground chicken, grated zucchini, Parmesan cheese, breadcrumbs, minced garlic, Italian seasoning, onion powder, paprika, salt, and pepper. Mix until well combined.

3. Using your hands, shape the mixture into small poppers, about 1 inch in diameter, and place them on the prepared baking sheet.

4. Bake the chicken zucchini poppers in the preheated oven for 15-20 minutes, or until they are cooked through and golden brown on the outside.

5. Once cooked, remove the poppers from the oven and let them cool slightly before serving.

6. Serve the chicken zucchini poppers warm as a delicious appetizer or snack.

Vegetable Fried Rice

Ingredients:

- 2 cups cooked rice (preferably day-old rice)
- 2 tablespoons vegetable oil
- 2 cloves garlic, minced
- 1 small onion, diced
- 1 carrot, diced
- 1 bell pepper, diced
- 1 cup frozen peas and carrots, thawed
- 2 eggs, lightly beaten
- 3 tablespoons soy sauce
- 1 tablespoon oyster sauce (optional)
- 1 teaspoon sesame oil
- Salt and pepper to taste
- Green onions, chopped, for garnish
- Sesame seeds, for garnish

Directions:

1. Heat 1 tablespoon of vegetable oil in a large skillet or wok over medium-high heat.

2. Add the minced garlic and diced onion to the skillet. Stir-fry for 1-2 minutes until fragrant and the onion is translucent.

3. Add the diced carrot and bell pepper to the skillet. Stir-fry for another 2-3 minutes until the vegetables are tender-crisp.

4. Push the vegetables to one side of the skillet, then add the remaining tablespoon of vegetable oil to the empty side.

5. Pour the lightly beaten eggs into the skillet. Allow them to cook undisturbed for a few seconds until they begin to set.

6. Use a spatula to scramble the eggs until fully cooked, then mix them with the vegetables in the skillet.

7. Add the cooked rice and thawed frozen peas and carrots to the skillet. Stir-fry for 2-3 minutes until the rice is heated through and evenly mixed with the vegetables and eggs.

8. Drizzle the soy sauce, oyster sauce (if using), and sesame oil over the rice mixture. Stir well to combine and evenly distribute the sauces.

9. Season with salt and pepper to taste. Stir-fry for another 1-2 minutes to allow the flavors to meld together.

10. Remove the skillet from the heat. Taste and adjust seasoning if necessary.

11. Transfer the vegetable fried rice to serving plates or bowls.

12. Garnish with chopped green onions and sesame seeds before serving.

Hearty Chicken and Rice Bowl

Ingredients:

- 1 cup long-grain white rice
- 2 cups chicken broth
- 1 tablespoon olive oil
- 2 boneless, skinless chicken breasts, diced
- Salt and pepper, to taste
- 1 teaspoon garlic powder
- 1 teaspoon paprika
- 1/2 teaspoon dried thyme
- 1/2 teaspoon dried oregano
- 1/2 teaspoon dried basil
- 1 bell pepper, diced
- 1 cup frozen corn kernels, thawed

- 1 cup canned black beans, drained and rinsed
- 1/2 cup diced tomatoes
- 1/4 cup chopped fresh cilantro
- Juice of 1 lime
- Optional toppings: avocado slices, sour cream, shredded cheese

Directions:

1. In a medium saucepan, combine the rice and chicken broth. Bring to a boil over medium-high heat, then reduce the heat to low, cover, and simmer for 18-20 minutes, or until the rice is tender and the liquid is absorbed.

2. Remove from heat and let it sit, covered, for 5 minutes.

3. While the rice is cooking, heat the olive oil in a large skillet over medium heat. Season the diced chicken breasts with salt, pepper, garlic powder, paprika, dried thyme, dried oregano, and dried basil.

4. Add the seasoned chicken to the skillet and cook for 6-8 minutes, or until cooked through and no longer pink in the center.

5. Add the diced bell pepper to the skillet with the cooked chicken and sauté for an additional 2-3 minutes, or until the bell pepper is tender-crisp.

6. Stir in the thawed corn kernels, black beans, diced tomatoes, chopped cilantro, and lime juice.

7. Cook for another 2-3 minutes, stirring occasionally, until heated through.

8. To assemble the bowls, divide the cooked rice among serving bowls. Top each bowl with the chicken and vegetable mixture.

9. Garnish with avocado slices, sour cream, shredded cheese, or any other desired toppings.

Heart Health

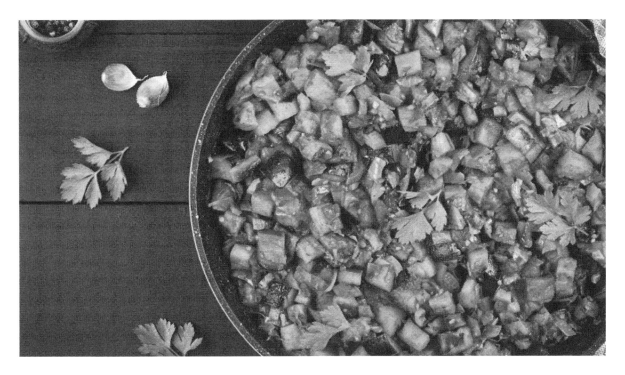

"The human heart, at whatever age, opens only to the heart that opens in return." –Maria Edgeworth

The heart is the center of our circulatory system, responsible for pumping life-giving blood and nutrients to every cell in our body. When our heart health is compromised, we may face a range of serious conditions, from high blood pressure and arrhythmia to heart attack and stroke. Nourishing our hearts with targeted herbs and heart-healthy recipes lowers our risk of cardiovascular disease, improves circulation, and promotes overall well-being.

Topical Treatments

Cilantro Gel Caps

Ingredients:

- Fresh cilantro leaves
- Empty gel capsules

Directions:

1. Wash and thoroughly dry fresh cilantro leaves.
2. Remove the stems from the cilantro leaves.
3. Open the empty gel capsules.
4. Fill each gel capsule with fresh cilantro leaves.
5. Seal the gel capsules tightly.
6. Store the cilantro gel capsules in an airtight container in the refrigerator until ready to use.
7. Take as needed, following the recommended dosage for cilantro supplements.

Dosage: 1 to 2 caps daily with food.

Garlic Gel Caps

Ingredients:

- Fresh garlic cloves
- Empty gel capsules

Directions:

- Peel and mince the fresh garlic cloves.
- Open the empty gel capsules.
- Fill each gel capsule with minced garlic, ensuring it's packed tightly but leaving a small amount of space at the top to seal the capsule.
- Seal the gel capsules tightly.

  Dosage: 1 to 2 caps daily with food
- Store the garlic gel capsules in an airtight container in the refrigerator until ready to use.
- Take as needed, following the recommended dosage for garlic supplements.

Herbal Brews and Drinks

Heart Strengthening Hawthorne Tea

Ingredients:

- 1 tablespoon dried hawthorn berries
- 1 teaspoon dried hawthorn leaves and flowers
- 1 cup water
- Optional: Honey or lemon for flavor

Directions:

1. In a small saucepan, bring the water to a boil.
2. Once boiling, add the dried hawthorn berries and leaves/flowers to the saucepan.
3. Reduce the heat to low and let the mixture simmer for 10-15 minutes.
4. After simmering, remove the saucepan from the heat and let the tea steep for an additional 5 minutes.
5. Strain the tea into a cup using a fine-mesh sieve or tea strainer to remove the hawthorn berries and leaves/flowers.
6. If desired, add honey or lemon to sweeten or flavor the tea.
7. Stir the tea well and enjoy it while it's warm.

Chamomile Health Shot

Ingredients:

- 1 tablespoon dried chamomile flowers
- 1 cup water
- 1 teaspoon honey (optional)
- 1/2 teaspoon fresh lemon juice (optional)

Directions:

1. In a small saucepan, bring the water to a boil.
2. Once boiling, remove the saucepan from the heat and add the dried chamomile flowers.
3. Cover the saucepan and let the chamomile steep in the hot water for about 5-10 minutes.
4. After steeping, strain the chamomile tea into a shot glass or small cup using a fine-mesh sieve or tea strainer.
5. If desired, stir in honey and fresh lemon juice to sweeten and enhance the flavor.
6. Let the chamomile health shot cool slightly before consuming.
7. Drink the chamomile health shot slowly and enjoy its potential calming and digestive benefits.

Switchel

Ingredients:

- 1 cup ginger, chopped
- 1/2 cup maple syrup (adjust to taste; molasses can be substituted for a more traditional flavor)
- 1/2 cup apple cider vinegar
- 2/3 cup lemon juice
- 6 cups water

Directions:

1. Fill a large saucepan about 2/3 full with water and add the chopped ginger.
2. Bring the water to a boil and allow the ginger to boil for approximately 2 minutes.
3. Remove the saucepan from the heat and let the ginger steep in the hot water for about 20 minutes.
4. In a large pitcher, combine the maple syrup, apple cider vinegar, and lemon juice.

5. Strain the ginger as you pour the steeped water into the pitcher.

6. Stir and mix all the ingredients well until fully combined.

7. Serve the switchel warm or over ice, according to your preference.

8. If desired, adjust the consistency by adding more water to dilute.

Wild Berry Hibiscus Latte

Ingredients:

- 1 tablespoon dried hibiscus flowers
- 1/2 cup mixed wild berries (such as strawberries, raspberries, blueberries)
- 1 cup milk (non-dairy)
- 1 tablespoon honey or maple syrup (optional, for sweetness)
- 1/2 teaspoon vanilla extract
- Fresh berries, for garnish (optional)

Directions:

1. In a small saucepan, combine the dried hibiscus flowers and mixed wild berries with 1 cup of water.

2. Bring the mixture to a simmer over medium heat and let it simmer for about 5-7 minutes, until the berries have softened and released their juices.

3. Use a spoon or masher to gently mash the berries and release more flavor.

4. Remove the saucepan from the heat and strain the berry and hibiscus mixture through a fine-mesh sieve into a clean bowl or measuring cup, pressing down on the solids to extract as much liquid as possible.

5. Discard the solids.

6. Rinse out the saucepan and return the strained berry-hibiscus liquid to it.

7. Add the milk, honey or maple syrup (if using), and vanilla extract to the saucepan with the berry-hibiscus liquid.

8. Heat the mixture over medium heat, stirring occasionally, until it is hot but not boiling.

9. Once heated through, remove the saucepan from the heat and pour the berry-hibiscus latte into mugs.

Greek Mountain Tea

Ingredients:

- 1 tablespoon dried Greek mountain tea leaves (Sideritis plant)
- 2 cups water
- Honey or lemon, to taste (optional)

Directions:

- In a small saucepan, bring 2 cups of water to a boil.
- Once the water is boiling, add the dried Greek mountain tea leaves to the saucepan.
- Reduce the heat to low and let the tea simmer for about 5-10 minutes, allowing the flavors to infuse into the water.
- Remove the saucepan from the heat and let the tea steep for an additional 5 minutes.
- Strain the tea through a fine-mesh sieve or tea strainer into a cup or teapot, discarding the used tea leaves.
- If desired, add honey or lemon to sweeten or flavor the tea.
- Stir well and serve the Greek mountain tea hot.

Heart Health Recipes

Carrot Pilaf with Coriander-Rich Chutney

Carrot Pilaf **Ingredients:**

- 1 cup basmati rice
- 2 cups water
- 2 tablespoons olive oil or ghee
- 1 small onion, finely chopped
- 2 cloves garlic, minced
- 2 cups grated carrots
- 1 teaspoon ground cumin
- 1/2 teaspoon ground coriander
- Salt and pepper, to taste
- Fresh cilantro, chopped, for garnish

Coriander-Rich Chutney **Ingredients:**

- 1 cup fresh coriander (cilantro) leaves
- 1/4 cup fresh mint leaves
- 2 green chilies, chopped
- 2 cloves garlic
- 1 tablespoon lemon juice
- Salt, to taste
- 2 tablespoons water (optional, for desired consistency)

Directions:

For the Carrot Pilaf:

1. Rinse the basmati rice under cold water until the water runs clear. Drain and set aside.

2. In a saucepan, heat the olive oil or ghee over medium heat. Add the chopped onion and cook until softened and translucent, about 5 minutes.

3. Add the minced garlic to the saucepan and cook for another minute until fragrant.

4. Stir in the grated carrots, ground cumin, and ground coriander.

For the Coriander-Rich Chutney:

8. In a blender or food processor, combine the fresh coriander leaves, mint leaves, chopped green chilies, garlic cloves, lemon juice, and salt.

9. Blend the ingredients until smooth, adding water as needed to

To Serve:

11. Serve the Carrot Pilaf hot, garnished with additional fresh cilantro if desired.

Cook for 2-3 minutes, until the carrots are slightly softened.

5. Add the rinsed basmati rice to the saucepan and stir to combine with the carrot mixture.

6. Pour in the water and season with salt and pepper. Bring to a boil, then reduce the heat to low, cover, and simmer for 15-20 minutes, or until the rice is tender and the liquid is absorbed.

7. Once cooked, fluff the rice with a fork and garnish with fresh chopped cilantro before serving.

reach your desired consistency.

10. Taste the chutney and adjust seasoning if necessary.

12. Serve the Coriander-Rich Chutney on the side as a flavorful accompaniment to the pilaf.

Mediterranean Fish Stew

Ingredients:

- 1 lb (450g) white fish filets (such as cod, halibut, or tilapia), cut into chunks
- 2 tablespoons olive oil
- 1 onion, finely chopped
- 3 cloves garlic, minced
- 1 red bell pepper, diced
- 1 yellow bell pepper, diced
- 1 can (14 oz/400g) diced tomatoes
- 1 cup (240ml) vegetable or fish broth
- 1/2 cup (120ml) dry white wine (optional)
- 1 teaspoon dried oregano
- 1 teaspoon dried basil
- 1 teaspoon dried thyme
- Salt and pepper, to taste
- Pinch of red pepper flakes (optional)
- 1/4 cup chopped fresh parsley, for garnish
- Crusty bread, for serving

Directions:

1. In a large pot or Dutch oven, heat the olive oil over medium heat. Add the chopped onion and cook until softened and translucent, about 5 minutes.

2. Add the minced garlic to the pot and cook for another minute until fragrant.

3. Stir in the diced red and yellow bell peppers and cook for 5-7 minutes, until they begin to soften.

4. Pour in the diced tomatoes (with their juices), vegetable or fish broth, and dry white wine (if using). Stir to combine.

5. Add the dried oregano, basil, thyme, salt, pepper, and red pepper flakes (if using). Stir well to incorporate the seasonings into the stew.

6. Bring the stew to a simmer, then reduce the heat to low and let it simmer gently for 10-15 minutes to allow the flavors to meld together.

7. Once the stew has simmered and the vegetables are tender carefully add the chunks of white fish to the pot.

8. Cover the pot and let the fish simmer in the stew for another 5-7 minutes, or until cooked through and opaque.

9. Taste the stew and adjust seasoning if necessary.

10. Ladle the Mediterranean Fish Stew into bowls, garnish with chopped fresh parsley, and serve hot with crusty bread for dipping

Aubergine and Lentil Bake

Ingredients:

- 2 large aubergines (eggplants), sliced into rounds
- 1 cup green or brown lentils, rinsed
- 2 cups vegetable broth
- 1 tablespoon olive oil
- 1 onion, finely chopped
- 2 cloves garlic, minced
- 1 red bell pepper, diced
- 1 can (14 oz/400g) diced tomatoes
- 1 teaspoon dried oregano
- 1 teaspoon dried basil
- Salt and pepper, to taste
- 1 cup grated cheese (such as mozzarella or cheddar), optional

- Fresh parsley, chopped, for garnish

Directions:

1. Preheat the oven to 375°F (190°C). Grease a baking dish with olive oil or cooking spray.

2. Place the sliced aubergines on a baking sheet lined with parchment paper. Brush both sides of the aubergine slices with olive oil and season with salt and pepper.

3. Bake in the preheated oven for 15-20 minutes, or until softened and lightly golden.

4. Remove from the oven and set aside.

5. In a medium saucepan, combine the rinsed lentils and vegetable broth. Bring to a boil over medium-high heat, then reduce the heat to low, cover, and simmer for 20-25 minutes, or until the lentils are tender and most of the liquid is absorbed.

6. Remove from heat and set aside.

7. In a large skillet, heat olive oil over medium heat. Add the chopped onion and cook until softened and translucent, about 5 minutes.

8. Add the minced garlic and diced red bell pepper, and cook for another 3-4 minutes.

9. Stir in the diced tomatoes (with their juices), dried oregano, dried basil, salt, and pepper. Cook for 5-7 minutes, allowing the flavors to meld together.

10. Add the cooked lentils to the skillet with the tomato mixture and stir to combine. Cook for an additional 2-3 minutes.

11. Layer half of the cooked aubergine slices on the bottom of the prepared baking dish. Spoon half of the lentil mixture on top of the aubergines. Repeat with another layer of aubergines and the remaining lentil mixture.

12. If desired, sprinkle grated cheese over the top of the lentil mixture.

13. Bake the aubergine and lentil bake in the preheated oven for 20-25 minutes, or until the cheese is melted and bubbly.

14. Remove from the oven and let it cool slightly before serving.

Turkey Meatballs with Hummus Dip

Ingredients:

For the Turkey Meatballs:
- 1 lb (450g) ground turkey
- 1/2 cup breadcrumbs
- 1/4 cup grated Parmesan cheese
- 1 egg
- 2 cloves garlic, minced

For the Hummus Dip:
- 1 can (15 oz/425g) chickpeas, drained and rinsed
- 2 tablespoons tahini
- 2 tablespoons lemon juice
- 2 cloves garlic, minced

- 1 teaspoon dried oregano
- 1 teaspoon dried basil
- Salt and pepper, to taste
- Olive oil, for cooking

- 2 tablespoons olive oil
- Salt, to taste
- Water, as needed for consistency

Directions:

1. Preheat the oven to 400°F (200°C). Line a baking sheet with parchment paper or lightly grease it with olive oil.

2. In a large mixing bowl, combine the ground turkey, breadcrumbs, grated Parmesan cheese, egg, minced garlic, dried oregano, dried basil, salt, and pepper. Mix until well combined.

3. Shape the turkey mixture into small meatballs, about 1 inch in diameter, and place them on the prepared baking sheet.

4. Drizzle or spray the meatballs with olive oil to help them brown in the oven.

5. Bake the turkey meatballs in the preheated oven for 15-20 minutes, or until they are cooked through and golden brown on the outside.

6. While the meatballs are baking, prepare the hummus dip. In a food processor, combine the drained and rinsed chickpeas, tahini, lemon juice, minced garlic, olive oil, and salt. Blend until smooth, adding water as needed to reach your desired consistency.

7. Taste the hummus and adjust seasoning if necessary.

8. Transfer the hummus dip to a serving bowl and garnish with a drizzle of olive oil and a sprinkle of paprika or chopped parsley, if desired.

9. Once the turkey meatballs are cooked, remove them from the oven and let them cool slightly.

10. Serve the turkey meatballs warm alongside the hummus dip.

Hypertension

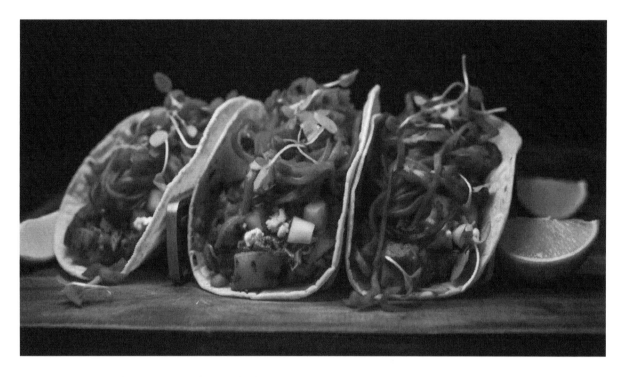

"The greatest medicine of all is to teach people how not to need it." –Hippocrates

Hypertension, or high blood pressure, is a silent killer that affects millions of people worldwide. When left untreated, hypertension can lead to serious complications, such as heart attack, stroke, and kidney damage. By adopting a heart-healthy lifestyle and incorporating targeted herbs and nutrients into our diets, we can help to lower blood pressure naturally, reduce our risk of complications, and promote overall cardiovascular health.

Topical Treatments

Ashwagandha Gel Caps

Ingredients:

- Ashwagandha powder (as per recommended dosage)
- Empty gel capsules

Directions:

- Measure out the desired amount of Ashwagandha powder according to the recommended dosage.
- Carefully open the empty gel capsules and separate them into halves.
- Using a small spoon or a capsule filling machine, fill each half of the gel capsules with the measured Ashwagandha powder.
- Once filled, carefully close the gel capsules by pressing the two halves together until they snap shut.

- Repeat the process until all the Ashwagandha powder is used or until you've filled the desired number of gel capsules.
- Store the filled gel capsules in a cool, dry place, away from direct sunlight or moisture.
- Label the container with the contents and the date of preparation for future reference.
- Take the Ashwagandha gel caps as directed by your healthcare provider or as per the recommended dosage on the packaging.

Dosage: Take 2 caps daily with food.

Herbal Brews and Drinks

Hibiscus Iced Tea

Ingredients:

- 1 cup boiling water
- 1 teaspoon whole cloves
- 4-5 pieces star anise
- 4 cups cold filtered water
- 5 bags hibiscus tea
- 8 bags green tea
- 6 ounces cranberry juice cocktail
- 1/2 fresh orange
- Seltzer water

Directions:

- Boil 1 cup of water in the microwave.
- Place the whole cloves and star anise in the boiling water.
- Cover with a lid or small dish and set it aside for about 10 minutes to steep.
- Pour the 4 cups of cold filtered water into a large pitcher with a lid.
- Add the hibiscus and green tea bags and press down lightly so they're submerged.
- Add the cranberry juice and a generous squeeze of the fresh orange juice. If desired, slice the orange half and add it to the pitcher.
- When the spices have finished steeping, add them along with the hot water to the pitcher.
- Cover the pitcher and let it stand on the counter for at least 2 hours, and up to 6 hours or until it's dark red in color.
- Remove the tea bags, and if desired, strain off the spices and orange slices.
- To serve, fill a glass with ice, add the tea until about 2/3 full, and top off with seltzer water.
- Keep the tea in the refrigerator for up to 5 days. Note: it should keep longer if you remove the spices and fruit.

Calming Onion Tea

Ingredients:

- 1 1/2 cups water
- 1 onion, chopped
- 2-3 cloves garlic, crushed
- 1 bay leaf
- Honey (to taste)
- Cinnamon powder (to taste)
- Lemon juice (to taste)

Directions:

- In a saucepan, bring 1 1/2 cups of water to a boil.
- Add the chopped onion, crushed garlic cloves, and bay leaf to the boiling water.
- Boil for some more time until the water changes color to a deeper hue, indicating that the flavors have infused well.
- Remove the saucepan from the heat and strain the liquid into a cup to remove the onion, garlic, and bay leaf.
- Add honey and cinnamon powder to taste. You may also add a dash of cinnamon while boiling the water for extra flavor.
- Squeeze in some fresh lemon juice to enrich the taste further.
- Stir well to combine all the ingredients.
- Enjoy

Rosemary and Peppermint Heart Blend

Ingredients:

- 16 oz (473 ml) Water
- 2 teaspoons Dried Mint
- 1 teaspoon Dried Rosemary
- Orange or lemon slices (optional, for garnish)

Directions:

- Bring the water to a boil in a saucepan or tea kettle.
- Optional: While the water is heating, use a mortar and pestle to bruise the rosemary slightly. This helps release more flavor, but it's not necessary if you prefer a milder taste.
- Combine the dried rosemary and mint in a tea strainer or tea infuser.
- Once the water reaches a boil, pour it over the rosemary and mint in a teapot or directly into teacups.
- Allow the herbs to steep in the hot water for about 5 minutes to

extract their flavors fully.

- After steeping, remove the tea strainer or infuser, or strain the tea into teacups if loose herbs were used.
- If desired, garnish each cup with a slice of orange or lemon for added flavor and presentation.

Pineapple, Beet, and Carrot Blood Pressure Blend

Ingredients:

- 1 large beet (peeled) or 2 small beets (peeled)
- 4 large carrots (peeled or unpeeled)
- Half of a pineapple with the core intact
- 2 medium oranges (peeled)

Directions:

- Wash all the fruits and vegetables thoroughly.
- Peel the beet(s) and carrots if desired. Cut them into smaller pieces to fit into your juicer chute.
- Remove the skin from the oranges and cut them into quarters.
- Cut the pineapple in half and remove the skin. Cut it into smaller pieces, ensuring the core remains intact as it contains valuable nutrients.
- Feed the beet(s), carrots, pineapple, and oranges through a juicer, processing them into a smooth juice.
- Stir the juice to ensure all flavors are well combined.
- Pour the juice into glasses and serve immediately.

Tropical Carrot Blend

Ingredients:

- 4 large carrots, peeled or unpeeled
- 1 cup pineapple chunks
- 1 medium orange, peeled and segmented
- 1 small mango, peeled and diced
- 1 tablespoon fresh lime juice
- 1 cup coconut water (optional, for added tropical flavor)

Directions:

- Wash all the fruits and vegetables thoroughly.
- Peel the carrots if desired and cut them into smaller pieces to fit into your juicer chute.
- Prepare the pineapple by cutting it into chunks, ensuring to remove the skin and core.
- Peel the orange and separate it into segments.
- Peel the mango and dice it into smaller pieces.
- Juice the carrots, pineapple chunks, orange segments, and mango pieces using a juicer.
- Once juiced, transfer the juice to a blender.
- Add fresh lime juice and coconut water (if using) to the blender.
- Blend the mixture until smooth and well combined.
- Taste the juice and adjust the sweetness or tartness by adding more lime juice if desired.
- Pour the juice into glasses over ice, if desired.

Hypertension Recipes

Chilli-Lime Salmon

Ingredients:

- 1 pound (about 454 grams) Yukon Gold potatoes, cut into 3/4-inch (about 2 cm) pieces
- 2 tablespoons (about 30 ml) extra-virgin olive oil, divided
- 3/4 teaspoon salt, divided (about 3.75 ml)
- 1/4 teaspoon ground pepper (about 1.25 ml)
- 2 teaspoons chili powder (about 10 ml)
- 1 teaspoon ground cumin (about 5 ml)
- 1/2 teaspoon garlic powder (about 2.5 ml)
- 1 lime, zested and quartered
- 2 medium bell peppers, any color, sliced
- 1 1/4 pounds (about 567 grams) center-cut salmon filet, skinned, if desired, and cut into 4 portions

Directions:

- Preheat the oven to 425 degrees F (about 220 degrees C). Coat a large rimmed baking sheet with cooking spray.
- In a medium bowl, toss the potatoes with 1 tablespoon of olive oil, 1/4 teaspoon of salt, and ground pepper until evenly coated. Transfer the potatoes to the prepared baking sheet and roast in the preheated oven for 15 minutes.
- Meanwhile, in a small bowl, combine the chili powder, ground cumin, garlic powder, and lime zest.
- In the same medium bowl used for the potatoes, add the sliced bell peppers. Toss the peppers with the remaining 1 tablespoon of olive oil and 1/2 tablespoon of the spice mixture until well coated.
- Coat the salmon filets evenly with the remaining spice mixture.
- After the initial 15 minutes of roasting the potatoes, remove the baking sheet from the oven. Add the bell peppers to the baking sheet and stir to combine with the potatoes.
- Return the baking sheet to the oven and roast for an additional 5 minutes.
- Remove the baking sheet from the oven again. Move some of the vegetables to the side to create space for the salmon filets.
- Place the seasoned salmon filets on the baking sheet.
- Return the baking sheet to the oven and roast until the salmon is just cooked through, about 6 to 8 minutes.
- Serve the Chilli-Lime Salmon with lime wedges for squeezing over

the top.

Veg and Black Bean Tacos

Ingredients:

- 1 tablespoon olive oil
- 1 small onion, diced
- 2 cloves garlic, minced
- 1 bell pepper, diced
- 1 zucchini, diced
- 1 cup (about 150g) corn kernels (fresh, canned, or frozen)
- 1 can (15 ounces/425g) black beans, drained and rinsed

- 1 teaspoon ground cumin
- 1 teaspoon chili powder
- Salt and pepper to taste
- 8 small corn or flour tortillas
- Toppings: diced tomatoes, shredded lettuce, chopped cilantro, sliced avocado, salsa, lime wedges, sour cream (optional)

Directions:

- Heat olive oil in a large skillet over medium heat.
- Add diced onion and minced garlic to the skillet. Cook, stirring occasionally, until onion is translucent and fragrant, about 2-3 minutes.
- Add diced bell pepper and zucchini to the skillet. Cook for another 4-5 minutes, or until vegetables are tender.
- Stir in corn kernels, black beans, ground cumin, chili powder, salt, and pepper. Cook for an additional 2-3 minutes, until heated through and well combined. Adjust seasoning to taste.

- While the filling is cooking, warm the tortillas according to package Directions. You can heat them in a dry skillet or wrap them in foil and warm them in the oven.
- Once the filling is ready and tortillas are warmed, assemble the tacos. Spoon some of the veg and black bean mixture onto each tortilla.
- Top with desired toppings such as diced tomatoes, shredded lettuce, chopped cilantro, sliced avocado, salsa, a squeeze of lime juice, and a dollop of sour cream if desired.

Hummus Sweet Potatoes

Ingredients:

- 4 medium sweet potatoes
- 1 can (15 ounces/425g) chickpeas (garbanzo beans), drained and rinsed
- 1/4 cup (60ml) tahini
- 2 cloves garlic, minced
- 2 tablespoons lemon juice

- 2 tablespoons olive oil
- 1/2 teaspoon ground cumin
- Salt to taste
- Optional toppings: chopped fresh parsley, paprika, sesame seeds, drizzle of olive oil

Directions:

1. Preheat the oven to 400°F (200°C). Line a baking sheet with parchment paper or aluminum foil for easy cleanup.
2. Scrub the sweet potatoes clean and pierce each one several times with a fork. Place them on the prepared baking sheet.
3. Bake the sweet potatoes in the preheated oven for 45-60 minutes, or until they are tender and easily pierced with a fork.
4. While the sweet potatoes are baking, prepare the hummus. In a food processor, combine the drained and rinsed chickpeas, tahini, minced garlic, lemon juice, olive oil, ground cumin, and a pinch of salt.
5. Process the mixture until smooth and creamy, scraping down the sides of the bowl as needed. If the hummus is too thick,

you can add a tablespoon or two of water to reach your desired consistency.
6. Once the sweet potatoes are done baking, remove them from the oven and let them cool slightly until they are easy to handle.
7. Slice each sweet potato lengthwise and gently press the ends towards the center to create an opening.
8. Spoon a generous amount of hummus into each sweet potato, filling the cavity.
9. Garnish the stuffed sweet potatoes with optional toppings such as chopped fresh parsley, a sprinkle of paprika, sesame seeds, and a drizzle of olive oil.

Tomato, Cucumber, and White Bean Salad

Ingredients:

- 2 cups cherry tomatoes, halved
- 1 English cucumber, diced
- 1 can (15 ounces/425g) white beans (such as cannellini or navy beans), drained and rinsed
- 1/4 cup red onion, thinly sliced

- 1/4 cup fresh parsley, chopped
- 2 tablespoons extra-virgin olive oil
- 1 tablespoon red wine vinegar or lemon juice
- 1 teaspoon Dijon mustard
- Salt and pepper to taste

- Optional toppings: crumbled feta cheese, olives, chopped fresh basil

Directions:

1. In a large mixing bowl, combine the cherry tomatoes, diced cucumber, white beans, sliced red onion, and chopped parsley.

2. In a small bowl, whisk together the extra-virgin olive oil, red wine vinegar or lemon juice, Dijon mustard, salt, and pepper to make the dressing.

3. Pour the dressing over the salad ingredients in the large mixing bowl.

4. Toss the salad gently until everything is evenly coated with the dressing.

5. Taste and adjust the seasoning with more salt and pepper if needed.

6. If desired, sprinkle crumbled feta cheese, olives, and chopped fresh basil over the salad for added flavor and garnish.

7. Serve the Tomato, Cucumber, and White Bean Salad immediately, or cover and refrigerate for later.

Quinoa, Chickpea, and Avocado Salad

Ingredients:

- 1 cup quinoa, rinsed
- 2 cups water or vegetable broth
- 1 can (15 ounces/425g) chickpeas (garbanzo beans), drained and rinsed
- 1 large avocado, diced
- 1 red bell pepper, diced
- 1/4 cup red onion, finely chopped
- 1/4 cup fresh cilantro or parsley, chopped
- Juice of 1 lemon or lime
- 2 tablespoons extra-virgin olive oil
- 1 teaspoon ground cumin
- Salt and pepper to taste
- Optional toppings: crumbled feta cheese, sliced cherry tomatoes, diced cucumber, chopped green onions

Directions:

1. In a medium saucepan, combine the rinsed quinoa and water or vegetable broth. Bring to a boil over medium heat.

2. Reduce the heat to low, cover, and simmer for 15-20 minutes, or until the quinoa is cooked and the liquid is absorbed. Remove from heat and let it sit, covered, for 5 minutes. Fluff with a fork and let it cool slightly.

3. In a large mixing bowl, combine the cooked quinoa, chickpeas, diced avocado, diced red bell pepper, finely chopped red onion, and chopped cilantro or parsley.

4. In a small bowl, whisk together the lemon or lime juice, extra-virgin olive oil, ground cumin, salt, and pepper to make the dressing.

5. Pour the dressing over the salad ingredients in the large mixing bowl.

6. Toss the salad gently until everything is evenly coated with the dressing.

7. Taste and adjust the seasoning with more salt and pepper if needed.

8. If desired, add optional toppings such as crumbled feta cheese, sliced cherry tomatoes, diced cucumber, or chopped green onions for extra flavor and garnish.

9. Serve the Quinoa, Chickpea, and Avocado Salad immediately, or cover and refrigerate for later.

IBS and Gastrointestinal Healing

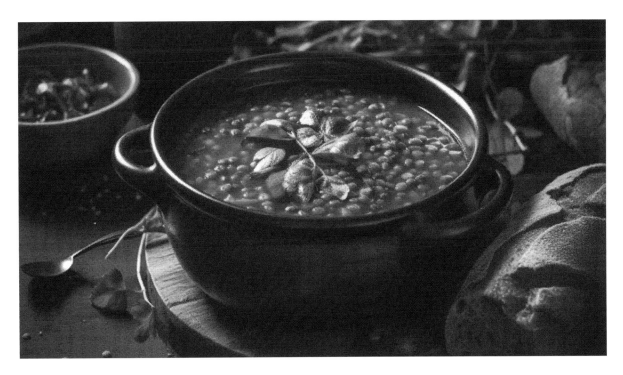

"The natural healing force within each one of us is the greatest force in getting well." —Hippocrates

Irritable Bowel Syndrome (IBS) and other gastrointestinal disorders can greatly impact our quality of life, causing uncomfortable symptoms like bloating, abdominal pain, and irregular bowel movements. While the exact causes of IBS and other gut health issues may vary, incorporating soothing herbs, probiotics, and gut-friendly recipes into our diets can help ease symptoms, reduce inflammation, and promote overall digestive health.

Topical Treatments

Herbal Gut Healing Caps

Ingredients:

- 1 tablespoon dried chamomile flowers
- 1 tablespoon dried peppermint leaves
- 1 tablespoon dried ginger root
- 1 tablespoon dried marshmallow root
- Empty gel capsules

Directions:

- Begin by ensuring your hands and all utensils are clean to prevent contamination.
- In a small bowl, mix together the dried chamomile flowers, peppermint leaves, ginger root, and marshmallow root. Ensure they are thoroughly combined.
- Carefully open the empty gel capsules and separate them into halves.
- Using a small spoon or a capsule filling machine, fill each half of the gel capsules with the herbal mixture.
- Once filled, carefully close the gel capsules by pressing the two halves together until they snap shut.
- Repeat the process until all the herbal mixture is used or until you've filled the desired number of gel capsules.
- Store the filled gel capsules in a clean, airtight container in a cool, dry place, away from direct sunlight or moisture.
- Label the container with the contents and the date of preparation for future reference.

- Take the herbal gut healing gel caps as directed by your healthcare   provider or as per your personal preference.

Herbal Brews and Drinks

Nourishing Gut Juice

Ingredients:

- 1 medium cucumber
- 2 stalks celery
- 1 inch fresh ginger root
- 1 medium apple
- 1 lemon, peeled
- 1 handful fresh parsley or cilantro
- 1-2 cups spinach or kale (optional, for extra greens)

Directions:

1. Wash all the fruits and vegetables thoroughly.
2. If not organic, consider peeling the cucumber and apple to reduce pesticide exposure.
3. Cut the cucumber, celery, ginger root, and apple into chunks that will fit into your juicer chute.
4. If using spinach or kale, tear the leaves into smaller pieces.
5. Juice all the ingredients, including the lemon (peeled).
6. Once juiced, stir the juice to ensure all flavors are well combined.
7. Taste the juice and adjust the flavor by adding more lemon if desired.
8. Pour the juice into glasses over ice if desired.

GI Healing Juice

Ingredients:

- 1 medium cucumber
- 2 stalks celery
- 1 inch fresh ginger root
- 1 medium apple
- 1/2 cup pineapple chunks (fresh or frozen)
- 1/2 lemon, peeled
- 1 small bunch of fresh mint leaves

Directions:

1. Wash all the fruits and vegetables thoroughly.
2. If not organic, consider peeling the cucumber and apple to reduce pesticide exposure.
3. Cut the cucumber, celery, ginger root, and apple into chunks that will fit into your juicer chute.
4. Add the pineapple chunks to the other ingredients.
5. Juice all the ingredients, including the lemon (peeled).
6. Once juiced, pour the juice into a glass.

Beet Celery Shots

Ingredients:

- 1 medium beet, washed and peeled
- 2 stalks celery, washed
- 1 small piece of ginger (about 1 inch), peeled (optional)

Directions:

1. Wash and peel the beet. Cut it into smaller pieces to fit into your juicer chute.
2. Wash the celery stalks and cut them into smaller pieces as well.
3. If using ginger, peel it and cut it into small chunks.
4. Juice the beet, celery, and ginger (if using) together using a juicer
5. Once juiced, pour the mixture into shot glasses.

Pear and Cucumber Gut Healing Juice

Ingredients:

- 2 ripe pears
- 1 cucumber
- 1 inch fresh ginger root
- 1/2 lemon, peeled
- 1 cup spinach or kale (optional, for extra greens)

Directions:

1. Wash all the fruits and vegetables thoroughly.
2. If not organic, consider peeling the cucumber to reduce pesticide exposure.
3. Core the pears and cut them into chunks.
4. Cut the cucumber into smaller pieces that will fit into your juicer chute.
5. Peel the ginger root and cut it into smaller chunks.
6. If using, tear the spinach or kale leaves into smaller pieces.
7. Juice all the ingredients, including the lemon (peeled).
8. Once juiced, stir the juice to ensure all flavors are well combined.
9. Taste the juice and adjust the flavor by adding more lemon if desired.
10. Pour the juice into glasses over ice if desired.

IBS and Gastrointestinal Healing Recipes

Spinach and Blueberry Plant Smoothie

Ingredients:

- 1 cup fresh spinach leaves
- 1/2 cup frozen blueberries
- 1 ripe banana
- 1/2 cup plain Greek yogurt (or dairy-free alternative)
- 1 tablespoon chia seeds (optional)
- 1 tablespoon honey or maple syrup (optional, for added sweetness)
- 1 cup almond milk or your choice of milk

Directions:

1. Wash the fresh spinach leaves thoroughly.
2. Peel the ripe banana and break it into chunks.
3. In a blender, combine the fresh spinach leaves, frozen blueberries, banana chunks, Greek yogurt, chia seeds (if using), and honey or maple syrup (if using).
4. Pour in the almond milk or your choice of milk.
5. Blend all the ingredients together until smooth and creamy. If the smoothie is too thick, you can add more milk until you reach your desired consistency.
6. Once blended, taste the smoothie and adjust the sweetness if needed by adding more honey or maple syrup.
7. Pour the smoothie into glasses and enjoy.

Anti-Inflammatory Beet Smoothie

Ingredients:

- 1 medium beet, cooked and peeled
- 1 cup (240 ml) unsweetened almond milk (or any milk of your choice)
- 1/2 cup (120 ml) Greek yogurt (or coconut yogurt for a dairy-free option)
- 1 ripe banana, peeled
- 1 tablespoon (15 ml) fresh ginger, grated
- 1 tablespoon (15 ml) ground flaxseeds
- 1 tablespoon (15 ml) honey or maple syrup (optional, for sweetness)
- 1/2 teaspoon ground turmeric
- 1/4 teaspoon ground cinnamon
- A pinch of black pepper (helps with turmeric absorption)
- Ice cubes (optional, for a colder smoothie)

Directions:

1. Prepare the beet by cooking it until tender. You can roast, boil, or steam the beet until easily pierced with a fork. Once cooked, allow it to cool slightly, then peel and chop it into chunks.
2. In a blender, combine the cooked beet chunks, almond milk, Greek yogurt, ripe banana, grated ginger, ground flaxseeds, honey or maple syrup (if using), ground turmeric, ground cinnamon, and a pinch of black pepper.
3. Blend the ingredients on high speed until smooth and creamy. If you prefer a colder smoothie, you can add a handful of ice cubes and blend again until well incorporated.
4. Taste the smoothie and adjust the sweetness or spice level if necessary, adding more honey, turmeric, or cinnamon according to your preference.
5. Once you're satisfied with the flavor and consistency, pour the smoothie into glasses and serve immediately.

No Bake FODMAP Peanut Butter Balls

Ingredients:

- 1 cup (240g) smooth peanut butter (make sure it's FOD-MAP-friendly)
- 1/4 cup (60ml) maple syrup or other FODMAP-friendly sweetener
- 1 teaspoon vanilla extract
- 1 1/2 cups (135g) rolled oats
- 1/4 cup (25g) unsweetened shredded coconut
- 1/4 cup (40g) mini dark chocolate chips (ensure they're FOD-MAP-friendly)
- A pinch of salt

Directions:

1. In a large mixing bowl, combine the smooth peanut butter, maple syrup, and vanilla extract. Stir until well combined.
2. Add the rolled oats, shredded coconut, mini dark chocolate chips, and a pinch of salt to the peanut butter mixture.
3. Stir until all the ingredients are evenly incorporated and form a thick, sticky dough.
4. Place the dough in the refrigerator for about 15-30 minutes to firm up slightly, which will make it easier to roll into balls.
5. Once the dough has chilled, remove it from the refrigerator. Using clean hands, scoop out about 1 tablespoon of the dough and roll it into a ball between your palms.
6. Repeat this process until all the dough is used, forming approximately 18-20 peanut butter balls.
7. Optional: Roll the peanut butter balls in additional shredded coconut or chopped nuts for extra flavor and texture.
8. Place the peanut butter balls on a baking sheet lined with parchment paper, spacing them apart so they don't stick together.
9. Transfer the baking sheet to the refrigerator and let the peanut butter balls chill for at least 30 minutes to firm up.
10. Once chilled, the peanut butter balls are ready to enjoy! Store any leftovers in an airtight container in the refrigerator for up to one week.

FODMAP Lentil Dahl

Ingredients:

- 1 cup (200g) red lentils, rinsed and drained
- 2 cups (480ml) low FODMAP vegetable broth
- 1 tablespoon garlic-infused oil
- 1 teaspoon ground cumin
- 1 teaspoon ground coriander
- 1/2 teaspoon ground turmeric
- 1/2 teaspoon ground ginger
- 1/4 teaspoon ground cinnamon
- 1/4 teaspoon ground cardamom
- 1/4 teaspoon cayenne pepper (adjust to taste)
- 1 tablespoon tomato paste (ensure it's FODMAP-friendly)
- 1 cup (240ml) canned coconut milk (ensure it's FODMAP-friendly)
- Salt and pepper to taste
- Fresh cilantro leaves, chopped, for garnish
- Cooked rice or quinoa, for serving

Directions:

1. In a large saucepan or pot, heat the garlic-infused oil over medium heat.
2. Add the ground cumin, ground coriander, ground turmeric, ground ginger, ground cinnamon, ground cardamom, and cayenne pepper to the pot. Cook the spices, stirring constantly, for about 1-2 minutes until fragrant.
3. Add the rinsed red lentils to the pot and stir to coat them in the spices.
4. Pour in the low FODMAP vegetable broth and tomato paste, stirring well to combine.
5. Bring the mixture to a gentle boil, then reduce the heat to low and let it simmer, uncovered, for about 20-25 minutes, stirring occasionally, until the lentils are tender and the mixture has thickened.
6. Once the lentils are cooked, stir in the canned coconut milk until well combined. Season the lentil dahl with salt and pepper to taste.
7. Continue to simmer the lentil dahl for an additional 5-10 minutes to allow the flavors to meld together.
8. Remove the pot from the heat. Taste and adjust the seasoning if needed.
9. Serve the lentil dahl hot, garnished with fresh chopped cilantro leaves.

Almond Cranberry Quinoa

Ingredients:

- 1 cup (180g) quinoa, rinsed
- 2 cups (480ml) water or low FODMAP vegetable broth
- 1/2 cup (60g) sliced almonds
- 1/2 cup (60g) dried cranberries
- 2 tablespoons (30ml) olive oil
- 2 tablespoons (30ml) freshly squeezed lemon juice
- 2 tablespoons (30ml) maple syrup
- 1 teaspoon Dijon mustard

- Salt and pepper to taste

Directions:

1. In a fine-mesh sieve, rinse the quinoa under cold water until the water runs clear. This helps remove any bitterness from the quinoa.

2. In a medium saucepan, combine the rinsed quinoa and water or low FODMAP vegetable broth. Bring the mixture to a boil over medium-high heat.

3. Once boiling, reduce the heat to low, cover the saucepan with a lid, and let the quinoa simmer for about 15-20 minutes, or until all the liquid is absorbed and the quinoa is tender.

4. While the quinoa is cooking, toast the sliced almonds in a dry skillet over medium heat until lightly golden and fragrant, stirring occasionally to prevent burning. This should take about 3-5 minutes. Once toasted, remove the almonds from the skillet and set aside.

5. In a small bowl, whisk together the olive oil, lemon juice, maple

- Fresh parsley or mint leaves for garnish (optional)

syrup, Dijon mustard, salt, and pepper to make the dressing.

6. Once the quinoa is cooked, fluff it with a fork and transfer it to a large mixing bowl.

7. Add the toasted sliced almonds and dried cranberries to the bowl with the quinoa.

8. Pour the dressing over the quinoa mixture and toss until everything is evenly coated in the dressing.

9. Taste the quinoa salad and adjust the seasoning if needed, adding more salt, pepper, or lemon juice according to your preference.

10. Garnish the Almond Cranberry Quinoa with fresh parsley or mint leaves if desired.

11. Serve the quinoa salad warm, at room temperature, or chilled, depending on your preference.

Sweet Chili Tofu

Ingredients:

- 1 block (about 14 ounces or 400g) firm tofu, pressed and drained
- 2 tablespoons (30ml) soy sauce or tamari (for gluten-free option)
- 2 tablespoons (30ml) rice vinegar
- 2 tablespoons (30ml) maple syrup or agave nectar
- 1 tablespoon (15ml) sweet chili sauce
- 1 tablespoon (15ml) sesame oil
- 2 cloves garlic, minced
- 1 teaspoon grated ginger
- 1 tablespoon (15ml) vegetable oil (for frying)
- Sesame seeds and chopped green onions for garnish (optional)

Directions:

1. Begin by pressing the tofu to remove excess moisture. To do this, place the block of tofu between paper towels or clean kitchen towels.

2. Place a heavy object on top, such as a cast iron skillet or a few cans, and let it sit for about 20-30 minutes.

3. While the tofu is pressing, prepare the marinade. In a small bowl, whisk together the soy sauce or tamari, rice vinegar, maple syrup or agave nectar, sweet chili sauce, sesame oil, minced garlic, and grated ginger until well combined.

4. Once the tofu has been pressed, cut it into cubes or slices, depending on your preference.

5. Place the tofu pieces in a shallow dish or a zip-top bag, and pour the marinade over them.

6. Gently toss the tofu to ensure all pieces are coated in the marinade. Let it marinate for at least 15-30 minutes, or longer if time allows, to allow the flavors to penetrate the tofu.

7. Heat the vegetable oil in a large skillet or frying pan over medium-high heat.

8. Once the oil is hot, add the marinated tofu pieces to the skillet, making sure they are in a single layer and not overcrowded. You may need to cook the tofu in batches depending on the size of your skillet.

9. Cook the tofu for about 3-4 minutes on each side, or until golden brown and crispy, flipping them halfway through cooking.

10. Once the tofu is cooked through and crispy on the outside, remove it from the skillet and transfer it to a serving plate.

11. Garnish the Sweet Chili Tofu with sesame seeds and chopped green onions, if desired.

Immune Health

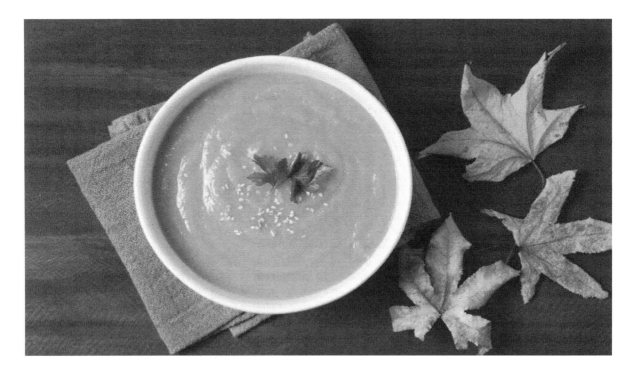

"The art of healing comes from nature, not from the physician." –Paracelsus

A strong, resilient immune system is the foundation of overall health and well-being, protecting our bodies from harmful pathogens, infections, and diseases. In today's stress-filled world, it's more important than ever to support our immune function with nourishing herbs, nutrient-dense foods, and healthy lifestyle practices. Incorporating immune-boosting remedies and recipes into our daily routines can help to strengthen our body's natural defenses, reduce the risk of illness, and promote lasting vitality.

Topical Treatments

Oregano Natural Throat Spray

Ingredients:

- 1 tablespoon dried oregano leaves (or 2 tablespoons fresh oregano leaves)
- 1 cup (240ml) filtered water
- 1 tablespoon honey (optional, for sweetness and soothing properties)
- 1-2 drops of peppermint essential oil (optional, for a cooling sensation)

Directions:

1. In a small saucepan, combine the dried or fresh oregano leaves with the filtered water.

2. Bring the mixture to a gentle boil over medium heat.

3. Once boiling, reduce the heat to low and let the mixture simmer for about 10-15 minutes to allow the oregano to infuse into the water.

4. After simmering, remove the saucepan from the heat and let the mixture cool slightly.

5. Strain the oregano leaves from the liquid using a fine mesh sieve or cheesecloth, pressing gently to extract as much liquid as possible.

6. If using honey for sweetness and added soothing properties, stir it into the strained oregano infusion until fully dissolved. You can adjust the amount of honey according to your taste preferences.

7. Optional: Add 1-2 drops of peppermint essential oil to the mixture for a cooling sensation and refreshing flavor.

8. Transfer the oregano throat spray to a clean spray bottle or glass jar with a tight-fitting lid for storage.

9. Store the throat spray in the refrigerator between uses to prolong its freshness and efficacy.

10. To use, shake the bottle well, then spray the oregano throat spray directly into the back of the throat as needed for soothing relief from soreness and irritation.

Immune Tonic with Honey and Garlic

Ingredients:

- 1/2 cup (120ml) raw honey
- 4-5 cloves of garlic, peeled and crushed
- Optional: 1-2 inches of fresh ginger, peeled and grated
- Optional: 1 lemon, juiced
- Optional: 1-2 teaspoons of ground turmeric

Directions:

- In a clean glass jar with a tight-fitting lid, combine the raw honey, crushed garlic cloves, and grated ginger (if using).
- If desired, add the lemon juice for additional vitamin C and flavor.
- Optionally, you can also add ground turmeric for its anti-inflammatory and immune-boosting properties.
- Stir the ingredients together until well combined.
- Seal the jar tightly with the lid and store it in a cool, dark place for at least 24 hours to allow the flavors to meld together and the garlic to infuse into the honey.
- After 24 hours, your immune tonic is ready to use. Shake the jar well before each use to ensure the ingredients are evenly distributed.
- To consume, take 1-2 teaspoons of the immune tonic daily, either on its own or mixed into warm water or herbal tea.

Herbal Brews and Drinks

Immunity Tea

Ingredients:

- 2 cups (480ml) water
- 1-inch piece of fresh ginger, sliced
- 1 cinnamon stick
- 4-5 whole cloves
- 2-3 slices of lemon
- 1-2 teaspoons of raw honey (optional)
- Optional: a pinch of cayenne pepper (for extra warmth and immune support)

Directions:

- In a small saucepan, bring the water to a boil over medium-high heat.
- Once boiling, add the sliced ginger, cinnamon stick, whole cloves, and lemon slices to the saucepan.
- Reduce the heat to low and let the tea simmer gently for about 10-15 minutes to allow the flavors to infuse into the water.
- After simmering, remove the saucepan from the heat and let the tea cool slightly.
- Strain the tea into mugs using a fine mesh sieve or tea strainer to remove the ginger, cinnamon, cloves, and lemon slices.
- If desired, stir in raw honey to sweeten the tea and enhance its soothing properties.
- Optionally, add a pinch of cayenne pepper for an extra kick and additional immune support.
- Stir the tea well to ensure the honey is fully dissolved.
- Serve the immunity tea warm

Holy Basil Chai

Ingredients:

- 2 cups (480ml) water
- 2 black tea bags or 2 tablespoons loose black tea leaves
- 1/2 cup (120ml) milk (dairy or non-dairy)
- 4-5 fresh holy basil leaves or 1 tablespoon dried holy basil leaves
- 2-3 whole cloves
- 2-3 green cardamom pods, lightly crushed
- 1 cinnamon stick
- 1-inch piece of fresh ginger, sliced
- 2-3 black peppercorns
- 1-2 tablespoons of honey or sweetener of choice (optional)

Directions:

- In a saucepan, bring the water to a boil over medium-high heat. Once the water is boiling, add the black tea bags or loose black tea leaves to the saucepan.
- Reduce the heat to low and let the tea steep for about 3-5 minutes, depending on your preference for tea strength.
- While the tea is steeping, add the milk to the saucepan, along with

the holy basil leaves (fresh or dried), cloves, crushed cardamom pods, cinnamon stick, sliced ginger, and black peppercorns.

- Let the tea simmer gently for an additional 5-7 minutes to allow the spices and holy basil to infuse into the tea.

- After simmering, remove the saucepan from the heat and strain the chai tea into mugs using a fine mesh sieve or tea strainer to remove the tea leaves and spices.

- If desired, stir in honey or sweetener of choice to sweeten the chai tea to your taste preferences.

Immune Booster Shots

Ingredients:

- 1 medium orange, juiced
- 1 lemon, juiced
- 1-inch piece of fresh ginger, grated
- 1 clove of garlic, minced
- 1/4 teaspoon ground turmeric
- 1/4 teaspoon ground black pepper
- 1 tablespoon raw honey or maple syrup (optional, for sweetness)

Directions:

- In a small bowl or jar, combine the freshly squeezed orange juice and lemon juice.
- Add the grated ginger, minced garlic, ground turmeric, and ground black pepper to the bowl with the citrus juices.
- Optional: Stir in raw honey or maple syrup to sweeten the immune booster shot to your taste preferences. This step is optional but can help balance out the flavors and add a touch of sweetness.
- Mix all the ingredients together until well combined.
- Transfer the immune booster shot mixture to a clean glass jar or

bottle with a tight-fitting lid for storage.

- Store the immune booster shot in the refrigerator for up to 3-4 days to keep it fresh.
- To consume, shake the jar well to mix the ingredients before pouring out a shot-sized portion (about 1-2 tablespoons) into a small glass.
- Drink the immune booster shot straight or dilute it with a bit of water if desired.

Pineapple and Mint Wellness Booster

Ingredients:

- 2 cups (480ml) fresh pineapple chunks
- 1/2 cup (120ml) coconut water or filtered water
- 1 tablespoon (15ml) freshly squeezed lime juice
- 1 tablespoon (15ml) raw honey or agave nectar (optional, for swe-

etness)

- 5-6 fresh mint leaves
- Ice cubes (optional)

Directions:

- In a blender, combine the fresh pineapple chunks, coconut water or filtered water, freshly squeezed lime juice, and raw honey or agave nectar (if using).
- Add the fresh mint leaves to the blender.
- Optional: If you prefer a colder drink, you can add a handful of ice cubes to the blender as well.
- Blend all the ingredients on high speed until smooth and well combined. If needed, you can add more water to reach your desired consistency.

- Once blended, taste the Pineapple and Mint Wellness Booster and adjust the sweetness or acidity levels if necessary, adding more honey or lime juice according to your preference.

- If desired, strain the mixture through a fine mesh sieve to remove any pulp or mint leaves, although this step is optional.

- Pour the Pineapple and Mint Wellness Booster into glasses and garnish with additional fresh mint leaves or a slice of lime for a decorative touch.

Immune Health Recipes

Elderberry Syrup

Ingredients:

- 1 cup dried elderberries
- 4 cups water
- 1 cinnamon stick
- 4 cloves
- 1-inch piece of fresh ginger, sliced
- 1 cup honey (raw honey is preferable, but any honey will work)

Directions:

1. In a medium saucepan, combine the dried elderberries, water, cinnamon stick, cloves, and fresh ginger slices.

2. Bring the mixture to a boil over medium-high heat.

3. Once boiling, reduce the heat to low and let the mixture simme

uncovered for about 30-45 minutes, or until the liquid has reduced by half.

4. Remove the saucepan from the heat and let the mixture cool slightly.

5. Once cooled, strain the mixture through a fine mesh sieve or cheesecloth into a clean bowl, pressing gently to extract as much liquid as possible.

6. Discard the elderberry solids and spices.

7. Allow the strained elderberry liquid to cool to lukewarm temperature.

8. Once cooled, stir in the honey until well combined. Adjust the amount of honey to your taste preferences, adding more or less as needed.

9. Transfer the elderberry syrup to clean glass bottles or jars with tight-fitting lids for storage.

10. Store the elderberry syrup in the refrigerator, where it will keep for several weeks to a few months.

To use, take 1-2 tablespoons of elderberry syrup daily as a natural immune booster.

Zinc-Laden Pumpkin Pesto

Ingredients:

- 1 cup (240g) canned pumpkin puree
- 1/2 cup (60g) raw pumpkin seeds (pepitas)
- 2 cloves garlic, peeled
- 1/4 cup (60ml) extra virgin olive oil
- 1/4 cup (15g) fresh basil leaves
- 1/4 cup (15g) fresh parsley leaves

- 2 tablespoons (30ml) lemon juice
- 1/4 cup (15g) grated Parmesan cheese (optional, omit for vegan version)
- Salt and black pepper to taste
- Optional: 1/4 teaspoon ground turmeric for extra zinc boost

Directions:

1. In a food processor or blender, combine the canned pumpkin puree, raw pumpkin seeds, peeled garlic cloves, extra virgin olive oil, fresh basil leaves, fresh parsley leaves, and lemon juice.

2. If using, add the grated Parmesan cheese to the mixture.

3. Optionally, add ground turmeric for an extra boost of zinc and additional health benefits.

4. Blend all the ingredients until smooth and well combined, scraping down the sides of the food processor or blender as needed.

5. If the pesto is too thick, you can add a bit more olive oil or water to reach your desired consistency.

6. Season the pumpkin pesto with salt and black pepper to taste, adjusting the seasoning as needed.

7. Once blended to your liking, transfer the pumpkin pesto to a clean glass jar or airtight container for storage.

8. Store the pesto in the refrigerator, where it will keep for up to one week.

Sweet Potato and Pumpkin Creamy Cold Soup

Ingredients:

- 2 cups (400g) sweet potatoes, peeled and diced
- 2 cups (400g) pumpkin puree (canned or homemade)
- 1 small onion, chopped
- 2 cloves garlic, minced
- 3 cups (720ml) vegetable broth
- 1 cup (240ml) coconut milk (canned, full-fat)
- 1 tablespoon (15ml) olive oil

- 1 teaspoon ground cumin
- 1/2 teaspoon ground cinnamon
- 1/4 teaspoon ground nutmeg
- Salt and black pepper to taste
- Juice of 1 lime
- Fresh cilantro or parsley leaves for garnish (optional)

Directions:

1. In a large pot or Dutch oven, heat the olive oil over medium heat. Add the chopped onion and minced garlic, and sauté until softened and fragrant, about 3-4 minutes.

2. Add the diced sweet potatoes to the pot, along with the ground cumin, ground cinnamon, and ground nutmeg. Stir to coat the sweet potatoes in the spices, and cook for another 2-3 minutes.

3. Pour in the vegetable broth, and bring the mixture to a boil. Once boiling, reduce the heat to low, cover the pot, and let it simmer for about 15-20 minutes, or until the sweet potatoes are tender and easily pierced with a fork.

4. Once the sweet potatoes are cooked, remove the pot from the heat and let the mixture cool slightly.

5. Using an immersion blender or regular blender, blend the soup until smooth and creamy.

6. Return the blended soup to the pot (if using a regular blender), and stir in the pumpkin puree and coconut milk until well combined.

7. Season the soup with salt and black pepper to taste. If the soup is too thick, you can add more vegetable broth or coconut milk to reach your desired consistency.

8. Squeeze in the lime juice, and stir to incorporate.

9. Transfer the soup to a large bowl or individual serving bowls, and enjoy.

Ginger and Tumeric Stuffed Potatoes

Ingredients:

- 4 large baking potatoes
- 2 tablespoons (30ml) olive oil
- 1 onion, finely chopped
- 2 cloves garlic, minced
- 1 tablespoon (15g) fresh ginger, grated
- 1 teaspoon ground turmeric
- 1/2 teaspoon ground cumin
- 1/4 teaspoon chili powder (optional)
- Salt and black pepper to taste
- 1/2 cup (120ml) vegetable broth or water
- 1/2 cup (120ml) coconut milk
- 1/4 cup (60g) plain Greek yogurt or sour cream
- Fresh cilantro or parsley leaves for garnish

Directions:

1. Preheat the oven to 400°F (200°C). Wash and scrub the potatoes, then pat them dry. Pierce the potatoes several times with a fork, then wrap each potato in foil. Place the wrapped potatoes on a baking sheet and bake for about 1 hour, or until tender when pierced with a fork.

2. While the potatoes are baking, heat the olive oil in a large skillet over medium heat. Add the chopped onion and sauté until softened and translucent, about 5 minutes.

3. Add the minced garlic, grated ginger, ground turmeric, ground cumin, chili powder (if using), salt, and black pepper to the skillet. Stir to combine and cook for another 1-2 minutes, until fragrant.

4. Pour in the vegetable broth or water and simmer for 5 minutes. Remove from heat and stir in the coconut milk. Set aside.

5. Once the potatoes are cooked, carefully remove the foil and let them cool slightly. Cut each potato in half lengthwise and scoop out most of the flesh, leaving a thin shell to hold the filling.

6. In a bowl, mash the potato flesh with a fork or potato masher. Stir in the ginger-turmeric mixture until well combined.

7. Spoon the filling back into the potato shells, and place them back on the baking sheet. Return the stuffed potatoes to the oven and bake for an additional 10-15 minutes, or until heated through.

8. Remove the stuffed potatoes from the oven and let them cool slightly. Top each potato with a dollop of Greek yogurt or sour cream and a sprinkle of fresh cilantro or parsley leaves.

9. Serve the Ginger and Turmeric Stuffed Potatoes

Chicken and Green Pea Curry

Ingredients:

- 1 1/2 pounds (680g) boneless, skinless chicken breasts or thighs, cut into bite-sized pieces
- 1 tablespoon (15ml) vegetable oil
- 1 large onion, finely chopped
- 3 cloves garlic, minced
- 1 tablespoon (15g) fresh ginger, grated
- 2 teaspoons ground cumin
- 1 teaspoon ground coriander
- 1 teaspoon turmeric
- 1/2 teaspoon cayenne pepper (optional)
- 1 (14.5 oz/400g) can diced tomatoes
- 1 cup (240ml) chicken broth
- 1 cup (150g) frozen green peas
- 1/2 cup (120ml) coconut milk
- Salt and black pepper to taste
- Fresh cilantro leaves for garnish

Directions:

1. Heat the vegetable oil in a large, deep skillet or Dutch oven over medium heat (350°F/175°C). Add the chopped onion and sauté until softened and translucent, about 5 minutes.

2. Add the minced garlic, grated ginger, ground cumin, ground coriander, turmeric, and cayenne pepper (if using) to the skillet. Stir to combine and cook for another 1-2 minutes, until fragrant.

3. Add the chicken pieces to the skillet and cook until browned on all sides, about 5-7 minutes.

4. Pour in the diced tomatoes and chicken broth, and bring the mixture to a simmer. Reduce the heat to low 250°F (120°C), cover the skillet, and let the curry simmer for 15-20 minutes, or until the chicken is cooked through.

5. Stir in the frozen green peas and coconut milk, and continue to simmer for another 5 minutes, or until the peas are heated through and the curry has thickened slightly.

6. Season the curry with salt and black pepper to taste.

7. Remove the skillet from heat and let the curry cool slightly. Garnish with fresh cilantro leaves.

8. Serve the Chicken and Green Pea Curry hot with rice or naan bread.

Inflammation Management

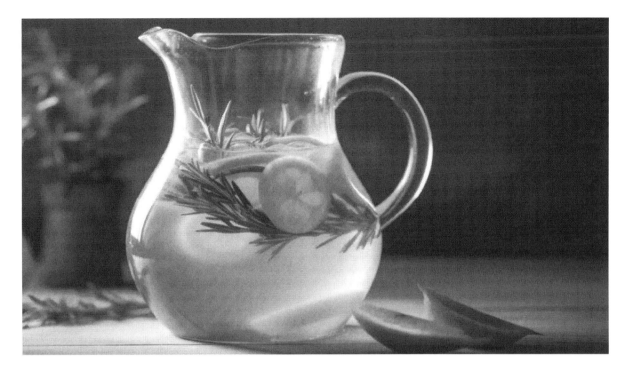

"Health is a state of complete harmony of the body, mind, and spirit." –B.K.S. Iyengar

Inflammation is a natural response of the body's immune system to injury, infection, or irritation. However, when inflammation becomes chronic, it can contribute to a wide range of health problems, from heart disease and cancer to autoimmune disorders and chronic pain. By adopting an anti-inflammatory lifestyle and incorporating powerful herbs and nutrient-rich foods into our diets, we can help to reduce systemic inflammation, alleviate symptoms, and promote overall well-being.

Topical Treatments

Cucumber and Aloe Topical Gel

Ingredients:

- 1/2 cup fresh cucumber juice
- 1/4 cup pure aloe vera gel
- 1 tablespoon vegetable glycerin
- 1 teaspoon witch hazel
- 5 drops lavender essential oil

Directions:

1. In a blender or food processor, puree fresh cucumber chunks until smooth.
2. Strain the puree through a fine-mesh sieve or cheesecloth to extract the juice.
3. In a small bowl, combine the cucumber juice, aloe vera gel, vegetable glycerin, witch hazel, and lavender essential oil.
4. Whisk until well combined.
5. Pour the mixture into a clean, airtight glass jar or bottle.
6. Store the gel in the refrigerator for up to 2 weeks.
7. To use, apply a small amount of the gel to clean, dry skin and gently massage until absorbed.
8. Use daily, or as needed, to help soothe inflammation, hydrate the skin, and promote a healthy, glowing complexion.

Basil and Rosemary Anti-Inflammatory Paste

Ingredients:

- 1/2 cup fresh basil leaves, finely chopped
- 1/4 cup fresh rosemary leaves, finely chopped
- 1/2 cup extra-virgin olive oil

- 2 tablespoons beeswax pastilles
- 10 drops peppermint essential oil
- 5 drops eucalyptus essential oil

Directions:

- In a small saucepan, combine the finely chopped basil leaves, rosemary leaves, and olive oil.
- Heat the mixture over low heat, stirring occasionally, for 20-30 minutes to infuse the oil with the herbs.
- Strain the infused oil through a fine-mesh sieve or cheesecloth into a clean, heat-resistant bowl. Press on the herbs to extract as much oil as possible.
- Return the infused oil to the saucepan and add the beeswax pastilles. Heat over low heat, stirring constantly, until the beeswax is fully melted and combined with the oil.

- Remove the saucepan from heat and let the mixture cool for 2-3 minutes. Stir in the peppermint and eucalyptus essential oils.
- Pour the mixture into a clean, airtight glass jar or tin. Allow the paste to cool completely and solidify at room temperature.
- To use, apply a small amount of the paste to the affected area and gently massage until absorbed. Use as needed to help reduce inflammation, alleviate pain, and promote healing.

Herbal Brews and Drinks

Anti-Inflammatory Bone Broth Shot

Ingredients:

- 1/2 cup high-quality, organic bone broth
- 1/2 teaspoon ground turmeric
- 1/4 teaspoon ground ginger

- 1/8 teaspoon black pepper
- 1/2 lemon, juiced
- Pinch of sea salt

Directions:

1. In a small saucepan, heat the bone broth over medium heat until steaming.
2. Whisk in the ground turmeric, ginger, and black pepper. Simmer for 1-2 minutes to allow the flavors to meld.
3. Remove the saucepan from heat and stir in the lemon juice and sea salt.

4. Pour the mixture into a small, heat-resistant glass or mug.
5. Allow the health shot to cool slightly before consuming.
6. Drink this anti-inflammatory bone broth health shot daily, preferably on an empty stomach.

Celery Shots

Ingredients:

- 1 bunch organic celery, washed and chopped
- 1 lemon, peeled

- 1-inch piece of fresh ginger, peeled
- Pinch of cayenne pepper (optional)

Directions:

1. In a high-speed blender or juicer, combine the chopped celery, peeled lemon, and peeled ginger. If using a blender, add a small amount of water to help with blending.
2. Blend or juice the ingredients until smooth and well combined.
3. If using a blender, strain the mixture through a fine-mesh sieve or

cheesecloth to remove the pulp.

4. Pour the celery juice into small, shot-sized glasses. If desired, add a pinch of cayenne pepper to each shot for an extra kick and metabolism boost.

Baking Soda and Water Sip

Ingredients:

- 1/2 teaspoon baking soda
- 1 cup (240ml) water (room temperature or slightly warm)

- 1/2 tablespoon (7.5ml) fresh lemon juice (optional)
- 1/2 tablespoon (7.5ml) honey or maple syrup (optional)

Directions:

1. In a glass or mug, combine the baking soda and water. Stir well until the baking soda is completely dissolved.

2. If desired, add fresh lemon juice and/or honey or maple syrup to taste. Stir to combine.

3. Sip the mixture slowly, allowing it to coat your digestive tract.

Notes:

- It is recommended to drink this mixture on an empty stomach, preferably in the morning or at least 2 hours after a meal.
- Some people may experience a slightly salty or soapy taste due to the baking soda. The addition of lemon juice, honey, or maple syrup can help improve the taste.
- If you are on a low-sodium diet or have high blood pressure, consult your doctor before consuming baking soda regularly.
- Baking soda can help neutralize stomach acid and may provide relief from indigestion, heartburn, or upset stomach. However, if you experience persistent or severe symptoms, consult a healthcare professional.
- Do not consume baking soda if you are pregnant, nursing, or have a history of heart or kidney problems without consulting your doctor first.

Parsley Shots

Ingredients:

- 1 cup (240ml) water
- 1 bunch fresh parsley, washed and roughly chopped (about 2 cups or 60g)
- 1/2 lemon, juiced (about 1 1/2 tablespoons or 22ml)
- 1/2 inch (1.25cm) piece of fresh ginger, peeled and grated (optional)
- 1/2 green apple, chopped (optional)
- 1/2 tablespoon (7.5ml) honey or maple syrup (optional)

Directions:

1. In a blender, combine the water, chopped parsley, lemon juice, ginger (if using), and green apple (if using). Blend on high speed until smooth, about 30-60 seconds.
2. If desired, add honey or maple syrup to taste and blend again briefly to combine.
3. Place a fine-mesh strainer over a bowl and pour the blended mixture through the strainer to remove any pulp or parsley bits.
4. Pour the strained liquid into shot glasses or small cups.
5. Serve the parsley shots immediately for the best flavor and nutritional benefits.

Turmeric Lemonade

Ingredients:

- 4 cups (960ml) water, divided
- 1/4 cup (60ml) freshly squeezed lemon juice (about 2 lemons)
- 1/4 cup (60ml) honey or maple syrup, or to taste
- 1 teaspoon ground turmeric
- 1/4 teaspoon ground black pepper (optional)
- 1/4 teaspoon ground ginger (optional)
- Lemon slices and fresh mint leaves for garnish (optional)

Directions:

- In a small saucepan, combine 1 cup (240ml) of water with the honey or maple syrup. Heat over medium heat 350°F (175°C, stirring occasionally, until the honey or maple syrup has dissolved completely.
- Remove from heat.
- Add the ground turmeric, black pepper (if using), and ginger (if using) to the warm honey mixture.
- Whisk until the spices are well combined and no lumps remain.
- Pour the turmeric mixture into a large pitcher, along with the freshly squeezed lemon juice and the remaining 3 cups (720ml) of water. Stir well to combine.
- Taste the lemonade and adjust the sweetness by adding more honey or maple syrup if desired.
- Refrigerate the turmeric lemonade for at least 30 minutes to chill and allow the flavors to meld.

Inflammation Management Recipes

Orange and Beet Salad

Ingredients:

- 4 medium beets, cooked, peeled, and diced (about 2 cups or 400g)
- 3 medium oranges, peeled and segmented (about 1 1/2 cups or 300g)
- 1/2 small red onion, thinly sliced
- 1/4 cup (60ml) extra-virgin olive oil
- 2 tablespoons (30ml) freshly squeezed lemon juice
- 1 tablespoon (15ml) honey or maple syrup
- 1/2 teaspoon Dijon mustard
- Salt and black pepper to taste
- 1/4 cup (40g) crumbled feta cheese (optional)
- 1/4 cup (40g) chopped walnuts, toasted (optional)
- Fresh mint leaves for garnish (optional)

Directions:

1. In a large bowl, combine the diced beets, orange segments, and thinly sliced red onion.

2. In a small bowl, whisk together the extra-virgin olive oil, lemon juice, honey or maple syrup, Dijon mustard, salt, and black pepper until well combined.

3. Pour the dressing over the beet and orange mixture, and toss gently to coat evenly.

4. If desired, top the salad with crumbled feta cheese and toasted chopped walnuts.

5. Garnish with fresh mint leaves, if using.

6. Serve the Orange and Beet Salad chilled or at room temperature.

Arugula Pesto Pasta

Ingredients:

- 8 ounces (225g) pasta (e.g., spaghetti, linguine, or fusilli)
- 2 cups (60g) fresh arugula, packed
- 1/2 cup (50g) grated Parmesan cheese
- 1/3 cup (40g) toasted pine nuts or walnuts
- 2 cloves garlic, minced
- 1/2 cup (120ml) extra-virgin olive oil
- Salt and black pepper to taste
- 1/4 cup (60ml) reserved pasta cooking water
- Cherry tomatoes, halved, for garnish (optional)
- Additional grated Parmesan cheese for serving (optional)

Directions:

1. Cook the pasta in a large pot of salted boiling water according to package Directions until al dente.

2. Before draining the pasta, reserve 1/4 cup (60ml) of the pasta cooking water.

3. While the pasta is cooking, prepare the pesto. In a food processor or blender, combine the arugula, Parmesan cheese, pine nuts or walnuts, minced garlic, salt, and black pepper. Pulse a few times to roughly chop the ingredients.

4. With the food processor or blender running, slowly pour in the extra-virgin olive oil through the feed tube.

5. Process until the pesto is smooth and well combined, scraping down the sides as needed.

6. Taste the pesto and adjust the seasoning with salt and black pepper if desired.

7. Drain the cooked pasta, reserving the 1/4 cup (60ml) of pasta cooking water.

8. In a large bowl or the pasta cooking pot, combine the drained pasta and the arugula pesto.

9. Toss well to coat the pasta evenly, adding some of the reserved pasta cooking water if needed to thin the pesto and help it adhere to the pasta.

10. If desired, garnish the pasta with halved cherry tomatoes and serve with additional grated Parmesan cheese on the side.

Kale and Sweet Potato Hash Browns

Ingredients:

- 2 medium sweet potatoes, peeled and grated (about 4 cups or 500g)
- 2 cups (70g) kale, stemmed and finely chopped
- 1 small onion, finely diced
- 2 cloves garlic, minced
- 2 large eggs, lightly beaten
- 1/3 cup (50g) all-purpose flour or gluten-free flour
- 1 teaspoon salt
- 1/2 teaspoon black pepper
- 1/4 teaspoon smoked paprika (optional)
- 2 tablespoons (30ml) vegetable oil, divided
- Sour cream or Greek yogurt for serving (optional)
- Hot sauce for serving (optional)

Directions:

1. In a large bowl, combine the grated sweet potatoes, chopped kale, diced onion, minced garlic, beaten eggs, flour, salt, black pepper, and smoked paprika (if using). Mix well to combine.

2. Heat 1 tablespoon (15ml) of vegetable oil in a large skillet.

3. Scoop about 1/4 cup (60ml) of the sweet potato mixture into the skillet for each hash brown.

4. Flatten the mixture slightly with a spatula to form a patty. Cook the hash browns in batches, making sure not to overcrowd the skillet.

5. Cook the hash browns for about 3-4 minutes on each side, or until they are golden brown and crispy.

6. Add more oil to the skillet as needed between batches.

7. Transfer the cooked hash browns to a plate lined with paper towels to absorb any excess oil.

8. Serve the Kale and Sweet Potato Hash Browns hot.

Pineapple and Cherry Smoothie

Ingredients:

- 2 cups (300g) frozen pineapple chunks
- 1 cup (150g) frozen pitted cherries
- 1 ripe banana, peeled and sliced
- 1 cup (240ml) unsweetened almond milk or coconut milk

- 1/2 cup (120ml) plain Greek yogurt or coconut yogurt
- 1 tablespoon (15ml) honey or maple syrup (optional)
- 1/2 teaspoon vanilla extract (optional)

- 1/2 cup (120ml) ice cubes (optional, for a thicker smoothie)
- Fresh mint leaves or pineapple wedges for garnish (optional)

Directions:

1. In a blender, combine the frozen pineapple chunks, frozen pitted cherries, sliced banana, almond milk or coconut milk, Greek yogurt or coconut yogurt, honey or maple syrup (if using), and vanilla extract (if using).

2. If you prefer a thicker smoothie, add the ice cubes to the blender.

3. Blend the ingredients on high speed for 1-2 minutes, or until the mixture is smooth and creamy.

4. If needed, stop the blender and scrape down the sides with a spatula to ensure all ingredients are well combined.

5. Taste the smoothie and adjust the sweetness by adding more honey or maple syrup if desired.

6. Pour the smoothie into glasses and garnish with fresh mint leaves or pineapple wedges, if desired.

Ginger Baked Pears

Ingredients:

- 4 firm, ripe pears (such as Bosc or Anjou)
- 1/4 cup (60ml) honey
- 1/4 cup (60ml) fresh lemon juice
- 1 tablespoon (15g) grated fresh ginger
- 1 teaspoon ground cinnamon

- 1/4 teaspoon ground nutmeg
- 1/4 teaspoon salt
- 2 tablespoons (30g) unsalted butter, cut into small pieces
- 1/4 cup (60ml) water

Directions:

1. Preheat the oven to 375°F (190°C).

2. Peel the pears, cut them in half lengthwise, and remove the cores with a spoon or melon baller.

3. In a small bowl, whisk together the honey, lemon juice, grated ginger, cinnamon, nutmeg, and salt.

4. Arrange the pear halves cut-side up in a baking dish. Drizzle the honey-ginger mixture evenly over the pears, making sure it fills the hollow cores.

5. Dot the top of each pear half with a small piece of butter.

6. Pour the water into the bottom of the baking dish around the pears.

7. Bake the pears in the preheated oven for 30-40 minutes, basting them with the pan juices every 10-15 minutes, until they are tender when pierced with a fork and lightly caramelized on top.

8. Remove the baking dish from the oven and let the pears cool slightly before serving.

Joint and Muscle Recovery

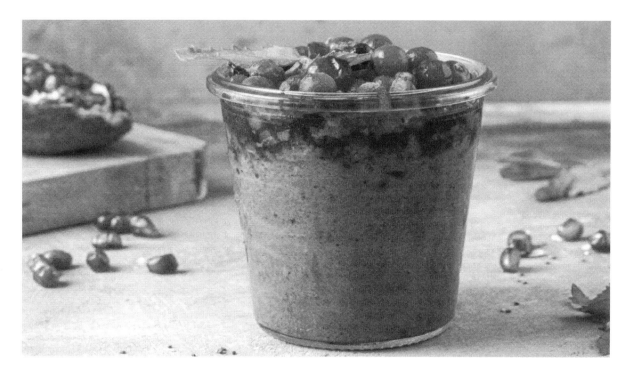

"It is health that is real wealth and not pieces of gold and silver." –Mahatma Gandhi

Joint and muscle pain can be debilitating, affecting our quality of life and ability to perform daily tasks. Whether caused by injury, overuse, or chronic conditions like arthritis, finding natural ways to support joint and muscle recovery is essential for maintaining mobility, flexibility, and overall well-being. Incorporating targeted herbs, nutrient-dense foods, and soothing remedies into our self-care routines helps to reduce inflammation, alleviate pain, and promote healing.

Topical Treatments

Mint and Rosemary Joint Rub

Ingredients:

- 1/2 cup (120ml) coconut oil, softened
- 1/4 cup (60ml) beeswax pellets
- 1/4 cup (60ml) shea butter
- 1 tablespoon (15ml) peppermint essential oil
- 1 tablespoon (15ml) rosemary essential oil
- 1 teaspoon vitamin E oil (optional, as a preservative)

Directions:

1. Create a double boiler by placing a heat-safe glass bowl on top of a pot filled with a few inches of water. Ensure the bottom of the bowl does not touch the water.

2. Heat the water in the pot over medium heat.

3. Add the coconut oil, beeswax pellets, and shea butter to the glass bowl. Stir occasionally until fully melted and combined.

4. Remove the bowl from the heat and let it cool slightly for 2-3 minutes.

5. Stir in the peppermint essential oil, rosemary essential oil, and vitamin E oil (if using).

6. Pour the mixture into a clean glass jar or tin and allow it to cool completely before sealing with a lid.

7. Apply as needed to sore joints and muscles, massaging gently into the skin.

Lavender Bath Soak

Ingredients:

- 1 cup (240g) Epsom salts
- 1/2 cup (120g) sea salt or Himalayan pink salt
- 1/2 cup (120g) baking soda
- 1/4 cup (60g) dried lavender buds
- 15-20 drops lavender essential oil

Directions:

1. In a large bowl, mix together the Epsom salts, sea salt or Himalayan pink salt, and baking soda.
2. Add the dried lavender buds and lavender essential oil to the salt mixture. Stir well to distribute the lavender evenly.
3. Transfer the mixture to an airtight glass jar or container.
4. To use, add 1/2 to 1 cup (120-240g) of the Lavender Bath Soak to warm running bath water. Soak in the bath for 20-30 minutes to relax and soothe the body.

Arnica Balm

Ingredients:

- 1/2 cup (120ml) olive oil or sweet almond oil
- 1/4 cup (60ml) beeswax pellets
- 1/4 cup (60ml) shea butter or cocoa butter
- 2 tablespoons (30ml) arnica-infused oil
- 1 teaspoon vitamin E oil (optional, as a preservative)

Directions:

1. Create a double boiler by placing a heat-safe glass bowl on top of a pot filled with a few inches of water. Ensure the bottom of the bowl does not touch the water.
2. Heat the water in the pot over medium heat.
3. Add the olive oil or sweet almond oil, beeswax pellets, and shea butter or cocoa butter to the glass bowl. Stir occasionally until fully melted and combined.
4. Remove the bowl from the heat and let it cool slightly for 2-3 minutes.
5. Stir in the arnica-infused oil and vitamin E oil (if using).
6. Pour the mixture into a clean glass jar or tin and allow it to cool completely before sealing with a lid.
7. Store the Arnica Balm in a cool, dry place.

Herbal Brews and Teas

Willow Bark and Chamomile Tea

Ingredients:

- 2 teaspoons (10g) dried willow bark
- 2 teaspoons (10g) dried chamomile flowers
- 2 cups (480ml) water
- Honey or lemon (optional, to taste)

Directions:

1. In a small saucepan, bring the water to a boil.
2. Remove the saucepan from heat and add the dried willow bark and chamomile flowers.
3. Cover the saucepan and let the herbs steep for 10-15 minutes.
4. Strain the tea into a mug or teapot, discarding the herbs.
5. Add honey or lemon to taste, if desired.
6. Drink the Willow Bark and Chamomile Tea while it's warm, up to 3 times daily.

Soothing Osteoarthritis Tea

Ingredients:

- 1 teaspoon (5g) dried ginger root
- 1 teaspoon (5g) dried turmeric root
- 1 teaspoon (5g) dried rosehips
- 1 cinnamon stick
- 2 cups (480ml) water
- Honey (optional, to taste)

Directions:

1. In a small saucepan, bring the water to a boil.
2. Remove the saucepan from heat and add the dried ginger root, turmeric root, rosehips, and cinnamon stick.
3. Cover the saucepan and let the herbs steep for 10-15 minutes.
4. Strain the tea into a mug or teapot, discarding the herbs and cinnamon stick.
5. Add honey to taste, if desired.
6. Drink the Soothing Osteoarthritis Tea while it's warm, up to 2-3 times daily.

Amish Meadow Tea

Ingredients:

- 1 tablespoon (15g) dried red clover blossoms
- 1 tablespoon (15g) dried chamomile flowers
- 1 tablespoon (15g) dried lemongrass
- 1 tablespoon (15g) dried peppermint leaves
- 4 cups (960ml) water
- Honey (optional, to taste)

Directions:

1. In a large saucepan or teapot, bring the water to a boil.
2. Remove the saucepan from heat and add the dried red clover blossoms, chamomile flowers, lemongrass, and peppermint leaves.
3. Cover the saucepan or teapot and let the herbs steep for 5-7 minutes.
4. Strain the tea into mugs or a serving teapot, discarding the herbs.
5. Add honey to taste, if desired.

Green Tea and Cherry Shots

Ingredients:

- 1 cup (240ml) strong brewed green tea, cooled
- 1/2 cup (120ml) cherry juice (fresh or bottled)
- 1 tablespoon (15ml) honey or agave syrup (optional, to taste)
- Ice cubes
- Fresh cherries for garnish (optional)

Directions:

1. In a small pitcher or bowl, whisk together the cooled green tea, cherry juice, and honey or agave syrup (if using) until well combined.
2. Fill shot glasses or small serving cups with ice cubes.
3. Pour the green tea and cherry mixture over the ice, filling each glass or cup.
4. Garnish each shot with a fresh cherry, if desired.

Hibiscus Cherry Tea

Ingredients:

- 2 tablespoons (30g) dried hibiscus flowers
- 1/2 cup (120g) fresh or frozen pitted cherries
- 4 cups (960ml) water
- Honey or agave syrup (optional, to taste)
- Ice cubes (for iced tea)

Directions:

1. In a large saucepan or teapot, bring the water to a boil.
2. Remove the saucepan from heat and add the dried hibiscus flowers and pitted cherries.
3. Cover the saucepan or teapot and let the mixture steep for 10-15 minutes.
4. Strain the tea into mugs or a serving pitcher, discarding the hibiscus flowers and cherries.
5. Add honey or agave syrup to taste, if desired.
6. Serve the Hibiscus Cherry Tea hot, or pour it over ice for a refreshing iced tea.

Joint and Muscle Recovery Recipes

Tart Cherry Smoothie

Ingredients:

- 1 cup (140g) frozen tart cherries
- 1 ripe banana, peeled and sliced
- 1 cup (240ml) unsweetened almond milk or coconut milk
- 1/2 cup (120g) plain Greek yogurt or coconut yogurt
- 1 tablespoon (15g) chia seeds
- 1 tablespoon (15ml) honey or maple syrup (optional, to taste)
- 1/2 teaspoon vanilla extract (optional)

Directions:

1. In a blender, combine the frozen tart cherries, sliced banana, almond milk or coconut milk, Greek yogurt or coconut yogurt, chia seeds, honey or maple syrup (if using), and vanilla extract (if using).
2. Blend the ingredients on high speed for 1-2 minutes, or until the mixture is smooth and creamy.
3. Taste the smoothie and adjust the sweetness by adding more honey or maple syrup if desired.

4. Pour the Tart Cherry Smoothie into glasses and serve immediately.

Tahini and Banana Smoothie

Ingredients:

- 2 ripe bananas, peeled and sliced
- 2 tablespoons (30g) tahini
- 1 cup (240ml) unsweetened almond milk or oat milk
- 1/2 cup (120ml) cold brewed coffee or regular coffee, cooled (op-
- tional)
- 1 tablespoon (15ml) honey or maple syrup (optional, to taste)
- 1/2 teaspoon ground cinnamon
- 1/2 cup (120ml) ice cubes

Directions:

1. In a blender, combine the sliced bananas, tahini, almond milk or oat milk, cold brewed coffee or cooled regular coffee (if using), honey or maple syrup (if using), ground cinnamon, and ice cubes.
2. Blend the ingredients on high speed for 1-2 minutes, or until the mixture is smooth and creamy.
3. Taste the smoothie and adjust the sweetness by adding more honey or maple syrup if desired.
4. Pour the Tahini and Banana Smoothie into glasses and serve immediately.

Ginger Chicken Meatballs

Ingredients:

- 1 pound (450g) ground chicken
- 1/2 cup (50g) breadcrumbs
- 1/4 cup (60ml) milk
- 1/4 cup (60g) finely chopped onion
- 2 cloves garlic, minced
- 1 tablespoon (15g) grated fresh ginger
- 1 large egg
- 1 teaspoon salt
- 1/4 teaspoon black pepper
- 2 tablespoons (30ml) vegetable oil

Directions:

1. In a large bowl, combine the breadcrumbs and milk. Let the mixture sit for 5 minutes to allow the breadcrumbs to absorb the milk.
2. Add the ground chicken, chopped onion, minced garlic, grated ginger, egg, salt, and black pepper to the bowl. Mix well until all ingredients are evenly combined.
3. Shape the mixture into meatballs, about 1 1/2 inches (4cm) in diameter.
4. Heat the vegetable oil in a large skillet over medium heat. Add the meatballs and cook for 6-8 minutes, turning them occasionally, until they are browned on all sides and cooked through.
5. Serve the Ginger Chicken Meatballs hot

Baked Salmon in Lemon Sauce

Ingredients:

- 4 salmon filets (about 6 ounces/170g each)
- Salt and black pepper to taste
- 1/4 cup (60ml) butter, melted
- 1/4 cup (60ml) freshly squeezed lemon juice
- 2 cloves garlic, minced
- 1 tablespoon (15ml) honey
- 1 teaspoon dried dill (or 1 tablespoon fresh dill, chopped)

Directions:

1. Preheat the oven to 400°F (200°C.
2. Season the salmon filets with salt and black pepper on both sides.
3. In a small bowl, whisk together the melted butter, lemon juice, minced garlic, honey, and dill.
4. Place the salmon filets in a baking dish, skin-side down (if applicable). Pour the lemon sauce over the salmon, ensuring each filet is well coated.
5. Bake the salmon for 12-15 minutes, or until it is cooked through and easily flakes with a fork.
6. Serve the Baked Salmon in Lemon Sauce hot.

Roasted Veggie and Egg Salad

Ingredients:

- 2 cups (300g) diced mixed vegetables (e.g., zucchini, bell peppers, red onion, cherry tomatoes)
- 1 tablespoon (15ml) olive oil
- Salt and black pepper to taste
- 4 large eggs, hard-boiled and chopped
- 2 cups (60g) mixed salad greens
- 1/4 cup (60g) crumbled feta cheese
- 1/4 cup (40g) chopped toasted walnuts
- Balsamic vinaigrette, to taste

Directions:

1. Preheat the oven to 425°F (220°C).

2. In a large bowl, toss the diced vegetables with olive oil, salt, and black pepper until evenly coated.

3. Spread the vegetables on a baking sheet lined with parchment paper. Roast for 20-25 minutes, or until the vegetables are tender and lightly caramelized, stirring halfway through.

4. In a large serving bowl, combine the mixed salad greens, chopped hard-boiled eggs, roasted vegetables, crumbled feta cheese, and chopped toasted walnuts.

5. Drizzle the salad with balsamic vinaigrette to taste, and toss gently to combine.

6. Serve the Roasted Veggie and Egg Salad immediately.

Protein-Packed Muesli

Ingredients:

- 2 cups (200g) old-fashioned rolled oats
- 1/2 cup (60g) chopped raw almonds
- 1/2 cup (60g) chopped raw walnuts
- 1/4 cup (40g) raw pumpkin seeds
- 1/4 cup (40g) raw sunflower seeds
- 1/4 cup (30g) ground flaxseed
- 1/4 cup (30g) vanilla protein powder (plant-based or whey)
- 1 teaspoon ground cinnamon
- 1/2 cup (80g) dried fruit (e.g., raisins, cranberries, chopped apricots)
- Milk, yogurt, or plant-based milk for serving

Directions:

1. In a large bowl, combine the rolled oats, chopped almonds, chopped walnuts, pumpkin seeds, sunflower seeds, ground flaxseed, vanilla protein powder, and ground cinnamon. Mix well to distribute the ingredients evenly.

2. Stir in the dried fruit until well combined.

3. Transfer the mixture to an airtight container or jar. Store in a cool, dry place for up to 2 weeks.

Kidney Health

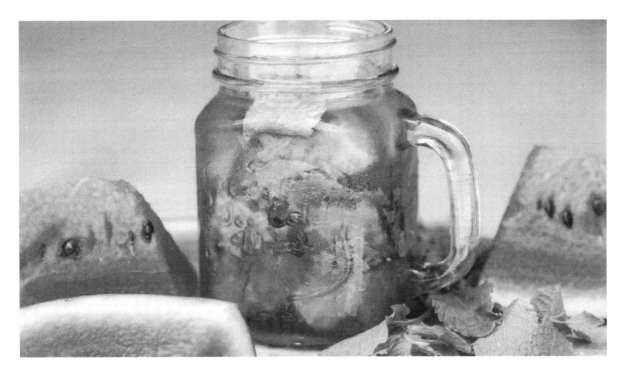

"The natural healing force within each one of us is the greatest force in getting well." –Hippocrates

Our kidneys play a vital role in maintaining overall health and well-being, filtering waste products from the blood, regulating blood pressure, and balancing essential nutrients and electrolytes. When our kidney function is compromised, it can lead to a range of health issues, from fatigue and swelling to more serious conditions like kidney disease. Supporting our kidney health with nourishing herbs, nutrient-rich foods, and cleansing remedies promotes optimal kidney function, reduces the risk of kidney problems, and maintains overall vitality.

Topical Treatments

Kidney Gel Caps

Ingredients:

- 1/2 cup (70g) cranberry extract powder
- 1/4 cup (30g) dried nettle leaf powder
- 1/4 cup (30g) dried dandelion leaf powder
- 1/4 cup (30g) dried parsley leaf powder
- 1/4 cup (40g) d-mannose powder
- 1/4 cup (30g) corn silk powder
- Empty vegetable gel capsules (size 00)

Directions:

1. In a large bowl, combine the cranberry extract powder, dried nettle leaf powder, dried dandelion leaf powder, dried parsley leaf powder, d-mannose powder, and corn silk powder. Mix well using a whisk or fork to ensure all ingredients are evenly distributed.

2. Set up a clean, dry work surface with the empty gel capsules and the powder mixture.

3. Fill each gel capsule with the powder mixture. You can do this by hand or use a capsule filling machine for more efficiency: a.

If filling by hand, separate the two halves of the capsule and carefully spoon the powder into the larger half. Pack the powder down gently, then replace the smaller half of the capsule and press together until it snaps shut. b. If using a capsule filling machine, follow the manufacturer's Directions for filling the capsules.

4. Store the filled capsules in an airtight container in a cool, dry place. They should remain potent for up to 6 months.

Suggested use: Take 2-3 capsules daily with water, preferably with meals.

Herbal Brews and Drinks

Cranberry Health Shot

Ingredients:

- 1 cup (240ml) unsweetened cranberry juice
- 1/4 cup (60ml) freshly squeezed lemon juice
- 1/4 cup (60ml) unsweetened apple juice
- 1-2 tablespoons (15-30ml) honey or maple syrup (optional)

Directions:

1. In a pitcher, whisk together the cranberry juice, lemon juice, apple juice, and honey or maple syrup (if using) until well combined.
2. Pour the mixture into small shot glasses or serving cups.
3. Serve the Cranberry Health Shots chilled, and consume immediately.

Watermelon Water

Ingredients:

- 4 cups (600g) diced seedless watermelon
- 1 cup (240ml) water
- 1/4 cup (60ml) freshly squeezed lime juice
- Fresh mint leaves for garnish (optional)

Directions:

1. In a blender, combine the diced watermelon, water, and lime juice. Blend until smooth.
2. Pour the mixture through a fine-mesh strainer into a pitcher to remove any pulp.
3. Chill the Watermelon Water in the refrigerator for at least 30 minutes.
4. Serve over ice, garnished with fresh mint leaves if desired.

Barley and Parsley Tea

Ingredients:

- 1/4 cup (50g) barley grains
- 1/4 cup (15g) fresh parsley, chopped
- 4 cups (960ml) water
- Honey or lemon (optional, to taste)

Directions:

1. In a large saucepan, combine the barley grains and water. Bring the mixture to a boil over high heat.
2. Reduce the heat to low and simmer for 30 minutes.
3. Add the chopped parsley to the saucepan and simmer for an additional 5 minutes.
4. Strain the tea through a fine-mesh strainer into a teapot or serving cups.
5. Add honey or lemon to taste, if desired. Serve the Barley and Parsley Tea hot.

Dandelion Root Kidney Tea

Ingredients:

- 2 tablespoons (20g) dried dandelion root
- 2 tablespoons (20g) dried nettle leaf
- 4 cups (960ml) water
- Honey or lemon (optional, to taste)

Directions:

1. In a large saucepan, bring the water to a boil over high heat.
2. Remove the saucepan from heat and add the dried dandelion root and nettle leaf.
3. Cover the saucepan and let the herbs steep for 10-15 minutes.
4. Strain the tea through a fine-mesh strainer into a teapot o serving cups.
5. Add honey or lemon to taste, if desired. Serve the Dandelion Root Kidney Tea hot or chilled.

Kidney Health Recipes

Cranberry and Ginger Chutney

Ingredients:

- 2 cups (200g) fresh or frozen cranberries
- 1/2 cup (100g) granulated sugar
- 1/4 cup (60ml) apple cider vinegar
- 1/4 cup (60ml) water
- 1 tablespoon (15g) grated fresh ginger
- 1/4 teaspoon ground cinnamon
- Pinch of salt

Directions:

1. In a medium saucepan, combine the cranberries, sugar, apple cider vinegar, water, grated ginger, cinnamon, and salt.
2. Bring the mixture to a boil over medium-high heat, stirring occasionally.
3. Reduce the heat to low and simmer for 15-20 minutes, or until the cranberries have burst and the chutney has thickened.
4. Remove from heat and let the chutney cool to room temperature.

Lemon Curry Chicken Salad

Ingredients:

- 2 cups (300g) cooked, diced chicken breast
- 1/2 cup (120g) plain Greek yogurt
- 1/4 cup (60g) mayonnaise
- 1 tablespoon (15ml) freshly squeezed lemon juice
- 1 teaspoon curry powder
- 1/4 teaspoon salt
- 1/4 teaspoon black pepper
- 1/4 cup (40g) diced red onion
- 1/4 cup (40g) diced celery
- 1/4 cup (40g) dried cranberries
- Lettuce leaves for serving

Directions:

1. In a large bowl, whisk together the Greek yogurt, mayonnaise, lemon juice, curry powder, salt, and black pepper until smooth.
2. Add the diced chicken, red onion, celery, and dried cranberries to the bowl. Mix well to coat the chicken and vegetables with the dressing.
3. Serve the Lemon Curry Chicken Salad on a bed of lettuce leaves or as a sandwich filling.

Roasted Asparagus Stew

Ingredients:

- 1 pound (450g) asparagus, trimmed and cut into 2-inch (5cm) pieces
- 1 tablespoon (15ml) olive oil
- Salt and black pepper to taste
- 1 onion, diced
- 2 cloves garlic, minced
- 1 teaspoon dried thyme
- 2 cups (480ml) vegetable broth
- 1 cup (240ml) canned diced tomatoes
- 1 (15-ounce/425g) can cannellini beans, drained and rinsed
- 1/4 cup (60ml) heavy cream

Directions:

1. Preheat the oven to 425°F (220°C).
2. On a baking sheet, toss the asparagus pieces with olive oil, salt, and black pepper. Roast for 10-12 minutes, or until tender and lightly caramelized.
3. In a large pot or Dutch oven, heat 1 tablespoon (15ml) of olive oil over medium heat. Add the diced onion and cook until softened, about 5 minutes.
4. Add the minced garlic and thyme to the pot. Cook for an additional 1-2 minutes, until fragrant.
5. Pour in the vegetable broth and diced tomatoes. Bring the mixture to a simmer and cook for 10 minutes.
6. Add the roasted asparagus, cannellini beans, and heavy cream to the pot. Stir to combine and cook for an additional 5 minutes, or until heated through.
7. Season the Roasted Asparagus Stew with salt and black pepper to taste. Serve hot.

Pineapple and Cranberry Sorbet

Ingredients:

- 3 cups (450g) frozen pineapple chunks
- 1 cup (100g) frozen cranberries
- 1/2 cup (120ml) simple syrup (or to taste)
- 1 tablespoon (15ml) freshly squeezed lime juice

Directions:

1. In a food processor or high-speed blender, combine the frozen pineapple chunks, frozen cranberries, simple syrup, and lime juice.

2. Blend the mixture until smooth and creamy, scraping down the sides as needed.

3. Taste the sorbet and adjust the sweetness by adding more simple syrup if desired.

4. Transfer the sorbet to a freezer-safe container and freeze for at least 2 hours, or until firm.

5. Scoop the Pineapple and Cranberry Sorbet into serving dishes and enjoy as a refreshing dessert.

Kids Remedies

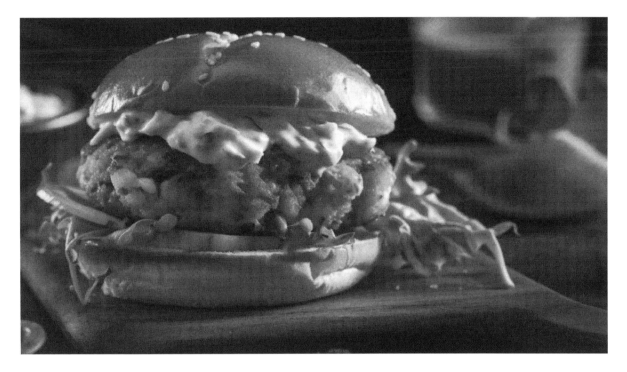

Children are the world's most valuable resource and its best hope for the future." –John F. Kennedy

Nurturing the health and well-being of our children is one of the most important responsibilities we have as parents and caregivers. From the food we provide to the habits we instill, every choice we make can have a lasting impact on their physical, mental, and emotional development. By incorporating kid-friendly, nutrient-dense recipes and natural remedies into their daily routines, we can help to support their growing bodies, boost their immune systems, and lay the foundation for a lifetime of healthy living.

Topical Treatments

Lavender Pillow Oil

Ingredients:

- 1/2 cup (120ml) carrier oil (e.g., sweet almond, jojoba, or fractionated coconut oil)
- 1/4 cup (10g) dried lavender buds
- 15-20 drops lavender essential oil

Directions:

1. In a small, clean jar, combine the carrier oil and dried lavender buds.

2. Seal the jar and place it in a sunny window for 1 to 2 weeks, shaking daily to infuse the oil with lavender.

3. After 1 to 2 weeks, strain the oil through a fine-mesh sieve or cheesecloth into a clean jar, discarding the lavender buds.

4. Add the lavender essential oil to the infused oil and shake well to combine.

5. To use, lightly mist a small amount of the Lavender Pillow Oil onto your pillow before bedtime to promote relaxation and restful sleep.

Honey and Ginger Cough Syrup

Ingredients:

- 1/2 cup (170g) raw honey
- 1/4 cup (60ml) water
- 1/4 cup (25g) grated fresh ginger
- 1/2 lemon, juiced

Directions:

1. In a small saucepan, combine the water and grated ginger. Bring the mixture to a boil, then reduce heat and simmer for 5 minutes.
2. Remove the saucepan from heat and let the ginger steep for 10 minutes.
3. Strain the ginger-infused water through a fine-mesh sieve into a clean jar, pressing on the ginger to extract as much liquid as possible.
4. Add the raw honey and lemon juice to the ginger-infused water. Stir until the honey is fully dissolved.
5. Store the Honey and Ginger Cough Syrup in the refrigerator for up to 2 weeks.
6. To use, take 1-2 tablespoons (15-30ml) as needed to soothe coughs and sore throats.

Calendula Gel

Ingredients:

- 1/4 cup (5g) dried calendula flowers
- 1/2 cup (120ml) boiling water
- 1 teaspoon vegetable glycerin
- 1/2 teaspoon xanthan gum

Directions:

1. Place the dried calendula flowers in a heat-safe bowl and pour the boiling water over them. Cover the bowl and let the flowers steep for 15-20 minutes.
2. Strain the calendula-infused water through a fine-mesh sieve into a clean bowl, pressing on the flowers to extract as much liquid as possible.
3. In a small bowl, whisk together the vegetable glycerin and xanthan gum until smooth.
4. Slowly pour the calendula-infused water into the glycerin mixture, whisking constantly to prevent lumps from forming.
5. Transfer the Calendula Gel to a clean jar or squeeze bottle and store it in the refrigerator for up to 2 weeks.
6. To use, apply the gel to minor cuts, scrapes, or skin irritations as needed.

Aloe Sunburn Gel

Ingredients:

- 1/2 cup (120ml) aloe vera gel (fresh or store-bought)
- 1/4 cup (60ml) witch hazel
- 10 drops peppermint essential oil
- 10 drops lavender essential oil

Directions:

1. In a small bowl, whisk together the aloe vera gel and witch hazel until smooth.
2. Add the peppermint and lavender essential oils, and whisk to combine.
3. Transfer the Aloe Sunburn Gel to a clean jar or squeeze bottle and store it in the refrigerator for up to 2 weeks.
4. To use, apply the gel to sunburned or irritated skin as needed to soothe and cool the skin.

Oatmeal Skin Mask

Ingredients:

- 1/2 cup (45g) colloidal oatmeal (or finely ground rolled oats)
- 1/4 cup (60ml) warm water
- 1 tablespoon (15ml) raw honey
- 1 tablespoon (15ml) plain yogurt

Directions:

- In a small bowl, mix together the colloidal oatmeal and warm water until a smooth paste forms.
- Add the raw honey and plain yogurt to the oatmeal mixture, and stir to combine.
- Apply the Oatmeal Skin Mask to clean, damp skin, avoiding the eye area.
- Leave the mask on for 10 to 15 minutes, then rinse off with lukewarm water and pat dry.
- Use the mask 1 to 2 times per week to soothe and nourish the skin.

Herbal Brews and Drinks

Allergy Nettle Tea

Ingredients:

- 2 tablespoons (10g) dried nettle leaves
- 1 tablespoon (5g) dried peppermint leaves
- 2 cups (480ml) boiling water
- Honey or lemon (optional, to taste)

Directions:

1. In a teapot or heatproof jar, combine the dried nettle leaves and dried peppermint leaves.
2. Pour the boiling water over the herbs and let the tea steep for 10-15 minutes.
3. Strain the tea through a fine-mesh sieve into cups or mugs.
4. Add honey or lemon to taste, if desired.
5. Drink the Allergy Nettle Tea hot, 1-2 cups per day during allergy season to help alleviate symptoms.

Apple and Carrot Juice

Ingredients:

- 2 medium apples, cored and cut into chunks
- 2 medium carrots, peeled and cut into chunks
- 1/2 inch (1.25cm) piece of fresh ginger (optional)
- Ice cubes (optional)

Directions:

1. In a juicer, process the apple chunks, carrot chunks, and ginger (if using).
2. If you don't have a juicer, blend the ingredients in a high-speed blender until smooth, then strain the mixture through a fine-mesh sieve or cheesecloth to separate the juice from the pulp.
3. Pour the juice over ice cubes, if desired.
4. Serve the Apple and Carrot Juice immediately for the best flavor and nutritional benefits.

Kid Friendly Camomile Tea

Ingredients:

- 2 tablespoons (10g) dried chamomile flowers
- 2 cups (480ml) boiling water
- 1-2 tablespoons (15 to 30ml) honey or agave syrup
- 1/2 cup (120ml) unsweetened apple juice (optional)

Directions:

1. In a teapot or heatproof jar, place the dried chamomile flowers.
2. Pour the boiling water over the flowers and let the tea steep for 5 to 7 minutes.
3. Strain the tea through a fine-mesh sieve into cups or mugs.
4. Stir in honey or agave syrup to taste, and add apple juice if desired for added sweetness and flavor.
5. Serve the Kid-Friendly Chamomile Tea warm or chilled, and enjoy as a soothing, caffeine-free beverage.

Peppermint Iced Tea

Ingredients:

- 4 cups (960ml) water
- 1/4 cup (15g) fresh peppermint leaves (or 2 tablespoons dried peppermint leaves)
- 2-3 tablespoons (30 to 45 ml) honey or agave syrup (optional, to taste)
- Ice cubes
- Fresh peppermint sprigs for garnish (optional)

Directions:

- In a saucepan, bring the water to a boil. Remove from heat and add the fresh or dried peppermint leaves.
- Cover the saucepan and let the tea steep for 5 to 7 minutes.
- Strain the tea through a fine-mesh sieve into a pitcher, discarding the peppermint leaves.
- Stir in honey or agave syrup to taste, if desired.
- Let the tea cool to room temperature, then refrigerate until chilled.
- Serve the Peppermint Iced Tea over ice cubes, garnished with fresh peppermint sprigs if desired.

Kid-Friendly Recipes

Super Veg Pasta

Ingredients:

- 8 oz / 225g whole wheat pasta
- 1 cup / 100g broccoli florets
- 1 cup / 100g sliced mushrooms
- 1 cup / 150g diced bell pepper
- 1 cup / 150g diced zucchini
- 2 cloves garlic, minced
- 2 tablespoons / 30ml olive oil
- 1/2 teaspoon / 2.5ml dried basil
- 1/2 teaspoon / 2.5ml dried oregano
- Salt and pepper to taste
- 1/4 cup / 30g grated Parmesan cheese

Directions:

- Cook pasta according to package Directions. Drain and set aside.
- In a large skillet, heat olive oil over medium-high heat. Add garlic and cook for 1 minute until fragrant.
- Add broccoli, mushrooms, bell pepper and zucchini. Season with basil, oregano, salt and pepper.
- Cook for 5-7 minutes, stirring frequently, until veggies are tender-crisp.
- Add cooked pasta and Parmesan cheese. Toss to combine.
- Serve immediately.

Sugar-Free Apple Crunch

Ingredients:

- 6 cups / 900g peeled, sliced apples (about 6 medium apples)
- 1 teaspoon / 5ml ground cinnamon
- 1/2 cup / 50g rolled oats
- 1/3 cup / 40g almond flour
- 1/4 cup / 30g chopped pecans or walnuts
- 3 tablespoons / 45 ml butter or coconut oil, melted
- 1 teaspoon / 5 ml vanilla extract

Directions:

- Preheat oven to 350°F. Grease a baking dish.
- Arrange sliced apples in prepared baking dish and sprinkle with cinnamon.
- In a bowl, mix together oats, almond flour, chopped nuts, melted butter and vanilla until crumbly.
- Spread oat mixture evenly over apples.
- Bake for 30-35 minutes until apples are tender and topping is golden brown.
- Let cool slightly before serving.

Tropical Fruit Yogurt

Ingredients:

- 1 cup / 240g plain Greek yogurt
- 1/2 cup / 75g diced fresh pineapple
- 1/2 cup / 90g diced mango
- 1/4 cup / 40g diced kiwi
- 2 tablespoons / 15g shredded coconut
- 1 tablespoon / 15 ml honey (optional)

Directions:

- In a bowl, mix together the yogurt, pineapple, mango, kiwi and shredded coconut.
- Drizzle with honey if desired for added sweetness.
- Divide mixture evenly into cups or bowls.
- Refrigerate for 30 minutes before serving to allow flavors to blend
- Garnish with extra fruit or coconut if desired.

Muesli With Apple and Banana

Ingredients:

- 2 cups / 180g old-fashioned rolled oats
- 1/2 cup / 60g sliced almonds
- 1/4 cup / 30g sunflower seeds
- 1/4 cup / 30g pumpkin seeds
- 1 apple, diced
- 1 banana, sliced
- 1 cup / 240 ml milk or non-dairy milk
- 1/4 cup / 60ml plain yogurt or dairy-free yogurt

- 2 tablespoons / 30ml honey (optional)

Directions:

- In a bowl, mix together oats, sliced almonds, sunflower seeds and pumpkin seeds.
- Add diced apple, sliced banana, milk and yogurt. Stir to combine.
- Drizzle with honey if desired for added sweetness.
- Allow to sit for 5 minutes to soften oats before serving.

Chickpea Fritters

Ingredients:

- 1 cup / 185g chickpea flour (or all-purpose flour for non-gluten-free)
- 1/2 cup / 120ml water
- 1/2 teaspoon / 2.5ml baking powder
- 1/2 teaspoon / 2.5ml cumin
- 1/4 teaspoon / 1.25ml cayenne pepper
- 1/2 teaspoon / 2.5ml salt
- 1/4 cup / 60ml olive oil or vegetable oil for frying
- 1 cup / 100g spinach, chopped
- 1 carrot, grated (about 1/2 cup / 65g)

Directions:

- In a bowl, whisk together chickpea flour, water, baking powder, cumin, cayenne and salt until a batter forms.
- Fold in chopped spinach and grated carrot.
- Heat oil in a skillet over medium heat to 350°F / 175°C.
- Scoop batter by heaping tablespoons and carefully drop into hot oil.
- Fry for 2-3 minutes per side until golden brown.
- Drain fritters on a paper towel-lined plate and serve warm.

Veggie Nuggets

Ingredients:

- 1 cup / 130g cooked brown rice
- 1/2 cup / 60g whole wheat breadcrumbs
- 1 cup / 100g finely chopped broccoli florets
- 1/2 cup / 65g grated carrot
- 1/3 cup / 45g peas
- 1 egg, beaten
- 1 teaspoon / 5ml onion powder
- 1/2 teaspoon / 2.5ml garlic powder
- 1/2 teaspoon / 2.5ml salt
- 1/4 teaspoon / 1.25ml black pepper
- Oil or cooking spray for baking

Directions:

- Preheat oven to 400°F / 200°C. Line a baking sheet with parchment paper.
- In a bowl, mix together cooked rice, breadcrumbs, broccoli, carrot, peas, egg, onion powder, garlic powder, salt and pepper.
- Form mixture into small nugget shapes using your hands and place on baking sheet.
- Lightly spray or brush nuggets with oil.
- Bake for 20-25 minutes, flipping halfway, until golden brown and crispy.
- Let cool for 5 minutes before serving.

Turkey Burgers and Beetroot Sauce

Ingredients:

Turkey Burgers

- 1 lb / 450g ground turkey
- 1 egg, beaten
- 1/3 cup / 40g breadcrumbs
- 2 tablespoons / 30ml olive oil

Beetroot Sauce

- 1 small beetroot, peeled and grated (about 1 cup / 100g)
- 1/2 cup / 120g plain Greek yogurt
- 1 garlic clove, minced
- 1 teaspoon / 5 ml dried oregano
- 1/2 teaspoon / 2.5ml salt
- 1/4 teaspoon / 1.25ml black pepper

- 1 tablespoon / 15 ml lemon juice
- 1 teaspoon / 5 ml honey
- 1/4 teaspoon / 1.25ml salt

Directions:

Burgers:

- In a bowl, mix together ground turkey, egg, breadcrumbs, 1 tablespoon olive oil, oregano, salt and pepper until combined.
- Form into 4 equal patties.

Beetroot Sauce:

- Make sauce by combining grated beetroot, yogurt, garlic, lemon juice, honey and salt. Mix well.
- Serve turkey burgers warm with beetroot sauce spooned over the top.
- Heat remaining 1 tablespoon olive oil in a skillet over medium heat.
- Cook patties for 4-5 minutes per side until cooked through.

Liver Health

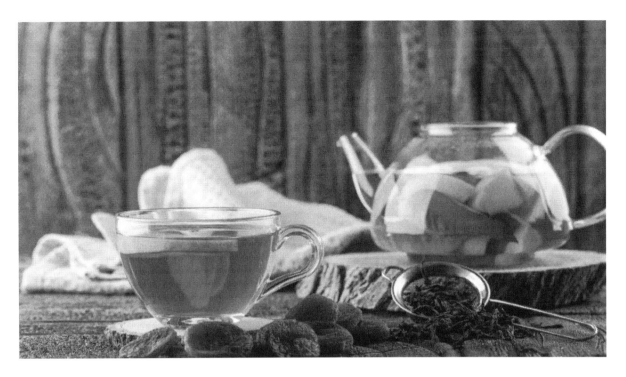

"The liver is a miraculous organ that deserves our care and respect." –Dr. Andrew Weil

The liver is a powerhouse organ, performing over 500 vital functions that are essential for our overall health and well-being. From filtering toxins and metabolizing fats to regulating blood sugar levels and producing essential proteins, the liver plays a crucial role in maintaining the body's delicate internal balance. By embracing a liver-friendly lifestyle centered around wholesome foods, detoxifying herbs, and mindful practices, we can support this hardworking organ and promote its optimal function.

Topical Treatments

Liver Capsules

Ingredients:

- 1 lb (450g) fresh beef liver
- 1 cup (240ml) filtered water or bone broth
- 1 tbsp (15ml) fresh lemon juice
- 1 tsp (5ml) apple cider vinegar
- 1/2 tsp (2.5ml) sea salt
- 500-600 empty gel capsules (size 00)

Directions:

1. Rinse the beef liver under cold water and pat dry with paper towels. Remove any visible membranes.
2. Cut the liver into small pieces and place in a blender or food processor. Add the water/broth, lemon juice, apple cider vinegar and salt.
3. Blend on high speed until completely pureed and smooth, stopping to scrape down sides as needed.
4. Carefully strain the liver puree through a fine mesh sieve or cheesecloth to remove any remaining solids or grit.
5. Using a capsule machine or by hand, fill the empty gel capsules with the strained liver puree mixture. Each 00 capsule holds around 0.8-1.0ml.
6. Once filled, preserve capsules by placing them in an airtight container and storing in the refrigerator for up to 2 weeks or freezer for up to 6 months.
7. For therapeutic liver support, take 4-6 capsules daily or as directed by your healthcare provider.

Herbal Brews and Drinks

Olive Oil and Lemon Shot

Ingredients:

- 1 tbsp (15ml) extra virgin olive oil
- 1 tbsp (15ml) fresh lemon juice
- 1/4 tsp (1.25ml) grated ginger (optional)

Directions:

1. In a small glass, combine the olive oil and lemon juice.
2. If using ginger, grate it directly into the mixture.
3. Stir briskly with a fork or small whisk to emulsify the ingredients.
4. Drink the shot quickly in one or two gulps.
5. Chase with water or herbal tea if desired.
6. Take on an empty stomach first thing in the morning.

Dandelion Liver Detox Tea

Ingredients:

- 1 tbsp (4g) dried dandelion root
- 1 tbsp (3g) dried dandelion leaf
- 1 tsp (1g) dried burdock root
- 1 tsp (2g) dried milk thistle
- 1 cup (240ml) filtered water

Directions:

1. In a tea pot or saucepan, combine all the dried herbs.
2. Pour the water over the herbs and allow to steep for 10-15 minutes.
3. Strain the tea through a fine mesh sieve.
4. Optionally, add honey or lemon to taste.
5. Drink 1 to 2 cups of this detox tea daily.

Milk Thistle Tea Blend

Ingredients:

- 1 tbsp (4g) dried milk thistle seeds
- 1 tsp (2g) dried dandelion root
- 1 tsp (1g) dried burdock root
- 1 cinnamon stick
- 1 cup (240ml) water

Directions:

1. In a small saucepan, combine all the dried ingredients.
2. Pour in the water and bring to a gentle simmer.
3. Reduce heat to low, cover and steep for 10 minutes.
4. Strain the tea through a fine mesh sieve.
5. Add honey to taste if desired.
6. Drink 1 to 2 cups of this liver supportive tea daily.

Lemon Liver Flush

Ingredients:

- 1/2 cup (120ml) fresh lemon juice
- 1/2 cup (120ml) cold-pressed olive oil
- 1 tbsp (15g) grated ginger (optional)

Directions:

- In the evening, prepare by eating a light vegetable soup for dinner. Avoid anything too heavy or fatty.
- Around 8pm, mix together the lemon juice, olive oil, and grated ginger if using.
- Drink the mixture, using a straw to bypass the taste buds if needed.
- Immediately after, lie down and remain completely still for at least 30 minutes.
- Go to sleep, resting diagonally if possible to encourage bile flow.
- Upon waking, drink another 8oz (240ml) of lemon water to flush the liver.

Liver Health Recipes

Parsnip, Pear, and Thyme Soup

Ingredients:

- 1 tbsp (15ml) olive oil or butter
- 1 onion, diced
- 1 lb (450g) parsnips, peeled and sliced
- 2 pears, peeled, cored and diced
- 4 cups (960ml) vegetable or chicken broth
- 1 tsp (5ml) fresh thyme leaves
- 1/2 cup (120ml) heavy cream or full-fat coconut milk
- Salt and pepper to taste

Directions:

1. In a large pot, heat the olive oil/butter over medium heat. Add the diced onion and sauté for 2 to 3 minutes until translucent.
2. Add the sliced parsnips, diced pears, broth, and thyme. Season with a pinch of salt and pepper.
3. Bring to a boil, then reduce heat and simmer for 20-25 minutes until parsnips are very soft.
4. Remove from heat and puree using an immersion blender until smooth and creamy.
5. Stir in the cream/coconut milk and adjust seasoning with more salt and pepper if needed.
6. Garnish with extra thyme leaves and serve warm.

Tropical Buckwheat Smoothie

Ingredients:

- 1 cup (170g) cooked buckwheat groats, cooled
- 1 cup (240ml) pineapple juice
- 1 banana
- 1/2 cup (70g) frozen mango chunks
- 1/4 cup (30g) shredded coconut
- 1 tbsp (15ml) fresh lime juice
- 1 tsp (5ml) vanilla extract

Directions:

1. In a blender, combine the cooked buckwheat groats, pineapple juice, banana, frozen mango, shredded coconut, lime juice and vanilla.
2. Blend on high speed until smooth and creamy, scraping down sides as needed.
3. Pour into glasses and enjoy immediately, or refrigerate until ready to serve.

Spirulina Breakfast Bowl

Ingredients:

- 1 cup (240g) Greek yogurt or coconut yogurt
- 1 banana, sliced
- 1/4 cup (40g) fresh or frozen blueberries
- 2 tbsp (14g) chia seeds
- 1 tbsp (8g) hemp seeds
- 1 tsp (3g) spirulina powder
- 1 tbsp (15ml) honey or maple syrup
- 1/4 cup (30g) granola

Directions:

1. In a bowl, layer the yogurt, sliced banana and blueberries.
2. In a small bowl, mix together the chia seeds, hemp seeds, spirulina powder and honey/maple syrup.
3. Sprinkle the seed mixture over the yogurt and fruit.
4. Top with granola.
5. Allow to sit for 5 minutes to let chia seeds soften before eating.

Kelp Noodle Rainbow Veggies

Ingredients:

- 8 oz (225g) kelp noodles, rinsed and drained
- 1 red bell pepper, julienned
- 1 yellow bell pepper, julienned
- 1 cup (100g) julienned carrots
- 1 cup (100g) thinly sliced purple cabbage
- 2 green onions, sliced
- 2 tbsp (30ml) rice vinegar
- 2 tbsp (30ml) toasted sesame oil
- 2 tbsp (30ml) low-sodium soy sauce or tamari
- 1 tbsp (8g) sesame seeds
- 1 tsp (3g) freshly grated ginger
- Salt and pepper to taste

Directions:

1. In a large bowl, combine the rinsed kelp noodles with the julienned bell peppers, carrots, cabbage, and sliced green onions.

2. In a small bowl, whisk together the rice vinegar, sesame oil, soy sauce/tamari, sesame seeds, and grated ginger.

3. Pour the dressing over the kelp noodle veggie mixture and toss well to coat evenly.

4. Season with salt and pepper to taste.

5. Let marinate for 10-15 minutes to allow flavors to meld.

6. Serve chilled or at room temperature.

Cashew Curry

Ingredients:

- 1 cup (150g) raw cashews, soaked
- 1 tbsp (15ml) coconut oil
- 1 onion, diced
- 3 cloves garlic, minced
- 1 tbsp (8g) grated ginger
- 2 tsp (5g) curry powder
- 1 tsp (3g) garam masala
- 1 cup (240ml) vegetable broth
- 1 cup (240ml) coconut milk
- 1 cup (150g) diced potato
- 1 cup (150g) diced cauliflower florets
- Salt and pepper to taste
- Chopped cilantro for garnish

Directions:

1. Soak the raw cashews in water for 4-6 hours or overnight. Drain and rinse.

2. In a blender, puree the soaked cashews with 1/2 cup fresh water until smooth and creamy.

3. In a saucepan, heat the coconut oil over medium heat. Add the onions and sauté for 2-3 minutes until translucent.

4. Add the garlic, ginger, curry powder and garam masala. Cook for 1 minute until fragrant.

5. Pour in the veggie broth, coconut milk, and cashew cream. Whisk to combine.

6. Add the diced potatoes and cauliflower. Season with salt and pepper.

7. Bring to a simmer and cook for 15-20 minutes, until veggies are fork tender.

8. Adjust seasoning if needed, garnish with cilantro.

9. Serve over basmati rice or quinoa.

Lung Health

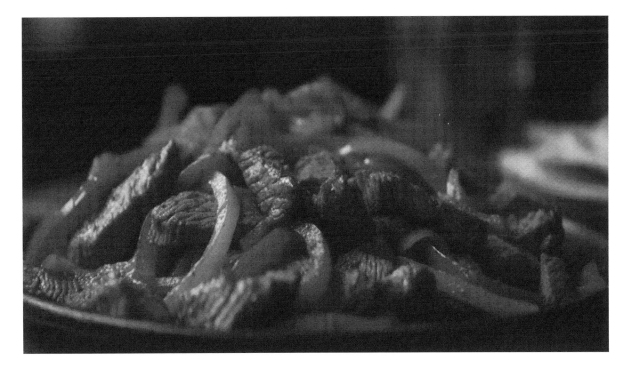

"Breath is the bridge which connects life to consciousness, which unites your body to your thoughts." —*Thich Nhat Hanh*

Our lungs work tirelessly to bring life-giving oxygen into our bodies and remove carbon dioxide with every breath we take. From the air we breathe to the foods we eat, the choices we make can have a profound impact on the health and function of our lungs. Incorporating lung-supportive herbs, nutrient-rich recipes, and breathwork practices into our daily routines help to strengthen our respiratory system, improve oxygenation, and promote overall vitality.

Topical Treatments

Lung Clearing Eucalyptus Steam

Ingredients:

- 3-4 drops eucalyptus essential oil
- 1 tsp (5ml) dried eucalyptus leaves (optional)
- 1 tbsp (15ml) dried peppermint leaves (optional)
- Bowl of steaming hot water

Directions:

1. Bring a pot of water to a boil, then carefully pour into a heat-safe bowl.
2. Add 3-4 drops of eucalyptus essential oil to the steaming water.
3. If using dried herbs, add 1 tsp eucalyptus leaves and 1 tbsp peppermint leaves to the bowl.
4. Lean over the bowl, draping a towel over your head to form a tent. This will contain the vapors.
5. Inhale the vapors deeply through your nose for 5-10 minutes.
6. Be careful not to burn your face on the hot steam.
7. Repeat 2 to 3 times per day to help clear mucus and open airways.

Oregano Lung Healing Capsules

Ingredients:

- 1/2 cup (60g) dried oregano leaf
- 500-600 empty vegetable capsules (size 00)

Directions:

- Grind the dried oregano leaf into a fine powder using a spice grinder, coffee grinder, or high-powered blender.
- Using a capsule machine or doing it manually, fill the empty vegetable capsules with the oregano powder. Size 00 capsules can hold around 0.5-0.7g powder each.
- Cap the filled capsules and store in an airtight container.
- For lung support, take 2 to 4 oregano capsules 2-3 times daily with food.
- Drink plenty of water.

Herbal Brews and Drinks

Oregano Lung Tea

Ingredients:

- 2 tsp (4g) dried oregano leaves
- 1 tsp (2g) dried thyme
- 1 tsp (2g) dried rosemary
- 1 cinnamon stick
- 1 tbsp (15ml) raw honey (optional)
- 1 cup (240ml) boiling water

Directions:

1. In a teapot or heatproof jar, combine the dried oregano, thyme, rosemary, and cinnamon stick.
2. Pour the boiling water over the herbs and cover with a lid. Allow to steep for 5-7 minutes.
3. Strain the tea through a mesh sieve into a mug.
4. Stir in raw honey if desired for added soothing effects.
5. Sip the tea slowly while hot.
6. You can drink 2-3 cups of this herbal lung tea per day.

Sea Moss Alkaline Water

Ingredients:

- 1/4 cup (10g) dried sea moss, rinsed
- 4 cups (960ml) spring water or filtered water
- 1 tbsp (15ml) fresh lemon juice

Directions:

1. Soak the dried sea moss in water for 12-24 hours to rehydrate it fully.
2. Drain and rinse the sea moss thoroughly under running water.
3. Place the rehydrated sea moss in a blender with 2 cups of fresh water. Blend until smooth and gel-like.
4. Pour the blended sea moss gel into a pitcher and add the remaining 2 cups of water along with lemon juice.
5. Stir or whisk vigorously to incorporate fully.
6. Drink 1-2 glasses per day for added minerals and alkalinity.
7. Store leftover sea moss drink in the fridge for up to 5 days.

Onion and Syrup Honey Tea

Ingredients:

- 1 yellow onion, thinly sliced
- 2 tbsp (30ml) raw honey
- 1 tbsp (15ml) fresh lemon juice
- 1 cinnamon stick
- 2 cups (480ml) water

Directions:

1. In a saucepan, combine the sliced onion, honey, lemon juice, cinnamon stick and water.
2. Bring mixture to a boil, then reduce heat and simmer uncovered for 15 minutes.
3. Remove from heat and allow to steep for 10 more minutes.
4. Strain the onion tea through a mesh sieve into a heat-safe pitcher or jar.
5. Sip warm or cool completely and refrigerate for iced tea.
6. Drink 1 cup morning and evening for soothing respirator support.

Licorice Root Iced Tea

Ingredients:

- 1/4 cup (25g) dried licorice root, chopped
- 1 tbsp (6g) dried marshmallow root (optional)
- 4 cups (960ml) water
- Raw honey or stevia to taste

Directions:

- Bring the 4 cups of water to a boil in a saucepan.
- Remove from heat and add the dried licorice root and marshmallow root if using.
- Allow to steep for 30 minutes to 1 hour to extract full flavor.
- Strain out the herbs using a mesh sieve.
- Allow tea to cool completely, then transfer to a pitcher and refrigerate until chilled.
- Sweeten with raw honey or stevia to taste when ready to drink.
- Sip this soothing licorice root tea throughout the day.

Lung Health Recipes

Orange and Strawberry Smoothie

Ingredients:

- 1 cup (150g) fresh strawberries, hulled
- 1 large orange, peeled and sectioned
- 1/2 cup (120ml) unsweetened almond milk or milk of choice
- 1/2 cup (120g) vanilla Greek yogurt
- 1 tbsp (15ml) honey or maple syrup (optional)

Directions:

1. Add the strawberries, orange sections, almond milk and Greek yogurt to a blender.
2. If desired, add 1 tbsp honey or maple syrup for added sweetness.
3. Blend on high speed until smooth and creamy, around 1 minute.
4. Pour into glasses and enjoy immediately.
5. Can top with extra strawberries, orange zest or granola if desired.

Tofu Breakfast Burritos

Ingredients:

- 8 oz (225g) firm tofu, drained and crumbled
- 1 tbsp (15ml) olive oil
- 1 tsp (3g) ground cumin
- 1 tsp (3g) chili powder
- 1/2 tsp garlic powder
- Salt and pepper to taste
- 4 large eggs or 1 cup (240ml) egg substitute
- 1/2 cup (50g) shredded cheddar cheese
- 4 medium tortillas or wraps
- Optional toppings: salsa, avocado, hot sauce, green onions

Directions:

1. In a non-stick skillet over medium heat, cook the crumbled tofu with olive oil, cumin, chili powder, garlic powder and salt/pepper for 3-4 minutes until spices are fragrant.
2. Push tofu to one side of the pan and crack in the eggs (or pour in egg substitute). Scramble the eggs gently, allowing them to mix with the tofu.
3. Remove from heat and stir in the shredded cheese.
4. Warm the tortillas/wraps briefly in the microwave for 15-30 seconds to make them pliable.
5. Spoon 1/4 of the tofu-egg mixture into each wrap. Top with desired toppings.
6. Fold up the bottom, then roll up tightly into a burrito. Serve warm.

Veggie Chickpea Sandwiches

Ingredients:

- 1 (15oz/425g) can chickpeas, rinsed and drained
- 1/2 cup (70g) shredded carrots
- 1/2 cup (50g) finely chopped bell pepper
- 2 green onions, sliced
- 1/4 cup (30g) all-purpose flour or chickpea flour
- 2 tbsp (30ml) tahini
- 1 tbsp (15ml) lemon juice
- 1 tsp (3g) ground cumin
- 1/2 tsp (2.5g) garlic powder
- Salt and pepper to taste

- 4 sandwich buns or pitas
- Desired toppings like lettuce, tomato, avocado

Directions:

1. In a bowl, mash the chickpeas with a potato masher or fork, leaving some chunks.
2. Add the shredded carrots, bell pepper, green onions, flour, tahini, lemon juice, cumin, garlic powder and salt/pepper. Mix well.
3. Form the mixture into 4 patties, packing them firmly together.
4. Cook the patties in a skillet over medium heat with a bit of oil for 3-4 minutes per side until golden brown.
5. Toast the buns/pitas and layer with desired toppings and a warm chickpea patty.

Beef and Broccoli Stir Fry

Ingredients:

- 1 lb (450g) beef sirloin, thinly sliced
- 1/4 cup (60ml) low-sodium soy sauce or tamari
- 2 tbsp (30ml) rice vinegar
- 1 tbsp (8g) cornstarch
- 2 tbsp (30ml) vegetable oil
- 4 cups (300g) broccoli florets
- 1 red bell pepper, sliced
- 3 cloves garlic, minced
- 1 tbsp (6g) freshly grated ginger
- Cooked rice or cauliflower rice, for serving

Directions:

1. In a bowl, toss the sliced beef with 2 tbsp soy sauce/tamari, rice vinegar and cornstarch until coated.
2. Heat vegetable oil in a wok or large skillet over high heat. Add the beef in a single layer and sear for 1-2 minutes until starting to brown.
3. Add the broccoli and bell pepper, stir fry for 2-3 minutes.
4. Add the garlic, ginger and remaining 2 tbsp soy sauce. Stir fry for 1 more minute.
5. Remove from heat and serve immediately over cooked rice or cauliflower rice.

Beetroot Waffles

Ingredients:

- 1 1/4 cups (155g) all-purpose flour
- 1 tsp (5g) baking powder
- 1/2 tsp (3g) baking soda
- 1/4 tsp salt
- 1 cup (240ml) milk or plant-based milk
- 1 egg
- 1/4 cup (60ml) melted coconut oil or butter
- 1 tsp (5ml) vanilla extract
- 1 cup (200g) grated raw beetroot
- Maple syrup or honey for serving

Directions:

1. In a bowl, whisk together the flour, baking powder, baking soda and salt.
2. In another bowl, whisk together the milk, egg, melted coconut oil/butter and vanilla.
3. Pour the wet ingredients into the dry and mix until just combined, being careful not to overmix.
4. Fold in the grated beetroot until evenly distributed.
5. Preheat your waffle iron and spray with non-stick cooking spray.
6. Pour batter onto the hot waffle iron in batches and cook 5-7 minutes until waffles are golden brown.
7. Serve the beetroot waffles warm, topped with maple syrup or honey.

Memory Boosters

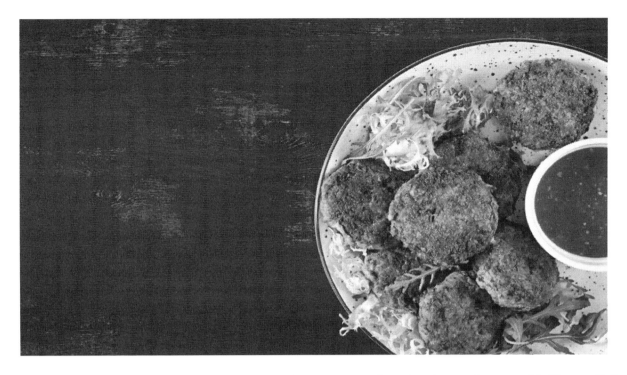

"Memory is the treasure house of the mind wherein the monuments thereof are kept and preserved." –Thomas Fuller

Our memories are the precious keepsakes of our lives, holding the stories, experiences, and knowledge that shape who we are. As we age, it's natural for our memory function to decline, but there are many ways we can support our brain health and maintain our cognitive sharpness. By incorporating memory-boosting herbs, brain-nourishing recipes, and mentally stimulating practices into our daily routines, we can help to enhance memory retention, improve recall, and keep our minds vibrant and agile.

Topical Treatments

Curcumin Caps

Ingredients:

- 1/2 cup (55g) turmeric powder
- 1/4 cup (35g) black pepper
- 500-600 vegetable capsules (size 00)

Directions:

1. In a small bowl, thoroughly mix together the turmeric powder and black pepper.

2. Using a capsule machine or by hand, fill each vegetable capsule with the turmeric-pepper mixture.

   Notes:

   Black pepper contains piperine which enhances absorption of curcumin.

   Can add coconut oil or lecithin powder to further increase bioavailability.

3. Cap the filled capsules tightly and store in an airtight container in a cool, dark place.

4. For inflammation support, take 2-3 curcumin capsules 1-2 times daily with meals.

- Start low and increase dose slowly as curcumin can cause digestive upset in some people.

Gingko Tonic

Ingredients:

- 1 tsp (2g) dried ginkgo biloba leaves
- 1/2 tsp (1g) dried gotu kola herb
- 1/2 tsp (1g) dried rosemary
- 1 cup (240ml) filtered water
- 1 tbsp (15ml) raw honey (optional)

Directions:

1. In a small saucepan, combine the dried ginkgo, gotu kola, and rosemary.
2. Pour in 1 cup of filtered water and bring to a gentle simmer over medium heat.
3. Reduce heat to low, cover, and allow to simmer for 10 minutes to extract the herbs.
4. Remove from heat and let the tonic steep for an additional 5 minutes.
5. Strain out the herbs using a fine mesh sieve.
6. Stir in raw honey if desired for added sweetness.
7. Drink the gingko tonic warm or refrigerate and enjoy chilled.

Brahmi Brain Tonic

Ingredients:

- 2 tsp (4g) dried brahmi (bacopa monnieri) leaf
- 1 tsp (2g) dried gotu kola herb
- 1/2 tsp (1g) dried ginkgo biloba leaf
- 1 cup (240ml) filtered water or milk
- 1-inch (2.5cm) piece fresh ginger, grated
- 1 tsp (5ml) ghee or coconut oil
- Raw honey to taste (optional)

Directions:

1. In a small saucepan, combine the brahmi, gotu kola, ginkgo biloba leaf and water/milk.
2. Add the grated ginger and ghee/coconut oil.
3. Bring mixture to a gentle simmer over medium heat.
4. Reduce heat to low, cover and allow to simmer for 15 minutes.
5. Remove from heat and let the tonic steep for 5 more minutes.
6. Strain the tonic through a fine mesh sieve, pressing on solids.
7. Sweeten with raw honey to taste if desired.
8. Drink the warm brahmi brain tonic daily for focus and cognitive support.

Herbal Brews and Drinks

Lemon and Rosemary Iced Tea

Ingredients:

- 4 cups (960ml) water
- 4 rosemary sprigs
- 4 lemon slices
- 2 tbsp (30ml) honey or agave nectar (optional)
- Ice cubes

Directions:

1. In a saucepan, bring the water to a boil. Remove from heat.
2. Add the rosemary sprigs and lemon slices. Cover and let steep for 15 minutes.
3. Remove the rosemary and lemon slices.
4. Stir in honey or agave if using for a touch of sweetness.
5. Allow the tea to cool completely, then pour into a pitcher filled with ice cubes.
6. Serve over ice, garnished with fresh rosemary sprig and lemon slice if desired.

Warm Sage Tea

Ingredients:

- 2 tsp (3g) dried sage leaves
- 1 cinnamon stick
- 1 cup (240ml) boiling water
- Honey to taste (optional)

Directions:

1. Place the dried sage and cinnamon stick in a mug or heat-proof cup.
2. Pour the boiling water over the herbs and let steep for 5-minutes.

3. Remove the cinnamon stick.

4. Sweeten with honey to taste if desired.

5. Sip the warm sage tea slowly while it's hot.

Macha Memory Latte

Ingredients:

- 1 tsp (2g) matcha green tea powder
- 1 cup (240ml) unsweetened almond milk or milk of choice
- 1 tsp (5ml) vanilla extract
- 1 tsp (5ml) honey or maple syrup
- 1/4 tsp ground cinnamon
- Tiny pinch of cardamom

Directions:

1. In a small saucepan, whisk together the matcha powder and 2-3 tbsp of the milk until dissolved.

2. Add the remaining milk and vanilla. Heat over medium, whisking frequently, until steaming hot but not boiling.

3. Remove from heat and whisk in the honey/maple syrup, cinnamon and cardamom until frothy.

4. Pour the matcha latte into a mug and enjoy immediately.

Memory Boosting Recipes

Ginger Miso Soup

Ingredients:

- 4 cups (960ml) vegetable or chicken broth
- 2 tbsp (30ml) white or yellow miso paste
- 1 tbsp (8g) grated fresh ginger
- 2 green onions, thinly sliced
- 8 oz (225g) silken tofu, cubed
- 2 tbsp (30ml) low-sodium soy sauce
- Sesame seeds for garnish

Directions:

1. In a saucepan, bring the broth to a simmer over medium heat.

2. In a small bowl, whisk together the miso paste with 1/2 cup of the hot broth until dissolved.

3. Pour the miso mixture back into the saucepan.

4. Add the grated ginger, green onions, tofu and soy sauce. Gently stir.

5. Allow to heat through for 2-3 minutes, do not boil.

6. Ladle soup into bowls and garnish with sesame seeds.

Blueberry Mint Granita

Here are the recipes:

Ginger Miso Soup

Ingredients:

- 4 cups (960ml) vegetable or chicken broth
- 2 tbsp (30ml) white or yellow miso paste
- 1 tbsp (8g) grated fresh ginger
- 2 green onions, thinly sliced
- 8 oz (225g) silken tofu, cubed
- 2 tbsp (30ml) low-sodium soy sauce
- Sesame seeds for garnish

Directions:

1. In a saucepan, bring the broth to a simmer over medium heat.

2. In a small bowl, whisk together the miso paste with 1/2 cup of the hot broth until dissolved.

3. Pour the miso mixture back into the saucepan.

4. Add the grated ginger, green onions, tofu and soy sauce. Gently stir.

5. Allow to heat through for 2-3 minutes, do not boil.

6. Ladle soup into bowls and garnish with sesame seeds.

Salmon Fish Cakes

Ingredients:

- 1 lb (450g) cooked salmon, flaked
- 2 eggs, lightly beaten
- 1/2 cup (60g) panko breadcrumbs
- 1/4 cup (35g) all-purpose flour
- 2 green onions, thinly sliced
- 2 tbsp (30ml) lemon juice

- 1 tbsp (8g) Dijon mustard
- Salt and pepper to taste
- Olive oil or butter for frying

Directions:

1. In a bowl, gently mix together the flaked salmon, eggs, panko, flour, green onions, lemon juice, mustard and salt & pepper until well combined.
2. Form the mixture into flat patty shapes, about 1/2 inch thick.
3. In a skillet, heat a thin layer of olive oil or butter over medium heat.
4. Cook the salmon cakes for 3-4 minutes per side until golden brown and heated through.
5. Transfer to a paper towel-lined plate.
6. Serve salmon cakes warm with lemon wedges and dipping sauce like tartar or remoulade.

Zucchini and Haloumi Fritters

Ingredients:

- 2 medium zucchinis, grated (about 2 cups/250g)
- 1/2 tsp salt
- 1 egg, lightly beaten
- 1/2 cup (65g) all-purpose flour
- 1/4 cup (30g) grated parmesan cheese
- 1 clove garlic, minced
- 1 tsp dried oregano
- 1/4 tsp black pepper
- 200g haloumi cheese, grated or cut into small cubes
- 2-3 tbsp olive oil or vegetable oil for frying

Directions:

1. Place the grated zucchini in a colander and sprinkle with 1/2 tsp salt. Let sit for 10 minutes to drain excess moisture, then squeeze out remaining liquid.
2. In a bowl, mix together the drained zucchini, beaten egg, flour, parmesan, garlic, oregano and black pepper until well combined.
3. Fold in the grated or cubed haloumi cheese.
4. Heat 2-3 tbsp oil in a skillet over medium heat.
5. Scoop heaping tablespoons of the zucchini mixture into the hot oil, flattening slightly into fritter shapes.
6. Fry for 2-3 minutes per side until golden brown.
7. Transfer fritters to a paper towel-lined plate and keep warm in oven at 200°F/95°C until all are cooked.
8. Serve the fritters warm with tzatziki or other dipping sauce.

Blueberry Mint Granita

Ingredients:

- 3 cups (480g) fresh blueberries
- 1/2 cup (120ml) water
- 1/4 cup (60ml) fresh mint leaves, packed
- 2 tbsp (30ml) honey or maple syrup

Directions:

1. In a blender, puree the blueberries, water, mint leaves and honey until smooth.
2. Pour the mixture into a shallow pan or baking dish.
3. Freeze for 1 hour, then use a fork to scrape and break up the frozen portions.
4. Return to freezer and continue freezing for 2 more hours, scraping with a fork every 30 minutes, until fully frozen into icy granita flakes.
5. Scoop granita into bowls or glasses to serve.

Raspberry Chia Brownies

Ingredients:

- 1 cup (120g) almond flour
- 1/2 cup (60g) unsweetened cocoa powder
- 1 tsp baking soda
- 1/4 tsp salt
- 1 cup (240ml) unsweetened applesauce
- 1/2 cup (120ml) maple syrup or honey
- 1/4 cup (60ml) melted coconut oil
- 1 tsp vanilla extract
- 1/4 cup (40g) chia seeds
- 1 cup (125g) fresh or frozen raspberries

Directions:

1. Preheat oven to 350°F (175°C). Grease an 8x8 inch baking pan.
2. In a bowl, whisk together the almond flour, cocoa powder, baking soda and salt.
3. In another bowl, mix the applesauce, maple syrup/honey, coconut oil and vanilla.
4. Pour the wet ingredients into the dry and mix until just combined.
5. Fold in the chia seeds and raspberries.
6. Spread batter evenly into the prepared baking pan.
7. Bake for 25-30 minutes until a toothpick inserted in the center comes out mostly clean.
8. Allow brownies to cool completely before cutting into squares.

Menopause and Perimenopause Support

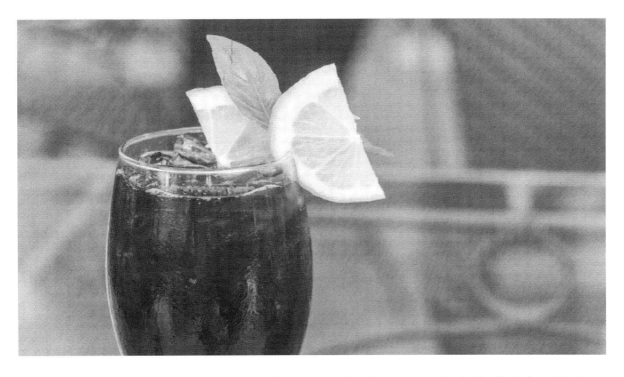

"Menopause is not a disease, but an opportunity for growth and transformation." –Dr. Christiane Northrup

Menopause and perimenopause are natural transitions in a woman's life, marking the end of her reproductive years and the beginning of a new chapter. While this time can bring physical and emotional challenges like hot flashes, mood swings, and sleep disturbances, it also presents an opportunity for self-discovery, personal growth, and renewed vitality. By incorporating hormone-balancing herbs, nourishing recipes, and self-care practices into our daily routines, we can help to ease menopausal symptoms, support our bodies' natural transitions, and embrace this transformative time with grace and resilience.

Topical Treatments

Vitamin E Hair Loss Oil

Ingredients:

- 1/2 cup organic jojoba oil
- 1/4 cup organic argan oil
- 2 vitamin E capsules
- 5 drops rosemary essential oil
- 5 drops lavender essential oil

Directions:

1. In a small, dark glass bottle, combine the jojoba oil and argan oil.
2. Pierce the vitamin E capsules with a clean pin and squeeze the contents into the oil mixture.
3. Add the rosemary and lavender essential oils to the bottle.
4. Replace the lid tightly and shake well to combine all ingredients.
5. Massage a small amount of the oil into your scalp and hair, focusing on the roots and ends.
6. Leave the oil on for at least 30 minutes, or overnight for deeper conditioning.
7. Wash your hair with a gentle, natural shampoo and style as usual.

8. Use this hair loss oil 2-3 times per week, or as needed, to help reduce hair loss, nourish your scalp, and promote healthy hair growth.

Licorice Root Hormone Balancing Tonic

Ingredients:

- 2 tablespoons dried licorice root
- 1 tablespoon dried spearmint leaves
- 2 cups water
- 1 lemon, juiced
- Raw honey (optional)

Directions:

1. In a medium saucepan, bring the water to a boil.
2. Add the dried licorice root and spearmint leaves to the boiling water, then reduce heat to a simmer.
3. Simmer the tonic for 10-15 minutes, then remove from heat and let it steep for an additional 5-10 minutes.
4. Strain the tonic through a fine-mesh sieve into a large mug or glass.
5. Stir in the lemon juice and raw honey (if using) until well combined.
6. Drink this hormone-balancing tonic daily, preferably in the morning or early afternoon, to help regulate estrogen levels, alleviate menopausal symptoms, and support overall endocrine health.

Sage Calming Facial Spray

Ingredients:

- 1/2 cup distilled water
- 1/4 cup aloe vera juice
- 1 tablespoon witch hazel
- 5 drops sage essential oil
- 5 drops lavender essential oil (optional)

Directions:

- In a small spray bottle, combine the distilled water, aloe vera juice, and witch hazel.
- Add the sage essential oil and lavender essential oil (if using) to the bottle.
- Replace the lid tightly and shake well to combine all ingredients.
- Mist the calming facial spray onto your face and neck, closing your eyes and inhaling deeply to enjoy the aromatherapeutic benefits.
- Use this spray throughout the day, as needed, to help reduce stress, balance emotions, and promote a sense of calm and well-being.

Herbal Brews and Drinks

Banana Peel Tea

Ingredients:

- 1 organic banana peel, washed and chopped
- 2 cups water
- 1 cinnamon stick (optional)
- Raw honey (optional)

Directions:

1. In a medium saucepan, bring the water to a boil.
2. Add the chopped banana peel and cinnamon stick (if using) to the boiling water, then reduce heat to a simmer.
3. Simmer the tea for 10-15 minutes, then remove from heat and let it steep for an additional 5-10 minutes.
4. Strain the tea through a fine-mesh sieve into a large mug or teapot.
5. Stir in raw honey (if using) until well combined.
6. Drink this soothing banana peel tea before bedtime to help support restful sleep, alleviate muscle cramps, and promote overall relaxation and well-being.

Spiced Cranberry Hormone Balancer

Ingredients:

- 2 cups unsweetened cranberry juice
- 1 cinnamon stick
- 1-inch piece of fresh ginger, sliced
- 1 tablespoon raw honey (optional)

Directions:

1. In a medium saucepan, combine the cranberry juice, cinnamon stick, and sliced ginger.
2. Bring the mixture to a simmer over medium heat, then reduce heat to low and let it simmer for 10-15 minutes.
3. Remove the saucepan from heat and let the mixture steep for an additional 5-10 minutes.
4. Strain the liquid through a fine-mesh sieve into a large mug or glass.
5. Stir in the raw honey (if using) until well combined.
6. Drink this spiced cranberry hormone balancer daily, preferably in the morning or early afternoon, to help regulate estrogen levels, alleviate menopausal symptoms, and support overall endocrine health.

Hot Flash Iced Coffee

Ingredients:

- 1 cup brewed coffee, chilled
- 1/2 cup unsweetened almond milk
- 1 teaspoon dried sage leaves
- 1 teaspoon dried peppermint leaves
- Ice cubes
- Raw honey (optional)

Directions:

1. In a small saucepan, combine the almond milk, sage leaves, and peppermint leaves.
2. Heat the mixture over medium heat until it begins to simmer, then remove from heat and let it steep for 5-10 minutes.
3. Strain the infused almond milk through a fine-mesh sieve into a blender.
4. Add the chilled coffee, ice cubes, and raw honey (if using) to the blender.
5. Blend on high until smooth and frothy.
6. Pour the hot flash iced coffee into a tall glass and enjoy immediately.
7. Drink this cooling beverage as needed to help alleviate hot flashes, boost energy levels, and promote overall well-being during menopause.

Black Cohosh Tea

Ingredients:

- 1 tablespoon dried black cohosh root
- 1 cup boiling water
- Raw honey (optional)

Directions:

1. Place the dried black cohosh root in a tea strainer or reusable tea bag.
2. Pour the boiling water over the black cohosh root and let it steep for 10-15 minutes.
3. Remove the tea strainer or tea bag and stir in raw honey (if using) until well combined.
4. Drink this black cohosh tea 1-2 times daily, or as directed by your healthcare provider, to help alleviate menopausal symptoms, regulate mood, and promote overall well-being.

Black Mulberry Iced Tea

Ingredients:

- 1/2 cup dried black mulberries
- 1 teaspoon dried lavender flowers
- 4 cups water
- Raw honey (optional)
- Ice cubes

Directions:

- In a medium saucepan, bring the water to a boil.
- Add the dried black mulberries and lavender flowers to the boiling water, then reduce heat to a simmer.
- Simmer the tea for 10-15 minutes, then remove from heat and let it steep for an additional 5-10 minutes.
- Strain the tea through a fine-mesh sieve into a large pitcher.
- Stir in raw honey (if using) until well combined.
- Refrigerate the tea until chilled, or serve over ice for an immediate cooling effect.
- Drink this black mulberry iced tea daily, or as desired, to help

regulate estrogen levels, reduce stress, and promote overall well-being during menopause and perimenopause.

Menopause and Perimenopause Recipes

Courgette, Basil, and Lentil Salad

Ingredients:

- 2 medium courgettes (zucchini), spiralized or julienned
- 1 cup cooked green or brown lentils
- 1/2 cup cherry tomatoes, halved
- 1/4 cup fresh basil leaves, chopped
- 2 tablespoons extra virgin olive oil
- 1 tablespoon fresh lemon juice
- 1 clove garlic, minced
- Salt and pepper to taste

Directions:

1. In a large bowl, combine the spiralized or julienned courgette, cooked lentils, cherry tomatoes, and chopped basil.
2. In a small bowl, whisk together the olive oil, lemon juice, minced garlic, salt, and pepper to create a dressing.
3. Pour the dressing over the courgette and lentil mixture, tossing gently to coat evenly.
4. Serve the salad immediately, or chill in the refrigerator for 30 minutes to allow the flavors to meld.
5. Enjoy this hormone-balancing salad as a light meal or side dish, 2-3 times per week, to help support overall well-being during menopause and perimenopause.

Miso Tofu with Stir Fried Ginger

Ingredients:

- 1 block firm tofu, drained and pressed
- 2 tablespoons white miso paste
- 1 tablespoon rice vinegar
- 1 tablespoon sesame oil
- 2 tablespoons coconut oil
- 2-inch piece of fresh ginger, peeled and julienned
- 2 cloves garlic, minced
- 2 green onions, sliced

Directions:

1. Cut the pressed tofu into 1/2-inch slices and set aside.
2. In a small bowl, whisk together the miso paste, rice vinegar, and sesame oil to create a marinade.
3. Brush the marinade evenly over the tofu slices and let them sit for 10-15 minutes.
4. In a large skillet or wok, heat the coconut oil over medium-high heat.
5. Add the julienned ginger and minced garlic to the skillet, stir-frying for 1-2 minutes until fragrant.
6. Add the marinated tofu slices to the skillet and cook for 3-4 minutes on each side, until golden brown and crispy.
7. Serve the miso tofu hot, garnished with sliced green onions, alongside your favorite vegetables or whole grains.
8. Enjoy this hormone-balancing, digestive-supportive dish 1-2 times per week, as part of a balanced diet for menopause and perimenopause.

Sweet Potato Rosti

Ingredients:

- 2 medium sweet potatoes, grated
- 1 small onion, grated
- 2 eggs, beaten
- 1 teaspoon ground turmeric
- 1/4 teaspoon black pepper
- Salt to taste
- 2 tablespoons coconut oil

Directions:

1. In a large bowl, combine the grated sweet potatoes, grated onion, beaten eggs, turmeric, black pepper, and salt. Mix well.
2. In a large skillet, heat the coconut oil over medium heat.
3. Scoop 1/4 cup portions of the sweet potato mixture into the skillet, flattening each portion with a spatula to create a thin, round rosti.
4. Cook the rostis for 3-4 minutes on each side, until golden brown and crispy.
5. Remove the rostis from the skillet and place them on a paper towel-lined plate to absorb excess oil.
6. Serve the sweet potato rostis hot, as a hormone-balancing, anti inflammatory side dish or snack.
7. Enjoy these rostis 1-2 times per week, as par

Mushroom and Fennel Hot Pot

Ingredients:

- 2 tablespoons olive oil
- 1 onion, diced
- 2 cloves garlic, minced
- 1 fennel bulb, thinly sliced
- 2 cups mixed mushrooms (shiitake, oyster, and cremini), sliced
- 4 cups vegetable or chicken broth
- 1 teaspoon dried thyme
- 1 bay leaf
- Salt and pepper to taste
- Fresh parsley, chopped (for garnish)

Directions:

1. In a large pot, heat the olive oil over medium heat.
2. Add the diced onion and minced garlic to the pot, sautéing until fragrant and translucent.
3. Add the sliced fennel and mushrooms to the pot, stirring to combine with the onion and garlic.
4. Pour in the vegetable or chicken broth and add the dried thyme and bay leaf.
5. Bring the hot pot to a boil, then reduce heat and let it simmer for 20-25 minutes, until the vegetables are tender.
6. Remove the bay leaf and season the hot pot with salt and pepper to taste.
7. Serve the mushroom and fennel hot pot garnished with chopped fresh parsley.
8. Enjoy this hormone-balancing, digestive-supportive dish 1-2 times per week, as part of a balanced diet for menopause and perimenopause.

Buckwheat and Turmeric Pancakes

Ingredients:

- 1 cup buckwheat flour
- 1 teaspoon baking powder
- 1/2 teaspoon ground turmeric
- 1/4 teaspoon salt
- 1 egg, beaten
- 1 cup unsweetened almond milk
- 1 tablespoon coconut oil, melted
- 1 tablespoon raw honey (optional)

Directions:

1. In a large bowl, whisk together the buckwheat flour, baking powder, turmeric, and salt.
2. In a separate bowl, combine the beaten egg, almond milk, melted coconut oil, and raw honey (if using).
3. Add the wet ingredients to the dry ingredients, stirring until just combined.
4. Heat a non-stick skillet or griddle over medium heat.
5. Scoop 1/4 cup portions of the batter onto the skillet, cooking the pancakes for 2-3 minutes on each side, until golden brown.
6. Serve the buckwheat and turmeric pancakes warm, topped with fresh berries, a drizzle of raw honey, or your favorite nut butter.
7. Enjoy these hormone-balancing, anti-inflammatory pancakes as a nourishing breakfast or brunch option, 1-2 times per week, as part of a balanced diet for menopause and perimenopause.

Fig and Ginger Bites

Ingredients:

- 1 cup dried figs, stemmed and chopped
- 1/2 cup raw almonds
- 1/4 cup raw pumpkin seeds
- 1 tablespoon fresh ginger, grated
- 1 tablespoon raw honey
- 1/2 teaspoon ground cinnamon
- Pinch of salt
- Unsweetened shredded coconut (for rolling)

Directions:

1. In a food processor, combine the chopped figs, almonds, pumpkin seeds, grated ginger, honey, cinnamon, and salt.
2. Pulse the mixture until it forms a sticky, cohesive dough.
3. Roll the dough into 1-inch balls, then roll each ball in the shredded coconut to coat.
4. Place the fig and ginger bites on a parchment-lined baking sheet and refrigerate for 30 minutes to set.
5. Store the energy bites in an airtight container in the refrigerator for up to 1 week.
6. Enjoy these hormone-balancing, digestive-supportive fig and ginger bites as a healthy snack or dessert, 1-2 per day, as part of a balanced diet for menopause and perimenopause.

Menstrual Support

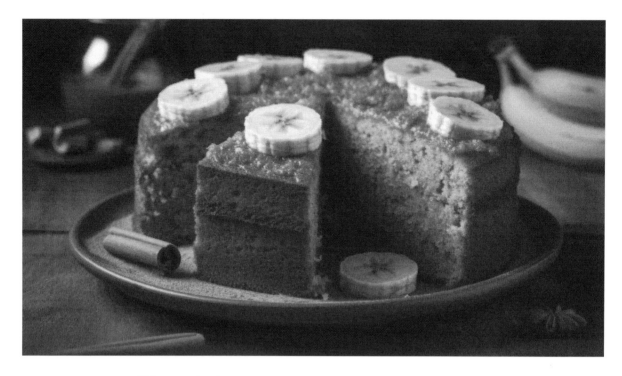

"Menstruation is not a curse, but a blessing in disguise." –Lara Owen

Menstrual health is an essential aspect of overall well-being for women throughout their reproductive years. From cramps and bloating to mood swings and fatigue, the symptoms associated with menstruation can range from mildly inconvenient to severely debilitating. By incorporating hormone-balancing herbs, nutrient-dense recipes, and self-care practices into our routines, we can help to alleviate menstrual discomfort, regulate our cycles, and promote overall reproductive health.

Topical Treatments

Menstrual Oil Rub

Menstrual Oil Rub

Ingredients:

- 1/2 cup (120ml) carrier oil (such as sweet almond, grapeseed or jojoba oil)
- 10 drops clary sage essential oil
- 5 drops lavender essential oil
- 5 drops rose geranium essential oil
- 2 drops chamomile essential oil

Directions:

1. In a glass bottle or jar, combine the carrier oil with all the essential oils.
2. Close the lid tightly and shake well to blend the oils together.
3. To use, massage a small amount of the menstrual oil rub onto the lower abdomen in a gentle circular motion.
4. You can also apply to the lower back, hips or inner thighs as needed for cramps or tension.
5. The oil blend can be used a few days before your period starts and during your cycle for soothing relief.
6. Store the remaining oil rub in a cool, dark place for up to 6 months.

Iron-Rich Liver Caps

Ingredients:

- 1/2 lb (225g) beef liver, frozen
- 1/4 cup (30g) vitamin C powder
- 500-600 vegetable capsules (size 00)

Directions:

1. Using a sharp knife, finely grate or shave the frozen beef liver into thin strips or flakes.
2. Spread the grated liver out on a parchment-lined baking sheet and freeze for 2 hours until completely frozen solid.
3. Transfer the frozen grated liver to a high-powered blender or spice grinder.
4. Add the vitamin C powder.
5. Pulse briefly until a fine powder forms, being careful not to overblend.
6. Using a capsule machine or manually, fill each vegetable capsule with the liver and vitamin C powder mixture until level.
7. Cap the filled capsules tightly and store in the freezer in an airtight container for up to 6 months.
8. Liver capsules with vitamin C help enhance iron absorption. Take as directed by your healthcare provider.

Herbal Brews and Drinks

Raspberry Leaf Iced Tea

Ingredients:

- 1/4 cup (10g) dried red raspberry leaves
- 4 cups (960ml) boiling water
- Honey or agave syrup to taste (optional)
- Ice cubes

Directions:

1. Place the dried raspberry leaves in a teapot or heat-safe pitcher.
2. Pour the boiling water over the leaves and let steep for 10-15 minutes.
3. Strain out the raspberry leaves using a fine mesh sieve.
4. Allow the tea to cool to room temperature, then refrigerate until chilled.
5. To serve, pour over ice cubes and sweeten with honey or agave if desired.
6. Garnish with fresh raspberries or lemon slices.

Fennel Seed Tea

Ingredients:

- 1 tbsp (8g) fennel seeds
- 1 cinnamon stick (optional)
- 1 cup (240ml) water

Directions:

1. In a small saucepan, lightly toast the fennel seeds over medium heat for 1-2 minutes until fragrant.
2. Add the water and cinnamon stick if using.
3. Bring to a boil, then reduce heat and simmer for 5 minutes.
4. Remove from heat, cover and let steep for 10 more minutes.
5. Strain the tea through a fine mesh sieve into a mug or teapot.
6. Drink fennel seed tea warm or allow to cool completely before refrigerating.

Ginger and Chamomile Warm Tea

Ingredients:

- 2 chamomile tea bags
- 1-inch (2.5cm) piece fresh ginger, sliced
- 1 cup (240ml) water
- Honey to taste (optional)

Directions:

1. In a small saucepan, bring the water to a simmer over medium heat.
2. Add the sliced fresh ginger and chamomile tea bags.
3. Remove from heat, cover and let steep for 7-10 minutes.
4. Remove the tea bags and ginger slices.
5. Stir in honey to taste if desired.
6. Sip the warm ginger chamomile tea slowly.

Basil, Carrot, and Lemon Shots

Ingredients:

- 4 large carrots, peeled and chopped
- 1 cup (25g) packed fresh basil leaves
- 1 lemon, juiced
- 1 inch (2.5cm) piece fresh ginger, peeled
- 1 tbsp (15ml) apple cider vinegar
- 1/2 tsp (2.5ml) honey (optional)

Directions:

1. In a blender, combine the chopped carrots, basil leaves, lemon juice, ginger, apple cider vinegar and honey if using.
2. Blend on high speed until completely smooth.
3. Strain the mixture through a mesh sieve or nut milk bag to remove pulp if desired.
4. Pour into shot glasses and drink immediately for best flavor and nutrients.

Kiwi and Kale Shot

Ingredients:

- 3 kiwi fruits, peeled
- 1 cup (30g) packed kale leaves, stems removed
- 1 tbsp (15ml) fresh lime juice
- 1 tsp (5ml) honey (optional)

Directions:

1. Add the peeled kiwi, kale leaves, lime juice and honey (if using) to a blender.
2. Blend on high speed until completely liquified, stopping to scrape down sides as needed.
3. Pour the bright green kiwi-kale shot into small glasses.
4. Drink immediately for a nutrient-packed refresher.

Menstrual Support Recipes

PMS Smoothie

Ingredients:

- 1 frozen banana
- 1 cup (165g) frozen mango chunks
- 1 cup (240ml) unsweetened almond milk
- 1 tbsp (10g) almond butter
- 2 tsp (6g) ground flaxseed
- 1 tsp (3g) pure maple syrup (optional)
- 1/4 tsp ground cinnamon

Directions:

1. Add all ingredients to a blender and blend on high speed until smooth and creamy.
2. If too thick, add a splash more almond milk to thin out.
3. Pour into a glass and enjoy this nourishing PMS smoothie.

Sweet Potato Pesto Bowl

Ingredients:

- 2 medium sweet potatoes, diced
- 1 cup (150g) cherry tomatoes, halved
- 1 cup (100g) cooked quinoa or brown rice
- 2 cups (60g) fresh basil leaves
- 1/4 cup (35g) toasted pine nuts
- 2 garlic cloves
- 2 tbsp (30ml) olive oil
- 2 tbsp (30g) grated parmesan
- Salt and pepper to taste

Directions:

1. Preheat oven to 400°F (200°C). Toss the diced sweet potatoes in a bit of oil and roast for 20-25 minutes until tender.
2. Make the pesto by blending the basil, pine nuts, garlic, olive oil, parmesan and a pinch of salt and pepper until smooth.
3. In a bowl, toss the roasted sweet potatoes with the cherry tomatoes and cooked quinoa or rice.
4. Add in a few spoonfuls of the pesto and gently mix to coat everything.
5. Serve the sweet potato pesto bowl warm or at room temperature with extra pesto on the side.

Turkey and Avo Burgers

Ingredients:

- 1 lb (450g) ground turkey
- 1 egg, lightly beaten
- 1/2 cup (30g) breadcrumbs
- 2 green onions, thinly sliced
- 2 tbsp (10g) grated parmesan
- 1 tsp dried oregano
- Salt and pepper to taste
- 1 large avocado, pitted and sliced
- 4 burger buns
- Desired toppings like lettuce, tomato, mayo

Directions:

1. In a bowl, gently mix together the turkey, egg, breadcrumbs, green onions, parmesan, oregano and salt & pepper until combined.
2. Form the mixture into 4 equal patties.
3. Heat a skillet or grill to medium-high heat and cook the turkey patties for 5-6 minutes per side until cooked through.
4. Toast the buns if desired. Layer the turkey burger on the bun with sliced avocado and desired toppings.

Chicken Korma

Ingredients:

- 1 lb (450g) boneless, skinless chicken breasts, cut into 1-inch pieces
- 2 tbsp (30ml) olive oil
- 1 onion, diced
- 4 cloves garlic, minced
- 1 tbsp (8g) grated ginger
- 2 tbsp (16g) korma curry paste
- 1 cup (240ml) coconut milk
- 1/2 cup (120ml) chicken or vegetable broth
- 1 tsp garam masala
- Salt to taste
- Chopped cilantro for garnish
- Cooked basmati rice for serving

Directions:

1. In a skillet, heat the olive oil over medium-high heat. Add the diced onions and cook for 2-3 minutes until translucent.
2. Add the minced garlic and grated ginger. Cook for 1 minute until fragrant.
3. Stir in the korma curry paste and mix well.
4. Add the chicken pieces and toss to coat with the korma sauce.
5. Pour in the coconut milk, broth and garam masala. Season with salt to taste.
6. Bring to a simmer and cook for 15-20 minutes, until chicken is fully cooked through.
7. Garnish with chopped cilantro.
8. Serve the chicken korma over basmati rice.

Bone Broth Hot Chocolate

Ingredients:

- 2 cups (480ml) beef or chicken bone broth
- 2 tbsp (16g) unsweetened cocoa powder
- 1 tbsp (15ml) maple syrup or honey
- 1 tsp (5ml) vanilla extract
- 1/4 tsp ground cinnamon
- Pinch of sea salt
- 1/4 cup (60ml) milk of choice (optional)

Directions:

1. In a saucepan, gently warm the bone broth over medium heat until steaming but not boiling.
2. Whisk in the cocoa powder until fully dissolved and no lumps remain.
3. Stir in the maple syrup, vanilla, cinnamon and salt until well combined.
4. If you want a richer, creamier hot chocolate, whisk in 1/4 cup milk of your choice.
5. Pour into mugs and enjoy the nourishing bone broth hot chocolate warm.
6. Can top with coconut whipped cream, cinnamon stick or shaved chocolate if desired.

Papaya Boat

Ingredients:

- 1 small papaya, halved lengthwise and seeded
- 1/2 cup (75g) fresh berries like blueberries, raspberries or strawberries
- 1 kiwi, peeled and sliced
- 2 tbsp (15g) unsweetened shredded coconut
- 1 tbsp (10g) sliced almonds
- 1 tbsp (15ml) honey or maple syrup
- Squeeze of fresh lime juice

Directions:

1. Using a spoon, hollow out a bit more of the papaya flesh, leaving a 1/2 inch border around the edges.
2. In a bowl, mix together the berries, kiwi slices, shredded coconut and sliced almonds.
3. Drizzle with honey and a squeeze of fresh lime juice. Toss gently to coat.
4. Spoon the fruit mixture evenly into the two papaya halves.
5. Serve the fresh papaya boats immediately or chill before eating.

Carrot Cake Bliss Balls

Ingredients:

- 1 cup (100g) grated carrots
- 1 cup (100g) pitted dates
- 1/2 cup (50g) rolled oats
- 1/2 cup (60g) walnuts
- 1 tsp ground cinnamon
- 1/4 tsp ground ginger
- 1/4 tsp ground nutmeg
- 1/4 cup (30g) shredded coconut for rolling

Directions:

1. In a food processor, pulse together the grated carrots, dates, oats, walnuts, cinnamon, ginger and nutmeg until a thick dough forms.
2. Scoop out heaping tablespoon amounts and roll into balls using your hands.
3. Roll each ball in the shredded coconut to fully coat the outside.
4. Place the carrot cake bliss balls on a plate or container and refrigerate for 30 minutes to set.
5. Store bliss balls in the fridge for up to 1 week or freeze for longer term storage.

Metabolism Boosters and Weight Loss Support

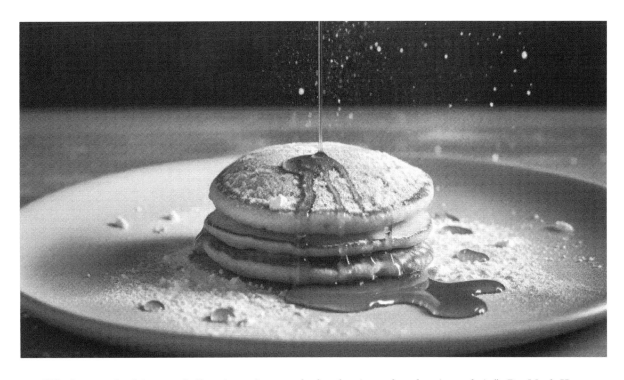

"The key to a healthy metabolism is to give your body what it needs, when it needs it." –Dr. Mark Hyman

A healthy metabolism is crucial for maintaining a healthy weight, sustaining energy levels, and promoting overall well-being. As we age or face various lifestyle challenges, our metabolism can slow down, making it more difficult to maintain a healthy body composition and feel our best. Incorporating metabolism-boosting foods, herbs, and lifestyle practices into our daily routine helps rev up our internal engines, support healthy weight management, and promote optimal vitality.

Topical Treatments

Spirulina and Cayenne Fat Burning Gel Caps

Ingredients:

- 1/2 cup (50g) spirulina powder
- 2 tbsp (12g) cayenne pepper powder
- 1 tbsp (7g) ginger powder
- 1 tsp (3g) black pepper
- 500-600 vegetable capsules (size 00)

Directions:

1. In a small bowl, mix together the spirulina powder, cayenne powder, ginger powder and black pepper until fully combined.

2. Using a capsule filling machine or doing it manually, fill each vegetable capsule with the spirulina-cayenne mixture. For size 00 capsules, fill each one with around 0.5-0.7 grams of powder.

3. Once all capsules are filled, cap them tightly.

4. Store the fat burning capsules in an airtight container in a cool, dry place away from direct light.

5. For fat burning support, take 2-4 capsules daily with water or juice, 20-30 minutes before meals. Start with a lower dose to assess tolerance.

6. Drink plenty of water throughout the day when supplementing

with these spicy capsules.

Herbal Brews and Drinks

Green Tea and Lemon Iced Tea

Ingredients:

- 4 green tea bags
- 4 cups (960ml) boiling water
- 1/4 cup (60ml) fresh lemon juice

- 2 tbsp (30ml) honey or agave nectar (optional)
- Ice cubes

Directions:

1. Steep the green tea bags in the boiling water for 5-7 minutes.
2. Remove tea bags and stir in the fresh lemon juice.
3. If desired, sweeten with honey or agave nectar to taste.
4. Allow tea to cool to room temperature, then refrigerate for 2 hours until chilled.
5. To serve, fill glasses with ice cubes and pour the lemon green tea over top.
6. Garnish with lemon slices if desired.

Apple Cider Vinegar and Cinnamon Gut Tonic

Ingredients:

- 1 cup (240ml) warm water
- 2 tbsp (30ml) apple cider vinegar
- 1 tbsp (15ml) honey

- 1 tsp (3g) ground cinnamon
- 1/4 tsp ground ginger (optional)

Directions:

1. In a mug or glass, combine the warm water and apple cider vinegar. Stir well.
2. Add in the honey and whisk until fully dissolved.
3. Sprinkle in the cinnamon and ginger if using. Whisk again to incorporate.
4. Drink the gut tonic 20-30 minutes before meals to support digestion.
5. Can also be refrigerated and consumed over ice.

Maca Powder Milk Tea

Ingredients:

- 1 cup (240ml) milk of choice (dairy, almond, oat etc.)
- 1-2 tsp (3-6g) maca powder
- 1 tsp (5ml) honey or maple syrup (optional)

- 1/4 tsp ground cinnamon
- 1/8 tsp ground nutmeg
- 1 black tea bag or 1 tsp loose leaf black tea

Directions:

1. In a small saucepan, gently warm the milk over medium heat until steaming and small bubbles form around the edges. Do not boil.
2. Remove milk from heat and whisk in the maca powder until fully dissolved.
3. If desired, sweeten with honey or maple syrup.
4. Add the cinnamon, nutmeg and black tea bag (or loose tea in an infuser). Allow to steep for 3-5 minutes.
5. Remove tea bag/infuser and give the milk tea a final whisk.
6. Pour into a mug and enjoy the maca milk tea warm.
7. Can top with an extra dusting of cinnamon if desired.

Energy Boosting Weight Loss Juice

Ingredients:

- 2 oranges, peeled and divided into segments
- 2 carrots, scrubbed and roughly chopped
- 1 beet, scrubbed and roughly chopped
- 1/2 lemon, peeled if desired

- 1-inch knob of fresh ginger, peeled
- 1 cup (30g) packed spinach or kale
- 1 tbsp chia seeds (optional)

Directions:

1. Feed the orange segments, carrots, beet, lemon, ginger and greens through a juicer one by one to extract the juice.
2. Stir in the chia seeds if using.

3. Give the juice a stir and pour into glasses over ice if desired.
4. Drink immediately for best flavor and nutrients.

Green and Orange Fat Burner

Ingredients:

- 2 oranges, peeled
- 1 grapefruit, peeled
- 1 lime, peeled
- 1 cup (30g) parsley leaves

- 1/4 cup (15g) cilantro leaves
- 1 tsp grated ginger
- Pinch of cayenne pepper (optional)

Directions:

1. In a blender, combine the peeled oranges, grapefruit, lime, parsley, cilantro and grated ginger.
2. Add a pinch of cayenne pepper if desired for an extra metabolism kick.
3. Blend on high speed until completely liquified and smooth.

4. Strain through a fine mesh sieve to remove any pulp or foam if desired.
5. Pour the green and orange juice into shot glasses.
6. Drink 1-2 fat burner shots daily before meals.

Metabolism Boosting Recipes

Metabolism Boosting Smoothie

Ingredients:

- 1 cup (240ml) unsweetened almond milk
- 1 cup (125g) frozen mixed berries
- 1 tbsp (8g) almond butter
- 1 tbsp (7g) chia seeds

- 1 tbsp (6g) ground flaxseeds
- 1 tsp (3g) cinnamon
- 1/2 tsp (1g) cayenne pepper

Directions:

1. Add all ingredients to a blender and blend on high speed until completely smooth and creamy.
2. If too thick, add a splash more almond milk to reach desired

consistency.
3. Pour into a glass and enjoy this metabolism boosting smoothie.

Pineapple Salsa Pork Tenderloin

Ingredients:

- 1 (1 lb) pork tenderloin
- 2 tsp olive oil
- 1 tsp chili powder
- 1 tsp ground cumin
- 1/2 tsp salt
- 1/4 tsp black pepper

- 1 cup diced pineapple
- 1/2 cup diced red onion
- 1/4 cup chopped cilantro
- 1 jalapeño, seeded and diced
- Juice of 1 lime
- Salt and pepper to taste

Directions:

1. Preheat oven to 400°F (205°C). Pat the pork tenderloin dry and season all over with chili powder, cumin, salt and black pepper.

2. Heat olive oil in an oven-safe skillet over high heat. Sear the tenderloin for 2-3 minutes per side until browned all over.

3. Transfer skillet to preheated oven and roast for 15-20 minutes until pork reaches 145°F (63°C) internally.

4. Meanwhile, make the pineapple salsa by combining pineapple, onion, cilantro, jalapeño and lime juice in a bowl. Season with salt and pepper.

5. Let pork rest for 5 minutes after roasting, then slice and serve with the fresh pineapple salsa spooned over the top.

Turkey Chili

Ingredients:

- 1 tbsp (15ml) olive oil
- 1 lb (450g) ground turkey
- 1 onion, diced
- 3 cloves garlic, minced
- 2 tbsp (16g) chili powder
- 1 tbsp (8g) ground cumin
- 1 tsp dried oregano
- 1 tsp salt
- 1/4 tsp cayenne (optional)
- 1 (14oz/400g) can diced tomatoes
- 1 (15oz/425g) can kidney beans, drained and rinsed
- 1 cup (240ml) low-sodium chicken or vegetable broth

Directions:

1. In a large pot or dutch oven, heat the olive oil over medium-high heat. Add the ground turkey and cook while crumbling with a wooden spoon until browned, about 5 minutes.

2. Add the onions and garlic, cook for 2 more minutes until fragrant.

3. Stir in the chili powder, cumin, oregano, salt and cayenne if using. Cook for 1 minute.

4. Pour in the diced tomatoes with their juices, drained beans and broth. Bring to a simmer.

5. Reduce heat and let the chili simmer for 20-25 minutes to allow flavors to meld, stirring occasionally.

6. Adjust seasoning if needed before serving.

High Protein Muffins

- 1/2 tsp baking soda
- 1/4 tsp salt
- 1 cup (240g) plain Greek yogurt
- 2 large eggs
- 1/4 cup (60ml) maple syrup
- 1/4 cup (60ml) milk of choice
- 1 tsp vanilla extract
- 1/2 cup (75g) fresh or frozen blueberries (optional)

Directions:

1. Preheat oven to 350°F (177°C) and spray a muffin tin with nonstick spray.

2. In a large bowl, whisk together the oat flour, protein powder, baking powder, baking soda and salt.

3. In another bowl, whisk together the Greek yogurt, eggs, maple syrup, milk and vanilla.

4. Pour the wet ingredients into the dry and mix until just combined, being careful not to overmix.

5. Gently fold in the blueberries if using.

6. Divide the batter evenly between the 12 muffin cups.

7. Bake for 18-20 minutes until a toothpick inserted in the center comes out clean.

8. Allow muffins to cool for 5 minutes before transferring to a wire rack.

Whole Wheat Pancakes

Ingredients:

- 1 cup (120g) whole wheat flour
- 2 tsp baking powder
- 1/4 tsp salt
- 1 cup (240ml) milk of choice
- 1 large egg
- 2 tbsp (30ml) melted butter or coconut oil
- 1 tbsp (15ml) maple syrup

Directions:

1. In a large bowl, whisk together the flour, baking powder and salt.

2. In another bowl, whisk together the milk, egg, melted butter/oil and maple syrup.

3. Pour the wet ingredients into the dry and mix just until combined (don't overmix).

4. Let the batter rest for 5-10 minutes.

5. Heat a nonstick skillet or griddle over medium heat.

6. For each pancake, pour 1/4 cup of the batter onto the skillet Cook until bubbles appear on the surface and the underside i lightly browned, 2-3 minutes.

7. Flip and cook for 1-2 minutes more until puffed and cooked through.

8. Serve the whole wheat pancakes warm with desired toppings.

Golden Milk Chia Pudding

Ingredients:

- 1 cup (240ml) unsweetened almond or coconut milk
- 1/4 cup (45g) chia seeds
- 1 tsp ground turmeric
- 1/4 tsp ground ginger
- 1/4 tsp ground cinnamon
- Pinch of black pepper
- 1-2 tbsp (15-30ml) maple syrup, to taste

Directions:

1. In a bowl or jar, whisk together the milk, chia seeds, turmeric, ginger, cinnamon and black pepper until fully combined.

2. Let the mixture sit for 5 minutes, then whisk again to break up any clumps.

3. Cover and refrigerate for at least 4 hours or overnight, whisking once halfway through.

4. Once thickened, stir in the maple syrup to taste.

5. Layer the golden milk chia pudding into cups or bowls with fruit, nuts, coconut, etc.

6. The pudding will keep for 4-5 days covered in the fridge.

Mobility and Muscle Flexibility

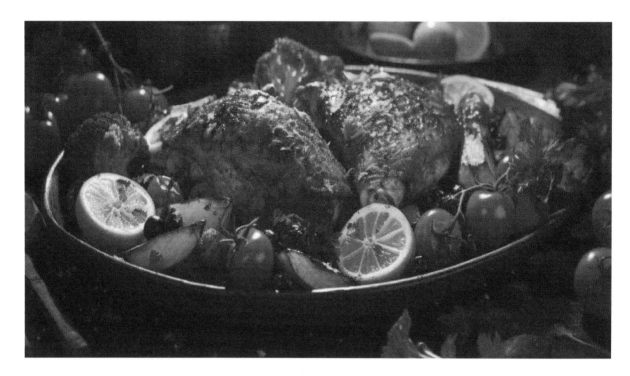

"Flexibility is the key to stability." –John Wooden

Maintaining mobility and muscle flexibility is essential for our overall physical health, allowing us to move with ease, prevent injuries and perform daily activities without discomfort. As we age or face various lifestyle challenges, our muscles can become tight, our joints can stiffen, and our range of motion can decrease, leading to pain, imbalances, and limitations in our physical abilities. By incorporating mobility-enhancing herbs, nourishing recipes, and regular stretching practices into our routines, we can help to support supple muscles, healthy joints, and optimal physical function.

Topical Treatments

Stinging Nettle Balm

Ingredients:

- 1/2 cup (120ml) olive oil or sweet almond oil
- 1/4 cup (25g) dried stinging nettle leaves
- 2 tbsp (30ml) beeswax pellets
- 10 drops tea tree essential oil
- 5 drops lavender essential oil

Directions:

1. In a double boiler or heatproof bowl, combine the olive/almond oil and dried nettle leaves. Gently warm over low heat for 30 minutes to infuse the oil.

2. Strain the nettle infused oil through a cheesecloth or fine mesh strainer to remove the leaves. Discard the leaves.

3. Return the infused oil to the double boiler and add the beeswax pellets. Heat and stir constantly until fully melted.

4. Remove from heat and stir in the tea tree and lavender essential oils.

5. Quickly pour the balm mixture into tins or jars and allow to fully set at room temperature.

6. To use, massage a small amount of the balm onto skin irritation like stings, rashes or eczema as needed.

Sore Muscle Balm

Ingredients:

- 1/2 cup (120ml) coconut oil
- 1/4 cup (60ml) olive oil
- 2 tbsp (30ml) beeswax pellets
- 10 drops peppermint essential oil
- 10 drops eucalyptus essential oil
- 5 drops rosemary essential oil

Directions:

1. In a double boiler, combine the coconut oil, olive oil and beeswax pellets. Heat on low, stirring frequently, until fully melted.
2. Remove from heat and stir in the peppermint, eucalyptus and rosemary essential oils.
3. Carefully pour the balm mixture into tins or jars. Allow to fully set at room temperature.
4. To use, massage the balm into sore, achy muscles after a workout. The cooling menthol helps soothe discomfort.
5. Store at room temperature for up to 6 months.

Cooling Joint Oil

Ingredients:

- 1/2 cup (120ml) fractionated coconut oil or sweet almond oil
- 10 drops peppermint essential oil
- 8 drops marjoram essential oil
- 5 drops copaiba essential oil

Directions:

- In a small glass bottle or jar, combine the fractionated coconut/almond oil with the peppermint, marjoram and copaiba essential oils.
- Secure the lid and gently roll the bottle to fully mix the oils together.
- To use, massage a few drops of the cooling joint oil blend onto sore, inflamed joints like knees, wrists, etc.
- The oils provide a cooling, anti-inflammatory effect to ease discomfort.
- Store at room temperature away from direct sunlight.

Herbal Brews and Drinks

Celery Joint Juice

Ingredients:

- 6 celery stalks
- 1 cucumber
- 1 lemon, peeled
- 1-inch piece fresh ginger
- 1 tbsp (5g) fresh parsley

Directions:

1. Wash and roughly chop the celery, cucumber, lemon, and ginger.
2. In a juicer, alternate feeding in the celery, cucumber, lemon, ginger, and parsley to extract the juice.
3. Stir the juice and pour over ice, if desired.
4. Drink immediately for best flavor and nutrients to support joint health.

Hot Carob Tea

Ingredients:

- 2 tsp (4g) roasted carob powder
- 1 cup (240ml) unsweetened almond milk (or milk of choice)
- 1 tbsp (15ml) maple syrup or honey (optional)
- 1/4 tsp ground cinnamon

Directions:

1. In a saucepan, whisk together the carob powder and almond milk until combined.
2. Heat over medium, whisking frequently, until hot but not boiling.
3. Remove from heat and stir in maple syrup/honey for sweetness, if desired.
4. Pour into a mug and dust the top with ground cinnamon.

Cucumber Fenugreek Morning Shot

Ingredients:

- 1/2 cucumber, chopped
- 1 tbsp (7g) fenugreek seeds, soaked
- 1 tbsp (15ml) fresh lemon juice
- 1 tsp (5ml) apple cider vinegar

Directions:

1. Add the chopped cucumber, soaked fenugreek seeds, lemon juice and vinegar to a blender.
2. Blend until completely liquified and no solids remain.
3. Strain through a fine mesh sieve if desired for smoother texture.
4. Pour into a shot glass and drink first thing in the morning.

Basil Fenugreek Sore Muscle Relief Drink

Ingredients:

- 1 cup (25g) fresh basil leaves
- 1-2 tbsp (7-14g) fenugreek seeds, soaked
- 1 tbsp (15ml) fresh lime juice
- 1 tsp (5g) raw honey (optional)
- 1 cup (240ml) water or coconut water

Directions:

1. In a blender, combine the basil, soaked fenugreek seeds, lime juice, honey (if using) and water.
2. Blend thoroughly until smooth and no solids remain.
3. For an icy cold beverage, blend in 1/2 cup ice cubes.
4. Drink this basil fenugreek mix for its anti-inflammatory properties after exercise.

For all recipes with soaked fenugreek, soak 1-2 tbsp seeds in water for 4-6 hours, then drain before using.

Mobility and Muscle Flexibility Recipes

Ashwagandha Smoothie

Ingredients:

- 1 banana
- 1 cup (240ml) unsweetened almond milk
- 1 tbsp (7g) almond butter
- 1 tsp (3g) ashwagandha powder
- 1 tsp (5ml) honey or maple syrup (optional)
- 1/4 tsp ground cinnamon
- 1/4 tsp ground ginger
- 1 cup (125g) ice cubes

Directions:

1. Add all ingredients to a blender and blend on high speed until completely smooth, about 1 minute.
2. Taste and adjust sweetness if needed by adding more honey/ maple syrup.
3. Pour into a glass and enjoy the ashwagandha smoothie immediately.

Green and Gold Salad

Ingredients:

- 4 cups (120g) mixed greens or baby spinach
- 1 avocado, diced
- 1 mango, diced
- 1/4 cup (35g) dried cranberries
- 1/4 cup (30g) sliced almonds
- 2 tbsp (30ml) olive oil
- 2 tbsp (30ml) apple cider vinegar
- 1 tsp Dijon mustard
- Salt and pepper to taste

Directions:

1. In a large bowl, combine the mixed greens, diced avocado, diced mango, dried cranberries and sliced almonds.
2. In a small bowl, whisk together the olive oil, apple cider vinegar, Dijon mustard and a pinch of salt and pepper.
3. Drizzle the dressing over the salad and gently toss to coat all the ingredients evenly.
4. Serve the Green and Gold Salad immediately for best freshness.

Tuna Potato Salad

Ingredients:

- 1 lb (450g) baby potatoes, boiled and quartered
- 1 (5oz/140g) can tuna, drained
- 1/2 cup (75g) diced celery
- 1/4 cup (35g) diced red onion
- 3 tbsp (45ml) mayonnaise
- 1 tbsp (15ml) Dijon mustard
- 2 tbsp (30ml) lemon juice
- 2 tbsp (10g) chopped fresh parsley
- Salt and pepper to taste

Directions:

1. In a large bowl, gently mix together the cooked potato quarters, drained tuna, diced celery and red onion.
2. In a small bowl, whisk together the mayonnaise, Dijon, lemon juice and parsley.
3. Pour the dressing over the tuna potato salad and gently toss to coat evenly.
4. Season with salt and pepper to taste.
5. Refrigerate for 30 minutes before serving to allow flavors to blend.

Herby Chicken With Couscous

Ingredients:

- 1 lb (450g) boneless, skinless chicken breasts
- 2 tbsp (30ml) olive oil
- 1 onion, diced
- 3 cloves garlic, minced
- 1 tsp dried thyme
- 1 tsp dried oregano
- 1/2 tsp paprika
- 1 cup (180g) couscous
- 1 1/4 cups (300ml) chicken or vegetable broth
- 1 cup (30g) fresh parsley, chopped
- Salt and pepper to taste

Directions:

1. Season the chicken breasts all over with salt, pepper and 1/2 tsp each of the dried thyme and oregano.
2. In a skillet, heat 1 tbsp olive oil over medium-high heat. Cook the chicken for 6-8 minutes per side until cooked through. Set aside.
3. In the same skillet, heat the remaining 1 tbsp olive oil. Sauté the onions until translucent, 2-3 minutes.
4. Add the garlic and cook for 1 minute until fragrant.
5. Stir in the remaining thyme, oregano, paprika and dry couscous. Toast for 1 minute.
6. Pour in the broth, bring to a boil, then cover and remove from heat. Let stand 5 minutes.
7. Fluff the couscous with a fork and fold in the fresh parsley.
8. Slice the chicken and serve over the herbed couscous.

Turkey Lettuce Wraps

Ingredients:

- 1 lb (450g) ground turkey
- 1 tbsp (15ml) olive oil
- 1 onion, diced
- 2 cloves garlic, minced
- 1 red bell pepper, diced
- 1 tbsp (8g) taco seasoning
- 1/4 cup (60ml) water
- 12 lettuce cups/leaves
- Desired toppings like avocado, salsa, cheese etc.

Directions:

1. In a skillet over medium-high heat, cook the ground turkey and break it up with a spoon until browned and crumbled. Drain any excess fat.
2. In the same skillet, heat the olive oil and sauté the diced onion for 2 minutes. Add the minced garlic and cook 1 minute more until fragrant.
3. Stir in the diced bell pepper and taco seasoning. Cook for 2 more minutes.
4. Add the water and turkey back to the skillet. Stir until everything is heated through.
5. Scoop portions of the turkey taco filling into the lettuce cups.
6. Top with desired toppings like avocado, salsa, cheese etc. Serve immediately.

Amla Date Bombs

Ingredients:

- 10 pitted medjool dates
- 1/2 cup (60g) dried amla (Indian gooseberry) powder
- 1/4 cup (30g) shredded unsweetened coconut
- 1 tbsp (7g) hemp seeds
- 1 tsp (3g) ground cinnamon
- Water or milk as needed

Directions:

1. In a food processor, pulse the dates until a thick paste forms, scraping down sides as needed.
2. Add the amla powder, shredded coconut, hemp seeds and cinnamon. Pulse to incorporate.
3. If needed, add 1-2 tbsp water or milk until a sticky dough comes together.
4. Scoop out 1.5 tbsp amounts and roll into balls with your hands.
5. Roll the balls in extra shredded coconut if desired.
6. Store the amla date bombs chilled for up to 2 weeks.

Mood Enhancers

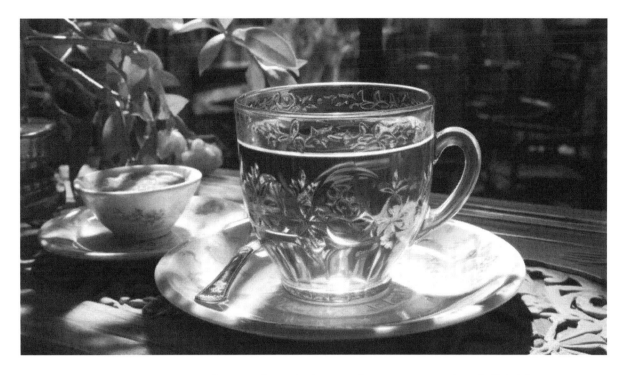

"Happiness is not something ready made. It comes from your own actions." –Dalai Lama

Our mood and emotional well-being play a crucial role in our overall quality of life, influencing our relationships, productivity, and daily experiences. In today's fast-paced, stress-filled world, it's common to experience occasional mood imbalances, such as anxiety, irritability, or low mood. By incorporating mood-supportive herbs, nutrient-dense recipes, and mindfulness practices into our daily routines, we can help to promote emotional balance, reduce stress, and cultivate a greater sense of happiness and well-being.

Topical Treatments

Witch Hazel Mood Spray

Ingredients:

- 1/2 cup (120ml) witch hazel extract
- 1/4 cup (60ml) distilled water
- 10 drops bergamot essential oil
- 5 drops clary sage essential oil
- 5 drops lavender essential oil

Directions:

1. In a small glass spray bottle, combine the witch hazel extract and distilled water.
2. Add the bergamot, clary sage and lavender essential oils.
3. Secure the spray top and gently shake to mix all the ingredients.
4. To use, mist over your face, neck and shoulders whenever you need an uplifting mood boost.
5. Avoid direct eye exposure. The witch hazel extract is astringent while the oils provide a calming, grounding aroma.

Summer Mood Lifting Body Mist

Ingredients:

- 1/2 cup (120ml) distilled water
- 1/4 cup (60ml) witch hazel or rose hydrosol
- 10 drops grapefruit essential oil
- 5 drops ylang ylang essential oil
- 2 drops patchouli essential oil

Directions:

1. In a small spray bottle, combine the water and witch hazel or rose hydrosol.
2. Add the grapefruit, ylang ylang and patchouli essential oils.
3. Secure the spray top and gently shake to fully blend the ingredients.
4. Mist over arms, legs and body after a shower or anytime for an uplifting, summery scent.
5. The citrusy grapefruit boosts mood while ylang ylang and patchouli provide grounding aromas.

Rose and Citrus Facial Mist

Ingredients:

- 1/2 cup (120ml) rose hydrosol
- 1/4 cup (60ml) distilled water
- 1 tbsp (15ml) vegetable glycerin (optional)
- 10 drops sweet orange essential oil
- 5 drops geranium essential oil

Directions:

1. In a small spray bottle, combine the rose hydrosol and distilled water.
2. If using vegetable glycerin, add it now for extra hydration.
3. Add the sweet orange and geranium essential oils.
4. Secure the spray top and gently shake to blend everything together.
5. Mist over clean face and neck after cleansing or anytime for a refreshing boost.
6. The rose helps soothe skin while orange and geranium uplift mood.

Herbal Brews and Drinks

Ginger Citrus Mocktail

Ingredients:

- 1 cup (240ml) freshly squeezed orange juice
- 1/2 cup (120ml) ginger ale or ginger beer
- 2 tbsp (30ml) fresh lemon juice
- 1 tbsp (15ml) honey or agave syrup (optional)
- Lemon and orange slices for garnish
- Ice cubes

Directions:

1. In a pitcher, combine the orange juice, ginger ale/beer, lemon juice, and honey/agave if using.
2. Stir well to combine the ingredients.
3. Fill glasses with ice cubes.
4. Pour the ginger citrus mocktail over the ice.
5. Garnish with lemon and orange slices.
6. Serve immediately.

Maca Root Sip Juice

Ingredients:

- 2 cups (480ml) almond milk (or milk of choice)
- 1 banana
- 1 tbsp (8g) maca powder
- 1 tbsp (15ml) honey or maple syrup
- 1 tsp (5ml) vanilla extract
- 1/4 tsp cinnamon

Directions:

1. Add all ingredients to a blender.
2. Blend on high speed until completely smooth.
3. Taste and adjust sweetness if desired.
4. Pour into glasses and drink the maca root sip juice chilled or at room temperature.

Rose Rooibos (Redbush) Tea

Ingredients:

- 4 cups (960ml) water
- 4 rooibos tea bags or 4 tsp loose rooibos
- 4 tsp (4g) dried rose petals or buds
- Honey, lemon or milk to serve (optional)

Directions:

1. In a saucepan or teapot, bring the water to a boil.
2. Remove from heat and add the rooibos tea bags or loose tea.
3. Add in the dried rose petals.
4. Cover and let steep for 5-7 minutes.
5. Strain out the tea bags/leaves and rose petals.
6. Sweeten with honey if desired, or add lemon or milk to taste.
7. Serve the rose rooibos tea hot or let cool and refrigerate for iced tea.

Mood Enhancing Recipes

Chia Banana Breakfast Shake

Ingredients:

- 1 ripe banana
- 1 cup (240ml) unsweetened almond milk or milk of choice
- 1/4 cup (40g) chia seeds
- 1 tbsp (15ml) maple syrup or honey (optional)
- 1 tsp (5ml) vanilla extract
- 1/4 tsp ground cinnamon

Directions:

1. In a blender, combine the banana, almond milk, chia seeds, maple syrup/honey (if using), vanilla, and cinnamon.
2. Blend on high speed until completely smooth and creamy, about 1 minute.
3. Pour into a glass and enjoy the chia banana shake immediately. Alternatively, you can refrigerate it overnight and drink it chilled.

Blueberry Baked Oats

Ingredients:

- 1 cup (80g) old-fashioned rolled oats
- 1 tsp baking powder
- 1/4 tsp salt
- 1 cup (240ml) unsweetened almond milk
- 1 egg
- 2 tbsp (30ml) maple syrup
- 1 tsp vanilla extract
- 1 cup (150g) fresh or frozen blueberries

Directions:

1. Preheat oven to 350°F (177°C). Grease an oven-safe dish.
2. In a bowl, mix together the oats, baking powder and salt.
3. In another bowl, whisk the almond milk, egg, maple syrup, and vanilla.
4. Pour the milk mixture into the oats mixture and stir to combine.
5. Gently fold in 3/4 of the blueberries, reserving some for the top.
6. Transfer to the prepared baking dish and top with remaining blueberries.
7. Bake for 30-35 minutes until set and lightly golden on top.
8. Allow to cool slightly before serving warm.

Avo and Black Bean Salad

Ingredients:

- 1 (15oz) can black beans, rinsed and drained
- 1 avocado, diced
- 1 cup (150g) cherry tomatoes, halved
- 1/2 red onion, finely diced
- 1 jalapeño, seeded and minced (optional)
- 1/4 cup (10g) chopped cilantro
- Juice of 1 lime
- 2 tbsp (30ml) olive oil
- 1 tsp ground cumin
- Salt and pepper to taste

Directions:

1. In a large bowl, gently mix together the black beans, avocado, cherry tomatoes, red onion, jalapeño (if using) and cilantro.
2. In a small bowl, whisk together the lime juice, olive oil, cumin, and salt and pepper.
3. Pour the dressing over the salad and toss gently to coat.
4. Let sit for 10 minutes to allow flavors to blend. Adjust seasoning if needed.

5. Serve the avocado and black bean salad chilled or at room temperature.

Tumeric Fried Eggs

Ingredients:

- 2 tbsp avocado oil or ghee
- 1/2 tsp ground turmeric
- 1/4 tsp ground cumin
- 1/4 tsp garlic powder
- Salt and pepper to taste
- 4 eggs
- Chopped cilantro for garnish

Directions:

1. Heat the avocado oil or ghee in a non-stick skillet over medium heat.
2. Once hot, sprinkle in the turmeric, cumin, garlic powder and a pinch each of salt and pepper.
3. Crack the eggs directly into the spiced oil and fry for 2-3 minutes until the whites are mostly set.
4. Optionally, flip the eggs and cook for 30 seconds more for runny yolks.
5. Remove eggs from heat to stop the cooking process.
6. Transfer turmeric fried eggs to plates and garnish with chopped cilantro.
7. Season with additional salt and pepper if desired. Serve immediately.

Coconut Fried Broccoli

Ingredients:

- 1 head broccoli, cut into florets
- 1/2 cup (60g) all-purpose flour or rice flour
- 1 tsp garlic powder
- 1/2 tsp salt
- 1/4 tsp black pepper
- 2 eggs, beaten
- 1 cup (80g) shredded unsweetened coconut
- Coconut oil or avocado oil for frying

Directions:

1. Set up three shallow bowls - one with flour mixed with garlic powder, salt and pepper, one with beaten eggs, and one with shredded coconut.
2. Dip the broccoli florets into the flour mixture first, coating well and shaking off excess.
3. Then dip into the beaten eggs letting any excess drip off.
4. Finally, coat the broccoli in the shredded coconut, pressing to adhere.
5. Heat 1/2 inch of coconut or avocado oil in a skillet over medium-high heat.
6. Working in batches, fry the coconut broccoli for 2-3 minutes per side until golden brown.
7. Transfer fried broccoli to a paper towel-lined plate. Season with more salt if desired.
8. Serve the coconut fried broccoli warm with your favorite dipping sauce.

Chili-Tempeh Stir-Fry

Ingredients:

- 1 (8oz) package tempeh, cubed
- 2 tbsp soy sauce or tamari
- 2 tsp rice vinegar
- 1 tsp sesame oil
- 1 tbsp cornstarch
- 2 tbsp avocado oil
- 1 onion, sliced
- 2 carrots, sliced
- 1 bell pepper, sliced
- 3 cloves garlic, minced
- 2 tsp chili garlic sauce
- 1 tsp ground ginger
- 4 cups cooked brown rice or quinoa

Directions:

1. In a bowl, toss the cubed tempeh with soy sauce, rice vinegar, sesame oil and cornstarch until coated.
2. Heat avocado oil in a large skillet or wok over high heat.
3. Add the tempeh in a single layer and fry for 2-3 minutes until browned on most sides. Remove tempeh from pan.
4. Add the onion, carrots, bell pepper and garlic. Stir-fry for 3 minutes.
5. Stir in the chili garlic sauce and ginger. Cook 1 minute more.
6. Return the fried tempeh to the pan and toss everything to combine.
7. Serve the chili-tempeh stir-fry immediately over brown rice or quinoa.

Crispy Sauerkraut Salad

Ingredients:

- 2 cups (280g) sauerkraut, drained and rinsed
- 1/2 cup (70g) all-purpose flour or rice flour
- 1 egg, beaten
- 1 cup (80g) panko breadcrumbs
- 1/4 cup (30g) walnuts, chopped
- 2 tbsp (30ml) olive oil or avocado oil
- 2 tbsp (30ml) apple cider vinegar
- 1 tbsp (15ml) whole grain mustard
- 1 tsp (5ml) honey
- Salt and pepper to taste

Directions:

1. Set up three shallow bowls - one with flour, one with beaten egg, and one with panko breadcrumbs mixed with chopped walnuts.
2. Working in batches, dredge the sauerkraut pieces first in flour, then the egg, and finally in the panko-walnut mixture, coating well.
3. Heat oil in a skillet over medium-high heat. Fry the breaded sauerkraut for 2 to 3 minutes per side until crispy and golden brown.
4. Transfer fried sauerkraut to a paper towel-lined plate and season lightly with salt.
5. Make the dressing by whisking together the vinegar, mustard and honey. Season with salt and pepper.
6. Arrange the crispy sauerkraut on a plate and drizzle with the dressing before serving.

Berry Banana Slushie

Ingredients:

- 1 ripe banana, frozen and roughly chopped
- 1 cup (150g) mixed frozen berries
- 1/2 cup (120ml) unsweetened almond milk or milk of choice
- 2 tbsp (30ml) honey or maple syrup (optional)
- 1 tsp (5ml) lemon juice
- 1/2 cup (120ml) cold water or ice cubes

Directions:

1. Add the frozen banana chunks, frozen mixed berries, almond milk, honey/maple syrup (if using), and lemon juice to a blender.
2. Pour in the cold water or add ice cubes if you want a thicker slushie texture.
3. Blend on high speed until smooth and slushy, stopping to scrape down sides as needed.
4. If too thick, add a splash more milk. If too thin, add a few more ice cubes.
5. Pour the berry banana slushie into glasses and serve immediately with spoons or straws.

Muscle Growth and Weight Gain

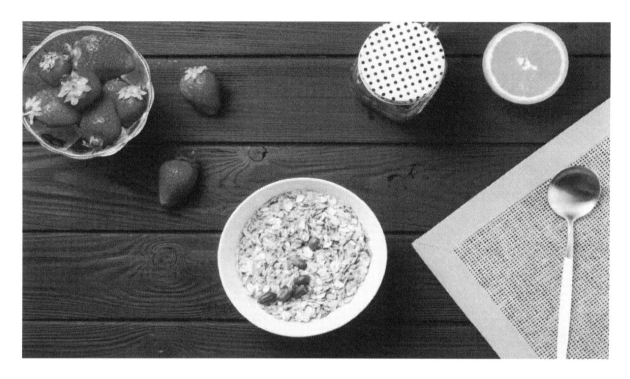

To keep the body in good health is a duty... otherwise we shall not be able to keep our mind strong and clear. –Buddha

Building lean muscle mass and achieving healthy weight gain can be important goals for those looking to improve their physical strength, athletic performance, or overall body composition. Whether you're recovering from illness, looking to support healthy aging, or simply striving to optimize your fitness, incorporating nutrient-dense foods, strength-training exercises, and targeted natural remedies into your routine can help to support muscle growth, healthy weight gain, and overall vitality.

Topical Treatments

Shatavari Gel Caps

Ingredients:

- 1/2 cup shatavari root powder
- 1/4 cup ashwagandha root powder
- 1/4 cup marshmallow root powder
- Empty gelatin or vegetarian capsules

Directions:

1. In a small bowl, mix together the shatavari root powder, ashwagandha root powder, and marshmallow root powder until well combined.

2. Fill each empty gelatin or vegetarian capsule with the herbal mixture, using a capsule filling machine or by hand.

3. Store the filled capsules in an airtight glass jar in a cool, dry place.

4. Take 2 capsules daily, preferably with food, to help support hormone balance, promote healthy muscle growth, and enhance overall vitality.

Licorice Powder Tonic

Ingredients:

- 1 teaspoon licorice root powder
- 1 cup warm water
- 1/4 teaspoon cinnamon
- Raw honey (optional)

Directions:

1. In a small saucepan, heat the water until warm but not boiling.
2. In a mug, combine the licorice root powder and cinnamon.
3. Pour the warm water over the herbs and spices, stirring to combine.
4. If desired, stir in a touch of raw honey for added sweetness and flavor.
5. Drink this licorice powder tonic once daily, preferably in the morning or before a meal, to help support healthy weight gain, reduce stress, and enhance overall physical performance.

Herbal Brews and Drinks

Bulletproof Coffee

Ingredients:

- 1 cup freshly brewed coffee
- 1 tablespoon MCT oil or coconut oil
- 1 tablespoon grass-fed, unsalted butter
- 1/4 teaspoon vanilla extract (optional)
- Pinch of cinnamon (optional)

Directions:

1. Brew a cup of high-quality coffee using your preferred method.
2. In a blender, combine the hot coffee, MCT oil or coconut oil, grass-fed butter, vanilla extract (if using), and cinnamon (if using).
3. Blend on high for 30 seconds to 1 minute, until the mixture is creamy and frothy.
4. Pour the bulletproof coffee into a mug and enjoy immediately.
5. Drink this energizing coffee blend once daily, preferably in the morning, to help support cognitive function, promote healthy weight gain, and enhance overall physical performance.

Early Morning Shot

Ingredients:

- 1/2 cup fresh spinach leaves
- 1/2 cup brewed green tea, cooled
- 1/2 ripe banana
- 1/2 teaspoon spirulina powder
- 1/4 teaspoon ginger powder
- Pinch of cayenne pepper (optional)

Directions:

1. In a high-speed blender, combine the spinach leaves, cooled green tea, banana, spirulina powder, ginger powder, and cayenne pepper (if using).
2. Blend on high until smooth and well combined.
3. Pour the mixture into a small glass or shot glass.
4. Drink this early morning shot once daily, upon waking, to help boost energy levels, promote healthy weight gain, and support overall vitality.

Herbal Brew for Weight Gain

Ingredients:

- 1 teaspoon fenugreek seeds
- 1/2 teaspoon fennel seeds
- 1/4 teaspoon ginger powder
- 1 cup water
- Raw honey (optional)

Directions:

1. In a small saucepan, combine the fenugreek seeds, fennel seeds, ginger powder, and water.
2. Bring the mixture to a boil, then reduce heat and simmer for 5-10 minutes.
3. Remove the saucepan from heat and let the herbal brew steep for an additional 5 minutes.
4. Strain the brew through a fine-mesh sieve into a mug.
5. If desired, stir in a touch of raw honey for added sweetness and flavor.
6. Drink this herbal brew once daily, preferably before a meal, to help stimulate appetite, promote healthy weight gain, and support overall well-being.

Chinese Jujube Tea

Ingredients:

- 5-6 dried Chinese jujube fruits (red dates)
- 2 cups water
- Raw honey (optional)

Directions:

1. In a small saucepan, combine the dried Chinese jujube fruits and water.
2. Bring the mixture to a boil, then reduce heat and simmer for 10-15 minutes.
3. Remove the saucepan from heat and let the tea steep for an additional 5 minutes.
4. Strain the tea through a fine-mesh sieve into a mug or teapot.
5. If desired, stir in a touch of raw honey for added sweetness and flavor.
6. Drink this Chinese jujube tea once daily, preferably in the morning or afternoon, to help promote healthy weight gain, reduce stress, and support overall physical performance.

Muscle Growth and Weight Gain Recipes

Frozen Berry Goat Yogurt Bowl

Ingredients:

- 1 cup (150g) frozen mixed berries
- 1/2 cup (120g) plain goat yogurt
- 2 tbsp (15g) sliced almonds
- 1 tbsp (10g) chia seeds
- 1 tsp (5ml) honey or maple syrup (optional)

Directions:

1. In a bowl, combine the frozen mixed berries and plain goat yogurt.
2. Top with sliced almonds, chia seeds, and a drizzle of honey or maple syrup if desired.
3. Let sit for 5 minutes to allow the frozen berries to thaw slightly.
4. Enjoy as a refreshing and nutritious yogurt bowl.

Strawberry Shortcake Oats

Ingredients:

- 1 cup (90g) rolled oats
- 1 cup (240ml) unsweetened almond milk or milk of choice
- 1 tsp (5ml) vanilla extract
- 1/4 tsp ground cinnamon
- 1 cup (150g) fresh strawberries, sliced
- 2 tbsp (15g) sliced almonds or coconut flakes
- 2 tbsp (30g) plain Greek yogurt or coconut yogurt (optional)

Directions:

1. In a small saucepan, combine the rolled oats, almond milk, vanilla extract, and ground cinnamon.
2. Cook over medium heat, stirring occasionally, until the oats have thickened and the liquid has been absorbed, about 5-7 minutes.
3. Remove from heat and transfer the oats to a bowl.
4. Top with fresh sliced strawberries, sliced almonds or coconut flakes, and a dollop of plain Greek yogurt or coconut yogurt (if desired).
5. Serve warm and enjoy this delicious strawberry shortcake-inspired oatmeal.

Chicken and Beet Bowl

Ingredients:

- 2 boneless, skinless chicken breasts
- 2 tbsp (30ml) olive oil, divided
- 1 tsp (3g) dried thyme
- Salt and pepper to taste
- 4 cups (300g) chopped kale or mixed greens
- 2 beets, peeled and diced
- 2 tbsp (30ml) balsamic vinegar
- 1 tbsp (15ml) Dijon mustard

Directions:

1. Season the chicken breasts with thyme, salt, and pepper.
2. In a skillet, heat 1 tbsp (15ml) olive oil over medium-high heat. Cook the chicken until browned and cooked through, about 6-8 minutes per side. Set aside.
3. In the same skillet, heat the remaining 1 tbsp (15ml) olive oil over medium heat.
4. Add the chopped kale or mixed greens and diced beets. Sauté for 3-4 minutes until slightly wilted.
5. In a small bowl, whisk together the balsamic vinegar and Dijon mustard.
6. Slice the cooked chicken breasts and place them over the greens and beets.
7. Drizzle the balsamic vinaigrette over the top.

Salmon and Avocado Mint and Lemon Bagels

Ingredients:

- 4 bagels, sliced in half
- 8 oz (225g) smoked salmon, torn into pieces
- 1 avocado, mashed
- 2 tbsp (30ml) fresh lemon juice
- 2 tbsp (10g) fresh mint leaves, finely chopped
- Salt and pepper to taste

Directions:

1. Toast the bagel halves until golden brown.
2. In a small bowl, combine the mashed avocado, lemon juice, chopped mint, and a pinch of salt and pepper. Mix well.
3. Spread the avocado mint mixture evenly over the toasted bagel halves.
4. Top with pieces of smoked salmon, distributing it evenly among the bagel halves.
5. If desired, you can add an extra squeeze of lemon juice over the top.
6. Serve the salmon and avocado mint and lemon bagels immediately, while the bagels are still warm.

Sundried Tomato and Herb Toasties

Ingredients:

- 8 slices of bread (sourdough or whole wheat)
- 4 oz (115g) cream cheese, softened
- 1/4 cup (35g) sundried tomatoes, chopped
- 2 tbsp (10g) fresh basil, finely chopped
- 1 tbsp (5g) fresh parsley, finely chopped
- 1 garlic clove, minced
- Salt and pepper to taste
- Butter or olive oil for cooking

Directions:

1. In a small bowl, mix together the cream cheese, chopped sundried tomatoes, fresh basil, fresh parsley, minced garlic, and a pinch of salt and pepper.
2. Spread the sundried tomato and herb mixture evenly on four slices of bread.
3. Top each with another slice of bread to form four sandwiches.
4. Heat a skillet or griddle over medium heat and melt a small amount of butter or olive oil.
5. Cook the sandwiches for 2-3 minutes per side, or until golden brown and crispy on the outside and the cheese has melted on the inside.
6. Cut the sundried tomato and herb toasties in half and serve warm.

Nutrient Boosters

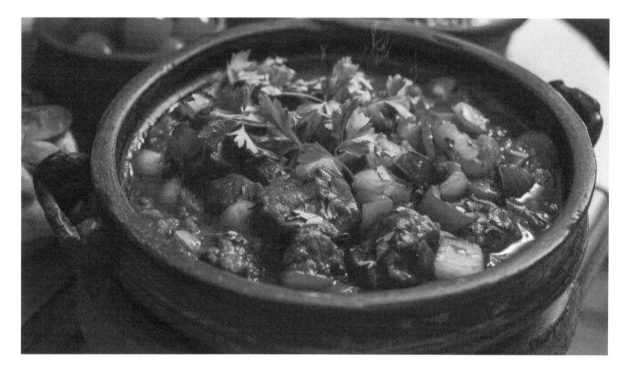

"When diet is wrong, medicine is of no use. When diet is correct, medicine is of no need." –Ayurvedic Proverb

Topical Treatments

Digestive Aloe Gel

Ingredients:

- 1/4 cup (60ml) aloe vera gel (from the inner leaf)
- 2 tbsp (30ml) freshly squeezed lemon juice
- 1 tsp (5ml) apple cider vinegar
- 1 tbsp (15ml) honey
- 1/8 tsp ground ginger

Directions:

1. Carefully extract the clear gel from an aloe vera leaf by slicing it lengthwise and scooping out the gel.
2. In a small bowl, mix together the aloe gel, lemon juice, apple cider vinegar, honey, and ground ginger until well combined.
3. Transfer the mixture to a clean jar or bottle with a lid.
4. Refrigerate the digestive aloe gel for up to one week.
5. To use, take 1-2 tbsp before meals or whenever you experience digestive discomfort.
6. The aloe gel may have a slightly bitter taste, but the lemon juice and honey help to balance the flavor.

Vitality Tonic

Ingredients:

- 1 cup (240ml) warm water
- 1 tbsp (15ml) fresh lemon juice
- 1 tbsp (15ml) apple cider vinegar
- 1 tsp (5ml) honey
- 1/2 tsp ground turmeric
- 1/4 tsp ground ginger
- Pinch of cayenne pepper (optional)
- Pinch of black pepper

Directions:

- In a mug or glass, combine the warm water, lemon juice, apple cider vinegar, honey, turmeric, ginger, cayenne pepper (if using), and black pepper.
- Stir well until the honey has fully dissolved and the ingredients are well combined.
- Drink the vitality tonic while it's still warm, or allow it to cool to your desired temperature.
- For best results, consume this tonic first thing in the morning on an empty stomach.
- The combination of ingredients is designed to support digestion, boost metabolism, and provide antioxidants for overall vitality.

Herbal Brews and Drinks

Revitalizer Juice

Ingredients:

- 1 mango, peeled and diced
- 1 cup (150g) fresh strawberries, hulled
- 1/2 cup (75g) fresh blueberries
- 1 cup (165g) fresh pineapple chunks
- 2 apples, cored and diced

Directions:

1. Add all the fruits to a blender.
2. Blend on high speed until smooth and well combined.
3. If the consistency is too thick, add a splash of water or orange juice to thin it out.
4. Taste and adjust sweetness if desired by adding honey or agave syrup.
5. Pour the health juice into glasses and serve immediately or refrigerate until ready to consume.

Morning Nutrition Shot

Ingredients:

- 4 cups (120g) loosely packed kale leaves, stems removed
- 1-inch (2.5cm) piece fresh ginger, peeled
- 2 apples, cored and quartered
- 3 celery stalks
- 1 cucumber
- 1/2 cup (15g) fresh parsley

Directions:

1. Wash all the produce thoroughly.
2. Feed the kale, ginger, apples, celery, cucumber, and parsley through a juicer, alternating between soft and hard ingredients.
3. Stir the juice well to combine.
4. If desired, you can strain the juice through a fine-mesh sieve to remove any foam or pulp.
5. Pour the fresh juice into glasses and enjoy immediately for maximum nutrient benefits.

Natural Medicine Ball Tea

Ingredients:

- 2 peppermint tea bags
- 2 peach herbal tea bags (or any fruity herbal tea)
- 1 cup (240ml) boiling water
- 1/4 cup (60ml) fresh lemon juice
- 2 tbsp (30ml) honey

Directions:

1. In a teapot or heatproof pitcher, place the peppermint and peach tea bags.
2. Pour the boiling water over the tea bags and let steep for 5 7 minutes.
3. Remove the tea bags, squeezing out any excess liquid.
4. Stir in the fresh lemon juice and honey until the honey is fully dissolved.

5. Pour the Medicine Ball Tea into mugs and enjoy while hot.

6. You can adjust the amount of honey to your desired sweetness level.

Goats Milk Morning Coffee

Ingredients:

- 4 cups (960ml) goat milk
- 1 tsp (2g) fennel seeds
- 1 tsp (2g) cumin seeds
- 3 cardamom pods
- 2 star anise pods
- 1-inch (2.5cm) piece fresh ginger, sliced
- 2 tsp (4g) licorice root powder or 1 stick of licorice root

Directions:

1. In a saucepan, combine the goat milk, fennel seeds, cumin seeds, cardamom pods, star anise pods, and sliced ginger.

2. If using licorice root powder, add it now. If using a licorice root stick, add it to the saucepan.

3. Bring the mixture to a gentle simmer over medium heat, stirring occasionally.

4. Once simmering, reduce the heat to low and let the tea steep for 10-15 minutes to allow the flavors to infuse.

5. Remove from heat and strain the tea through a fine-mesh sieve to remove the spices and ginger.

6. Serve the aromatic goat milk tea hot or allow it to cool to your desired drinking temperature.

7. You can sweeten the tea with a little honey or your preferred sweetener if desired.

Adaptogen Iced Coffee

Ingredients:

- 1 cup (240ml) strong brewed coffee, cooled
- 1 tsp (3g) ashwagandha powder
- 1 tsp (3g) reishi powder
- 1 tsp (3g) maca powder
- 1 tbsp (15ml) maple syrup or honey (optional)
- 1 cup (240ml) unsweetened almond milk or milk of choice
- Ice cubes

Directions:

1. In a blender, combine the cooled brewed coffee, ashwagandha powder, reishi powder, maca powder, and maple syrup or honey (if using).

2. Blend until the powders are fully incorporated and the mixture is smooth.

3. Add the almond milk or milk of choice and blend again briefly to combine.

4. Fill glasses with ice cubes and pour the adaptogen iced coffee over the ice.

5. Stir gently and enjoy immediately.

Nutrient Boosting Recipes

Tumeric Coconut Thai Curry

Ingredients:

- 2 tbsp (30ml) coconut oil or avocado oil
- 1 onion, diced
- 3 garlic cloves, minced
- 1 tbsp (8g) grated fresh ginger
- 2 tsp (5g) ground turmeric
- 1 tsp (3g) ground coriander
- 1 tsp (3g) ground cumin
- 1/4 tsp cayenne pepper (or to taste)
- 1 (14oz/400ml) can coconut milk
- 1 cup (240ml) vegetable or chicken broth
- 1 lb (450g) boneless, skinless chicken breasts or thighs, cut into bite-sized pieces
- 2 cups (300g) mixed vegetables (e.g., bell peppers, carrots, broccoli)
- 2 tbsp (30ml) fresh lime juice
- Salt and pepper to taste
- Chopped fresh cilantro for garnish

Directions:

1. In a large skillet or dutch oven, heat the coconut oil or avocado oil over medium heat.

2. Add the diced onion and sauté for 2-3 minutes until translucent.

3. Add the minced garlic and grated ginger, and cook for 1 more minute until fragrant.

4. Stir in the turmeric, coriander, cumin, and cayenne pepper, an

cook for another minute to toast the spices.

5. Pour in the coconut milk and vegetable or chicken broth, and bring the mixture to a simmer.

6. Add the chicken and mixed vegetables, and continue to simmer for 10-15 minutes, or until the chicken is cooked through and the

vegetables are tender.

7. Remove from heat and stir in the fresh lime juice. Season with salt and pepper to taste.

8. Garnish with chopped fresh cilantro before serving.

9. Serve hot over steamed rice or cauliflower rice.

Goats Cheese Salad

Ingredients:

- 4 cups (120g) mixed greens or arugula
- 1 pear or apple, thinly sliced
- 1/4 cup (30g) toasted walnuts
- 4 oz (115g) goat cheese, crumbled
- 2 tbsp (30ml) olive oil
- 2 tbsp (30ml) balsamic vinegar
- 1 tsp (5ml) honey or maple syrup
- Salt and pepper to taste

Directions:

1. In a large bowl, combine the mixed greens or arugula, sliced pear or apple, toasted walnuts, and crumbled goat cheese.

2. In a small bowl, whisk together the olive oil, balsamic vinegar, honey or maple syrup, and a pinch of salt and pepper to make the dressing.

3. Drizzle the dressing over the salad and toss gently to coat all the ingredients.

4. Serve the goat cheese salad immediately, or refrigerate until ready to serve.

Pan-Fried Feta

Ingredients:

- 8 oz (225g) feta cheese, cut into 1/2-inch thick slices
- 1/2 cup (60g) all-purpose flour or gluten-free flour
- 2 eggs, beaten
- 1 cup (80g) panko breadcrumbs or gluten-free breadcrumbs
- 1/4 cup (30g) grated Parmesan cheese
- 1 tsp (3g) dried oregano
- 1/2 tsp (1.5g) garlic powder
- Salt and pepper to taste
- 2 tbsp (30ml) olive oil or avocado oil for frying

Directions:

1. Set up three shallow bowls: one with flour, one with beaten eggs, and one with panko breadcrumbs mixed with grated Parmesan, dried oregano, garlic powder, salt, and pepper.

2. Dredge the feta slices in the flour, dip them in the beaten eggs, and then coat them with the seasoned breadcrumb mixture, pressing gently to adhere.

3. Heat the olive oil or avocado oil in a large skillet over medium-high heat.

4. Working in batches, pan-fry the breaded feta slices for 2-3 minutes per side, or until golden brown and crispy.

5. Transfer the pan-fried feta to a paper towel-lined plate to drain any excess oil.

6. Serve the pan-fried feta warm, with a drizzle of honey or your favorite dipping sauce on the side.

Fennel and Olive Moroccan Stew

Ingredients:

- 2 tbsp (30ml) olive oil
- 1 large onion, diced
- 4 cloves garlic, minced
- 1 fennel bulb, sliced (reserve fronds for garnish)
- 2 tsp (5g) ground cumin
- 1 tsp (3g) ground coriander
- 1 tsp (3g) paprika
- 1/2 tsp ground cinnamon
- 1/4 tsp cayenne pepper (or to taste)
- 1 (14oz/400g) can diced tomatoes
- 2 cups (480ml) vegetable or chicken broth
- 1 (15oz/425g) can chickpeas, drained and rinsed
- 1 cup (150g) green olives, pitted
- Salt and pepper to taste
- Chopped fresh parsley for garnish

Directions:

1. In a large pot or dutch oven, heat olive oil over medium heat.

2. Add the diced onion and sauté for 2-3 minutes until translucent.

3. Add the minced garlic and sliced fennel, and cook for 2 more

minutes.

4. Stir in the cumin, coriander, paprika, cinnamon, and cayenne pepper until fragrant, about 1 minute.

5. Pour in the diced tomatoes with their juices and the vegetable or chicken broth.

6. Add the chickpeas and green olives.

7. Season with salt and pepper to taste.

8. Bring the stew to a simmer and cook for 15-20 minutes, until the fennel is tender.

9. Adjust seasoning if needed.

10. Garnish with chopped fresh parsley and reserved fennel fronds before serving.

Coriander Chili Curry

Ingredients:

- 2 tbsp (30ml) coconut oil or vegetable oil
- 1 onion, diced
- 4 cloves garlic, minced
- 2 tbsp (16g) grated fresh ginger
- 2 tbsp (16g) ground coriander
- 2 tsp (5g) ground cumin
- 1 tsp (3g) paprika
- 1 tsp (3g) garam masala
- 1-2 tsp (3-6g) chili powder or cayenne pepper, to taste
- 1 (14oz/400ml) can diced tomatoes
- 1 (13.5oz/400ml) can coconut milk
- 1 lb (450g) boneless, skinless chicken thighs or breasts, cut into bite-sized pieces
- 1 cup (150g) diced potatoes
- Salt and pepper to taste
- Chopped fresh cilantro for garnish

Directions:

1. In a large skillet or pot, heat the coconut oil or vegetable oil over medium heat.

2. Add the diced onion and sauté for 2-3 minutes until translucent.

3. Add the minced garlic and grated ginger, and cook for 1 more minute until fragrant.

4. Stir in the ground coriander, cumin, paprika, garam masala, and chili powder or cayenne pepper to taste. Cook for 1 minute to toast the spices.

5. Pour in the diced tomatoes with their juices and the coconut milk. Bring to a simmer.

6. Add the chicken and diced potatoes, and season with salt and pepper to taste.

7. Reduce heat to low, cover, and simmer for 20-25 minutes, until chicken is cooked through and potatoes are tender.

8. Adjust seasoning if needed and garnish with chopped fresh cilantro before serving.

9. Serve over basmati rice or naan bread.

Oral Health

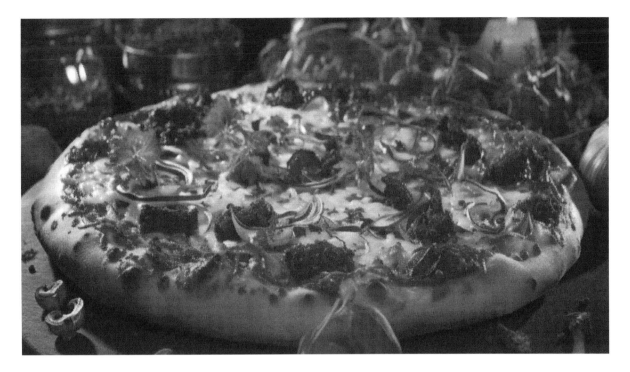

"A smile is the prettiest thing you can wear." –Unknown

Oral health is an essential component of overall well-being, playing a crucial role in our ability to eat, speak, and express ourselves with confidence. Poor oral hygiene can lead to a range of issues, from cavities and gum disease to systemic inflammation and chronic health problems. Incorporating natural, holistic practices and remedies into our daily oral care routines can help prevent dental issues, promote healthy gums and teeth, and maintain a vibrant, beautiful smile for years to come.

Topical Treatments

Herbal Mouthwash

Ingredients:

- 1 cup (240ml) distilled water
- 1/4 cup (60ml) vodka or witch hazel (as a preservative)
- 2 tbsp (30ml) vegetable glycerin
- 1 tsp (5ml) salt
- 10 drops peppermint essential oil
- 5 drops tea tree essential oil
- 5 drops clove essential oil

Directions:

1. In a small saucepan, heat the distilled water until just simmering, then remove from heat and allow to cool slightly.

2. In a glass jar or bottle, combine the vodka or witch hazel, vegetable glycerin, salt, peppermint essential oil, tea tree essential oil, and clove essential oil.

3. Pour the slightly cooled distilled water into the jar and stir well to combine all ingredients.

4. Use a funnel or pour carefully to transfer the mouthwash into a clean, airtight bottle or container.

5. To use, take a small amount into your mouth, swish around for 30 seconds to 1 minute, and spit out. Do not swallow.

6. Store the herbal mouthwash at room temperature, away from direct sunlight, for up to 6 months.

Homemade Natural Toothpaste

Ingredients:

- 1/2 cup (120g) coconut oil, softened
- 2-3 tbsp (20-30g) baking soda
- 1 tsp (5ml) salt
- 10-15 drops peppermint essential oil (or essential oil of your choice)

Directions:

1. In a small bowl, combine the softened coconut oil and baking soda. Mix well until a smooth paste forms.
2. Add the salt and peppermint essential oil (or your preferred essential oil), and stir to incorporate.
3. If the toothpaste is too thick, you can add a little water to thin it out to your desired consistency.
4. Transfer the homemade toothpaste to a clean, airtight container.
5. To use, apply a small amount to your toothbrush and brush as usual.
6. Store the natural toothpaste at room temperature, away from direct sunlight, for up to 6 months.

Herbal Teething Gum Cream

Ingredients:

- 1/4 cup (60ml) coconut oil
- 2 tbsp (30ml) olive oil
- 1 tbsp (15ml) beeswax pellets
- 10 drops chamomile essential oil
- 5 drops clove essential oil
- 5 drops lavender essential oil

Directions:

- In a double boiler or a heat-safe bowl placed over a saucepan of simmering water, melt the coconut oil, olive oil, and beeswax pellets together, stirring occasionally until fully combined and liquefied.
- Remove the mixture from heat and let it cool slightly, about 2-3 minutes.
- Add the chamomile, clove, and lavender essential oils, and stir well to incorporate.
- Carefully pour the herbal gum cream into a clean, airtight container or small jar.
- Allow the cream to cool and solidify completely before use.
- To use, gently massage a small amount of the cream onto your baby's gums with a clean finger, as needed for teething relief.
- Store the herbal teething gum cream at room temperature, away from direct sunlight, for up to 6 months.

Herbal Brews and Drinks

Gum Health Juice

Ingredients:

- 2 large cucumbers
- 4 celery stalks
- 1 bunch radishes (around 10-12)
- 1 bunch parsley
- 2-inch piece of fresh ginger, peeled

Directions:

1. Wash the cucumbers, celery stalks, radishes, parsley, and peel the ginger.
2. Roughly chop the ingredients into smaller pieces for easier juicing.
3. Feed the chopped ingredients through a juicer, alternating between soft and hard ingredients.
4. Stir the juice well to combine all the flavors.
5. If desired, strain the juice through a fine-mesh sieve to remove any foam or pulp.
6. Pour the fresh juice into a glass and enjoy immediately for maximum nutrient benefits.

Toothache Clove Tea

Ingredients:

- 1/2 cup (120ml) fresh aloe vera gel (from the inner leaf)
- 1 cup (165g) diced honeydew melon
- 1/4 cup (60ml) fresh lime juice
- 1 cup (240ml) coconut water

Directions:

1. Carefully extract the clear gel from an aloe vera leaf by slicing it lengthwise and scooping out the gel.
2. In a blender, combine the fresh aloe vera gel, diced honeydew melon, fresh lime juice, and coconut water.
3. Blend on high speed until smooth and well-combined.
4. If desired, strain the juice through a fine-mesh sieve to remove any foam or pulp.
5. Pour the refreshing aloe, honeydew, lime, and coconut water juice into glasses and serve chilled.

Aloe Plaque Destroyer

Ingredients:

- 1/4 cup (60ml) fresh aloe vera gel (from the inner leaf)
- 1/4 cup (60ml) raw honey
- 4 cups (960ml) filtered cold water
- 1/2 cup (120ml) fresh lemon juice
- Fresh mint leaves for garnish (optional)

Directions:

1. Carefully extract the clear gel from an aloe vera leaf by slicing it lengthwise and scooping out the gel.
2. In a large pitcher or jar, combine the fresh aloe vera gel, raw honey, filtered cold water, and fresh lemon juice.
3. Stir well until the honey is fully dissolved.
4. Taste and adjust the sweetness or tartness to your preference by adding more honey or lemon juice.
5. Add fresh mint leaves to the pitcher for extra flavor and aroma, if desired.
6. Serve the aloe lemonade over ice, garnished with a mint sprig or lemon slice.

Aloe Charcoal Tooth Whitener

Ingredients:

- 1/4 cup (60ml) fresh aloe vera gel (from the inner leaf)
- 2 tbsp (16g) activated charcoal powder
- 1 tsp (5ml) coconut oil
- 1 tsp (5ml) baking soda
- 5-10 drops of peppermint essential oil (optional)

Directions:

- Carefully extract the clear gel from an aloe vera leaf by slicing it lengthwise and scooping out the gel.
- In a small bowl, mix together the fresh aloe vera gel, activated charcoal powder, coconut oil, and baking soda until well combined into a smooth paste.
- If desired, add 5-10 drops of peppermint essential oil for a refreshing minty flavor.
- To use, dip your toothbrush into the mixture and gently brush your teeth for 1-2 minutes, paying extra attention to any stained or discolored areas.
- Spit out the mixture and rinse your mouth thoroughly with water.
- Store any remaining tooth whitener in an airtight container in the refrigerator for up to 1 week.

Oral Health Recipes

Loaded Sweet Potato Soup

Ingredients:

- 1 medium butternut squash, peeled, seeded, and cubed
- 2 large sweet potatoes, peeled and cubed
- 2 tablespoons coconut oil
- 1 onion, diced
- 2 cloves garlic, minced
- 1 teaspoon ground cumin
- 1 teaspoon ground coriander
- 1/2 teaspoon ground ginger
- 4 cups vegetable or chicken broth
- 1 (13.5 oz) can full-fat coconut milk
- Salt and pepper, to taste
- Chopped fresh cilantro for garnish

Directions:

1. In a large pot or Dutch oven, melt the coconut oil over medium heat.
2. Add the diced onion and sauté for 2-3 minutes until translucent.
3. Add the minced garlic, cumin, coriander, and ginger. Cook for 1 minute, stirring frequently.
4. Add the cubed squash, sweet potatoes, and broth. Bring to a boil.
5. Reduce heat to low, cover, and simmer for 20-25 minutes, or until the squash and sweet potatoes are tender.
6. Remove from heat and puree the soup using an immersion blender or a regular blender (in batches if needed).
7. Stir in the coconut milk and season with salt and pepper to taste.
8. Garnish with chopped fresh cilantro before serving.

Grain-Free Pizzas

Ingredients (for the crust):

- 1 cup (120g) almond flour
- 1/2 cup (60g) tapioca flour
- 1 teaspoon baking powder
- 1/2 teaspoon salt

Toppings of your choice (e.g., tomato sauce, cheese, veggies, etc.)

- 2 large eggs
- 2 tablespoons olive oil
- 2 tablespoons water

Directions:

1. Preheat the oven to 400°F (200°C). Line a baking sheet with parchment paper.
2. In a bowl, whisk together the almond flour, tapioca flour, baking powder, and salt.
3. In another bowl, beat the eggs, olive oil, and water together.
4. Pour the wet ingredients into the dry ingredients and stir until a dough forms.
5. Divide the dough into two equal portions and shape each into a flat circle or rectangle on the prepared baking sheet.
6. Bake the crusts for 10-12 minutes until lightly golden brown.
7. Remove the crusts from the oven and top with your desired toppings.
8. Return to the oven and bake for an additional 8-10 minutes, or until the toppings are heated through and any cheese has melted

Pecan Butter Ice Cream Brie and Strawberry Bits

Ingredients:

- 1 cup (240ml) unsweetened almond milk
- 1/2 cup (125g) pecan butter
- 1/4 cup (60ml) maple syrup
- 1 teaspoon vanilla extract
- 1/4 teaspoon salt

Directions:

1. In a blender, combine the unsweetened almond milk, pecan butter, maple syrup, vanilla extract, and salt. Blend until smooth and well combined.
2. Pour the mixture into an ice cream maker and churn according to
the manufacturer's Directions.
3. Once the ice cream has reached your desired consistency, transfer it to an airtight container and freeze for at least 2 hours before serving.

Crunchy Fruit Salad

Ingredients:

- 2 apples, cored and diced
- 2 pears, cored and diced
- 1 cup (150g) fresh blueberries
- 1 cup (150g) fresh raspberries
- 1/2 cup (70g) chopped pecans or walnuts
- 1/4 cup (30g) unsweetened shredded coconut
- 2 tablespoons (30ml) fresh lemon juice
- 1 tablespoon (15ml) honey (optional)

Directions:

1. In a large bowl, gently toss together the diced apples, diced pears, blueberries, and raspberries.
2. Add the chopped pecans or walnuts and shredded coconut to the fruit mixture.
3. Drizzle the fresh lemon juice over the salad and gently toss to coat.
4. If desired, add a tablespoon of honey to the salad for a touch of sweetness.
5. Serve the crunchy fruit salad chilled or at room temperature.

Skin Health

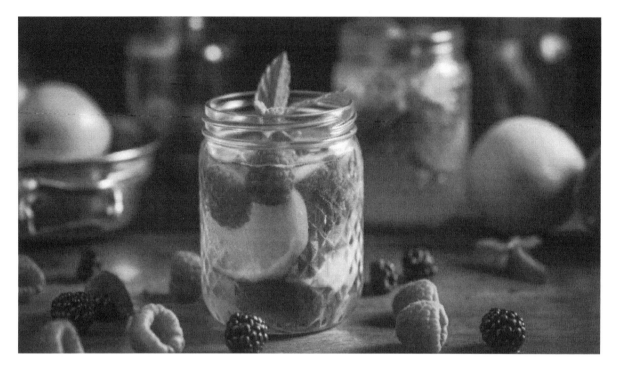

"Your skin is your friend. You like your skin. Your skin likes you. It protects you from the elements and literally keeps you together. You in turn do your best to protect it from any kind of damage. "–Zakiya Kassam

The skin is our body's largest organ, serving as a protective barrier against the environment and playing a crucial role in our overall health and well-being. From exposure to sun damage and pollution to the effects of stress and hormonal changes, our skin faces numerous challenges that can lead to premature aging, dryness, and various skin conditions. Nourishing our skin with gentle, natural ingredients and adopting a holistic skincare routine helps maintain a healthy, radiant complexion and promote resilient, youthful-looking skin.

Topical Treatments

Green Tea Facial Toner

Ingredients:

- 1/2 cup (120ml) brewed green tea, cooled
- 1/4 cup (60ml) witch hazel
- 1 tablespoon (15ml) apple cider vinegar
- 1 teaspoon (5ml) vegetable glycerin (optional)

Directions:

1. Brew a strong cup of green tea and allow it to cool completely.
2. In a clean bottle or container, combine the cooled green tea, witch hazel, and apple cider vinegar.
3. If using, add the vegetable glycerin, which can help hydrate and soften the skin.
4. Close the container and shake well to combine all the ingredients.
5. To use, apply the green tea toner to a cotton pad and gently wipe over your face and neck after cleansing.
6. Store the remaining toner in the refrigerator for up to 2 weeks.

Natural Avocado Skin Mask

Ingredients:

- 1 ripe avocado, mashed
- 2 tablespoons (30ml) plain yogurt
- 1 tablespoon (15ml) honey
- 1 teaspoon (5ml) lemon juice

Directions:

1. In a small bowl, mash the avocado until it forms a smooth paste.
2. Add the plain yogurt, honey, and lemon juice to the mashed avocado.
3. Mix all the ingredients together until well combined and smooth.
4. Apply the avocado mask evenly to your clean face, avoiding the eye area.
5. Leave the mask on for 15-20 minutes, allowing the nourishing ingredients to absorb into your skin.
6. Rinse off the mask with lukewarm water and gently pat your face dry.
7. Follow up with your regular moisturizer.

Rosewater Facial Mist

Ingredients:

- 1/2 cup (120ml) pure rosewater
- 1/4 cup (60ml) distilled water
- 1 tablespoon (15ml) vegetable glycerin (optional)
- 2-3 drops of vitamin E oil (optional)

Directions:

1. In a clean spray bottle, combine the pure rosewater and distilled water.
2. If using, add the vegetable glycerin, which can help hydrate and soften the skin, and the vitamin E oil, which provides antioxidant benefits.
3. Close the spray bottle and shake gently to mix the ingredients.
4. To use, mist the rosewater facial mist over your clean face and neck after cleansing or anytime you need a refreshing boost of hydration.
5. Allow the mist to absorb into your skin before applying any other skincare products.
6. Store the remaining facial mist in the refrigerator for up to 2 weeks.

Cucumber and Yogurt Face Mask

Ingredients:

- 1/2 cucumber, peeled and grated
- 1/2 cup (120g) plain Greek yogurt
- 1 tablespoon (15ml) honey
- 1 teaspoon (5ml) lemon juice

Directions:

1. In a small bowl, combine the grated cucumber, plain Greek yogurt, honey, and lemon juice. Mix well until all the ingredients are fully incorporated.
2. Gently apply the cucumber and yogurt face mask mixture evenly over your clean, dry face, avoiding the eye area.
3. Leave the mask on for 15-20 minutes, allowing the cooling and hydrating properties of the ingredients to work their magic.
4. Rinse off the mask with lukewarm water, using gentle circular motions to remove any residue.
5. Pat your face dry with a clean towel.
6. Follow up with your regular moisturizer or serum.

Sea Salt Scalp Scrub

Ingredients:

- 1/2 cup (120g) coarse sea salt
- 1/4 cup (60ml) coconut oil, melted
- 10-15 drops of essential oil (optional, such as lavender, rosemary, or peppermint)

Directions:

- In a small bowl, combine the coarse sea salt and melted coconut oil. Mix well until the salt is fully coated with the oil.
- If desired, add 10-15 drops of your favorite essential oil for added benefits and aroma.
- Before shampooing, section your hair and apply the sea salt scalp scrub directly to your scalp using your fingertips.
- Gently massage the scrub into your scalp for 2-3 minutes, paying extra attention to any areas with buildup or flakiness.
- Rinse thoroughly with warm water, making sure to remove all the salt and oil from your hair and scalp.
- Follow up with your regular shampoo and conditioner routine.

Herbal Brews and Drinks

Glowing Skin Tea

Ingredients:

- 1 tbsp (3g) dried chamomile flowers
- 1 tbsp (3g) dried jasmine flowers
- 1 tsp (2g) dried dandelion root
- 1 tsp (2g) dried peppermint leaves
- 1 cup (240ml) boiling water

Directions:

1. In a teapot or heat-safe vessel, combine the dried chamomile flowers, jasmine flowers, dandelion root, and peppermint leaves.
2. Pour the boiling water over the herbs.
3. Cover and let the tea steep for 5-7 minutes.
4. Strain the tea into cups, discarding the loose herbs.
5. Enjoy the tea hot or allow it to cool to your desired temperature.

Oily Skin Neutralizing Tea

Ingredients:

- 1 tsp (2g) shatavari root powder
- 1 tsp (3g) ground turmeric
- 1 cinnamon stick
- 1-inch (2.5cm) piece of fresh ginger, sliced
- 4 cardamom pods, lightly crushed
- 1/4 tsp (1g) black pepper
- 1 cup (240ml) boiling water

Directions:

1. In a small saucepan, combine the shatavari root powder, turmeric, cinnamon stick, sliced ginger, crushed cardamom pods, and black pepper.
2. Pour the boiling water over the spices and herbs.
3. Let the mixture simmer on low heat for 5-7 minutes, allowing the flavors to infuse.
4. Remove from heat, cover, and let the tea steep for an additional 3-5 minutes.
5. Strain the tea into a cup or teapot, discarding the loose herbs and spices.
6. Enjoy the tea hot or allow it to cool to your desired temperature.

Balanced Skin Tea

Ingredients:

- 1 tsp (2g) dried dandelion root
- 1 tsp (2g) dried nettle leaf
- 1 tsp (2g) dried burdock root
- 1 tsp (3g) dried chamomile flowers
- 1 tsp (3g) dried schizandra berries
- 1 cup (240ml) boiling water

Directions:

1. In a teapot or heat-safe vessel, combine the dried dandelion root, nettle leaf, burdock root, chamomile flowers, and schizandra berries.
2. Pour the boiling water over the herbs.
3. Cover and let the tea steep for 10-12 minutes to allow the herbs to fully infuse their flavors and beneficial compounds.
4. Strain the tea into cups, discarding the loose herbs.
5. Enjoy the tea hot or allow it to cool to your desired temperature

Skin Detox Juice

Ingredients:

- 2 medium beetroots, roughly chopped
- 2 oranges, peeled
- 3 carrots, roughly chopped
- 1 red apple, cored and quartered
- 1 cucumber, roughly chopped
- 3 celery stalks, roughly chopped

Directions:

1. Feed the chopped beetroots, oranges, carrots, red apple, cucumber, and celery through a juicer, alternating between soft and hard ingredients.
2. Stir the juice well to combine the flavors.
3. If desired, strain the juice through a fine-mesh sieve to remove any foam or pulp.
4. Pour the fresh juice into glasses and enjoy immediately for maximum nutrient benefits.

Golden Glow Shots

Ingredients:

- 3 large carrots, roughly chopped
- 1 cup (165g) fresh pineapple chunks
- 1 mango, peeled and chopped
- 2 oranges, peeled
- 1-inch (2.5cm) piece of fresh turmeric, peeled
- 1 lime, juiced

Directions:

1. In a blender, combine the chopped carrots, pineapple chunks, chopped mango, oranges, and fresh turmeric.
2. Add the freshly squeezed lime juice.
3. Blend on high speed until completely smooth and liquified.
4. If desired, strain the mixture through a fine-mesh sieve to remove any foam or pulp.
5. Pour the health shot into shot glasses or small glasses.
6. Drink immediately for a nutrient-packed and refreshing boost.

Hibiscus Sun Tea

Ingredients:

- 2 cups (480ml) boiling water
- 4 hibiscus tea bags or 4 tbsp (12g) loose hibiscus tea
- 1 orange, juiced (about 1/2 cup or 120ml)
- 2 tbsp (30ml) agave nectar or honey

Directions:

1. In a teapot or heat-safe pitcher, steep the hibiscus tea bags or loose tea in the boiling water for 5-7 minutes.
2. Remove the tea bags or strain out the loose tea leaves.
3. Stir in the freshly squeezed orange juice and agave nectar or honey until fully combined.
4. Allow the cocktail to cool to your desired drinking temperature.
5. Pour the hibiscus tea, orange, and agave morning cocktail into glasses filled with ice cubes.
6. Garnish with orange slices or mint leaves, if desired.

Skin Health Recipes

Skin Rich Breakfast Recipe

Ingredients:

- 1/2 cup (80g) fresh or frozen blueberries
- 1/2 avocado, mashed
- 1 tablespoon (15ml) flaxseed oil
- 1 tablespoon (15ml) honey
- 1 tablespoon (7g) chia seeds
- 1/2 cup (120g) plain Greek yogurt
- 1/4 cup (30g) sliced almonds

Directions:

1. In a small bowl, mash the avocado until smooth.
2. Add the flaxseed oil, honey, and chia seeds to the mashed avocado and mix well.
3. Gently fold in the Greek yogurt until well combined.
4. Layer the avocado mixture with the fresh or frozen blueberries in a bowl or jar.
5. Top with sliced almonds.
6. Enjoy this skin-rich breakfast recipe immediately or refrigerate until ready to serve.

Sesame Tuna Salad

Ingredients:

- 2 (5 oz) cans tuna, drained
- 1/4 cup (40g) diced red onion
- 2 tablespoons (30ml) sesame oil
- 2 tablespoons (30ml) rice vinegar
- 1 tablespoon (15ml) soy sauce
- 1 tablespoon (15ml) sesame seeds
- 1/4 cup (35g) diced celery
- Salt and pepper to taste

Directions:

1. In a medium bowl, combine the drained tuna, diced red onion, sesame oil, rice vinegar, soy sauce, and sesame seeds.
2. Gently mix in the diced celery.
3. Season with salt and pepper to taste.
4. Serve the sesame tuna salad chilled or at room temperature on a bed of greens or in a sandwich.

Baby Kale Salad with Strawberry Dressing

Baby Kale Salad with Strawberry Dressing

Ingredients for the Salad:

- 5 cups (100g) baby kale or mixed greens
- 1 cup (150g) fresh strawberries, sliced

Ingredients for the Strawberry Dressing:

- 1/2 cup (75g) fresh strawberries
- 2 tablespoons (30ml) olive oil
- 1 tablespoon (15ml) balsamic vinegar
- 1/4 cup (30g) sliced almonds
- 1/4 cup (30g) crumbled feta cheese

- 1 tablespoon (15ml) honey
- Salt and pepper to taste

Directions:

1. In a blender or food processor, combine all the ingredients for the strawberry dressing (strawberries, olive oil, balsamic vinegar, honey, salt, and pepper). Blend until smooth and well combined.
2. In a large salad bowl, combine the baby kale or mixed greens, sliced strawberries, sliced almonds, and crumbled feta cheese.
3. Drizzle the strawberry dressing over the salad and gently toss to coat the greens evenly.
4. Serve the baby kale salad with strawberry dressing immediately or refrigerate until ready to serve.

Strawberry and Cheese Salad

Ingredients:

- 1 lb (450g) fresh strawberries, hulled and sliced
- 1 head of romaine lettuce, chopped
- 1/2 cup (60g) crumbled feta cheese

For the Vinaigrette:

- 1/4 cup (60ml) olive oil
- 2 tablespoons (30ml) balsamic vinegar
- 1/2 cup (60g) toasted pecans or walnuts
- 1/4 cup (30g) thinly sliced red onion

- 1 tablespoon (15ml) honey
- Salt and pepper to taste

Directions:

1. In a large salad bowl, combine the sliced strawberries, chopped romaine lettuce, crumbled feta cheese, toasted pecans or walnuts, and sliced red onion.
2. In a small bowl or jar, whisk together the ingredients for the vinaigrette (olive oil, balsamic vinegar, honey, salt, and pepper) until well combined.
3. Drizzle the vinaigrette over the salad and gently toss to coat the ingredients evenly.
4. Serve the strawberry and cheese salad immediately or refrigerate until ready to serve.

Sleep Improvement

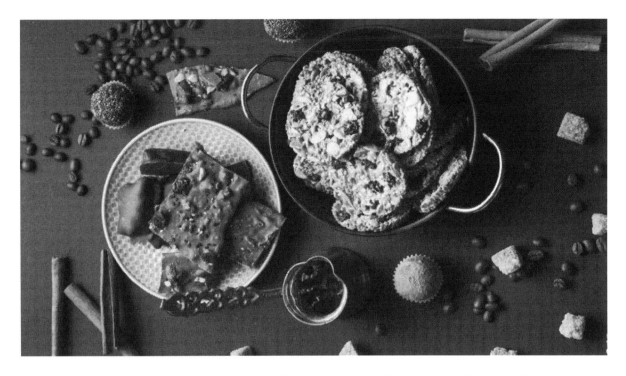

"Sleep is the golden chain that ties health and our bodies together." –Thomas Dekker

Quality sleep is essential for our physical, mental, and emotional well-being, playing a vital role in our ability to heal, regenerate, and function optimally. In today's fast-paced, often stressful world, many people struggle with sleep issues, from difficulty falling asleep to restless nights and daytime fatigue. By incorporating natural sleep-supportive remedies, creating a soothing bedtime routine, and adopting healthy sleep habits, we can help to improve the quality and quantity of our sleep, promoting better overall health and vitality.

Topical Treatments

Valerian Root Tincture

Ingredients:
- 1/2 cup (60g) dried valerian root
- 1 cup (240ml) vodka or brandy (80-proof or higher)

Directions:
1. Place the dried valerian root in a clean glass jar or bottle with a tight-fitting lid.
2. Pour the vodka or brandy over the valerian root, ensuring that the root is fully submerged.
3. Seal the jar or bottle tightly and give it a gentle shake.
4. Store the jar in a cool, dark place and shake it once a day for 4-6 weeks.
5. After the steeping period, strain the tincture through a cheesecloth or fine-mesh strainer to remove the valerian root.
6. Transfer the strained tincture into a clean, dark-colored bottle with a dropper or lid.
7. To use, take 1-2 droppers full (about 30-60 drops) of the valerian root tincture as needed, up to 30 minutes before bedtime.

Deep Sleep Pillow Spray

Ingredients:

- 1/2 cup (120ml) distilled water
- 2 tablespoons (30ml) witch hazel
- 10 drops lavender essential oil
- 5 drops chamomile essential oil
- 5 drops clary sage essential oil

Directions:

1. In a small spray bottle, combine the distilled water and witch hazel.
2. Add the lavender, chamomile, and clary sage essential oils.
3. Secure the spray bottle lid and gently shake to mix the ingredients.
4. To use, lightly mist your pillow and bedding with the deep sleep spray 10-15 minutes before bedtime.
5. The calming aromas of the essential oils can help promote relaxation and better sleep.

Jasmine Bath and Foot Soak

Ingredients:

- 1/2 cup (120ml) Epsom salts
- 1/4 cup (60ml) dried jasmine buds or petals
- 2 tablespoons (30ml) coconut oil or olive oil
- 10 drops lavender essential oil (optional)

Directions:

- In a large bowl or foot basin, combine the Epsom salts and dried jasmine buds or petals.
- Add the coconut or olive oil and lavender essential oil (if using).
- Fill a bathtub or foot basin with warm water, and add the jasmine salt mixture.
- Stir the water gently to help dissolve the salts and distribute the oils and jasmine.
- Soak your feet or immerse yourself in the jasmine bath for 20-30 minutes, allowing the calming aromas and minerals to work their magic.
- After soaking, pat your skin dry and follow up with a moisturizer or body oil if desired.

Herbal Brews and Drinks

Nutmeg Plant Milk

Ingredients:

- 1 cup (150g) raw cashews, soaked in water for 4-6 hours and drained
- 4 cups (960ml) filtered water
- 1/4 tsp ground nutmeg
- 1 tsp vanilla extract
- 2-3 dates or 1-2 tbsp maple syrup (optional, for sweetening)

Directions:

1. In a high-speed blender, combine the soaked cashews, filtered water, ground nutmeg, and vanilla extract.
2. If you want a sweetened nutmeg milk, add 2-3 dates or 1-2 tbsp of maple syrup.
3. Blend on high speed for 1-2 minutes until the mixture is smooth and creamy.
4. Strain the mixture through a nut milk bag or a fine-mesh strainer to remove any remaining solids.
5. Transfer the nutmeg plant milk to an airtight bottle or jar and refrigerate for up to 5 days.
6. Shake well before serving and enjoy chilled or warm.

Lavender Chamomile Blend Tea

Ingredients:

- 1 tbsp (4g) dried lavender buds
- 1 tbsp (3g) dried chamomile flowers
- 1 cup (240ml) boiling water

Directions:

1. In a teapot or heat-safe mug, combine the dried lavender buds and chamomile flowers.
2. Pour the boiling water over the herbs and let it steep for 5-7 minutes.
3. Strain the tea into a cup or remove the tea infuser.
4. Add honey or lemon if desired.
5. Enjoy the calming lavender chamomile blend tea hot or iced.

Deep Sleep Tea

Ingredients:

- 1 tsp (2g) dried valerian root
- 1 tsp (2g) dried passionflower
- 1 tsp (2g) dried lemon balm
- 1 cup (240ml) boiling water

Directions:

1. In a teapot or heat-safe mug, combine the dried valerian root, passionflower, and lemon balm.
2. Pour the boiling water over the herbs and let it steep for 10-15 minutes.
3. Strain the tea into a cup or remove the tea infuser.
4. Add honey or lemon if desired.
5. Drink the deep sleep tea about 30 minutes before bedtime to promote relaxation and better sleep.

Lemongrass Warm Brew

Ingredients:

- 4 stalks fresh lemongrass, bruised or sliced
- 4 cups (960ml) water
- Honey or stevia to taste (optional)

Directions:

1. In a saucepan, combine the fresh lemongrass stalks and water.
2. Bring the mixture to a boil over high heat.
3. Once boiling, reduce the heat to low and let it simmer for 10-15 minutes, allowing the lemongrass to infuse its flavor.
4. Remove the saucepan from heat and let it steep for an additional 5-10 minutes.
5. Strain the lemongrass warm brew into mugs or a serving pitcher, discarding the lemongrass stalks.
6. Add honey or stevia to sweeten if desired.
7. Serve the lemongrass warm brew hot or let it cool to room temperature before refrigerating and serving over ice.

Sleep Improvement Recipes

Bedtime Bowl

Ingredients:

- 1/2 cup (120g) plain Greek yogurt
- 1 banana, sliced
- 1 tbsp (10g) chia seeds
- 1 tbsp (10g) hemp seeds
- 1 tsp (3g) ground cinnamon
- 1 tsp (5ml) honey or maple syrup (optional)

Directions:

1. In a bowl, combine the plain Greek yogurt and sliced banana.
2. Sprinkle the chia seeds, hemp seeds, and ground cinnamon over the top.
3. Drizzle with honey or maple syrup if you prefer a sweeter taste.
4. Gently mix the ingredients together until well combined.
5. Cover the bowl and refrigerate for at least 30 minutes to allow the chia seeds to soften and absorb the flavors.
6. Enjoy the Bedtime Bowl chilled or at room temperature before going to bed.

Nightcap Oats

Ingredients:

- 1/2 cup (40g) old-fashioned rolled oats
- 1 cup (240ml) unsweetened almond milk or milk of choice
- 1 tbsp (10g) ground flaxseeds or chia seeds
- 1 tsp (3g) vanilla extract
- 1/4 tsp ground nutmeg
- 1 tbsp (15ml) honey or maple syrup (optional)

Directions:

1. In a small saucepan, combine the rolled oats, almond milk, ground flaxseeds or chia seeds, vanilla extract, and ground nutmeg.
2. Cook over medium heat, stirring frequently, until the mixture thickens and the oats are fully cooked, about 5-7 minutes.
3. Remove from heat and stir in honey or maple syrup if desired.
4. Transfer the Nightcap Oats to a bowl and let cool slightly before enjoying.
5. Serve warm or at room temperature as a comforting bedtime snack.

Serene Sleep Smoothie

Ingredients:

- 1 banana, frozen
- 1/2 cup (120ml) unsweetened almond milk or milk of choice
- 1 tbsp (10g) almond butter or peanut butter
- 1 tsp (3g) ground cinnamon
- 1/4 tsp ground nutmeg
- 1 tsp (5ml) honey or maple syrup (optional)

Directions:

1. In a blender, combine the frozen banana, almond milk, almond butter or peanut butter, ground cinnamon, and ground nutmeg.
2. If desired, add honey or maple syrup for a touch of sweetness.
3. Blend on high speed until smooth and creamy.
4. Pour the Serene Sleep Smoothie into a glass and enjoy before bedtime.
5. The combination of nutrients and warm spices in this smoothie may help promote relaxation and better sleep.

Raw Cherry Chocolate Sleep Bars

Ingredients:

- 1 cup (140g) raw almonds
- 1 cup (140g) pitted dates
- 1/2 cup (60g) dried cherries
- 1/4 cup (20g) unsweetened shredded coconut
- 2 tbsp (12g) cocoa powder
- 1/4 tsp ground cinnamon
- Pinch of sea salt

Directions:

1. In a food processor, pulse the almonds until they form a coarse flour-like consistency.
2. Add the pitted dates, dried cherries, shredded coconut, cocoa powder, cinnamon, and sea salt. Pulse until the mixture starts to come together and form a dough-like consistency.
3. Line a baking pan or dish with parchment paper.
4. Transfer the cherry chocolate mixture to the prepared pan and press it down firmly with your hands or a spatula to form a compact, even layer.
5. Refrigerate for at least 2 hours or until firm.
6. Once set, remove the bars from the pan and cut them into desired portions using a sharp knife.
7. Enjoy the raw cherry chocolate sleep bars as a bedtime snack or store them in an airtight container in the refrigerator for up to a week.

Bedtime Bites

Ingredients:

- 1 cup (90g) rolled oats
- 1/2 cup (65g) almond flour
- 1/4 cup (30g) ground flaxseeds
- 1/4 cup (60ml) honey or maple syrup
- 1/4 cup (60ml) creamy almond butter or peanut butter
- 1/4 cup (30g) dried tart cherries or cranberries
- 1 tsp (5ml) vanilla extract
- 1/2 tsp ground cinnamon

Directions:

1. Preheat your oven to 350°F (175°C) and line a baking sheet with parchment paper.
2. In a large bowl, mix together the rolled oats, almond flour, ground flaxseeds, honey or maple syrup, almond butter or peanut butter, dried cherries or cranberries, vanilla extract, and cinnamon until well combined.
3. Scoop out the mixture by heaping tablespoons and roll into small balls, placing them on the prepared baking sheet.
4. Bake for 12-15 minutes, or until lightly golden and set.
5. Remove the bedtime bites from the oven and let them cool completely on the baking sheet.
6. Store the cooled bites in an airtight container in the refrigerator for up to a week.

Stress Relief

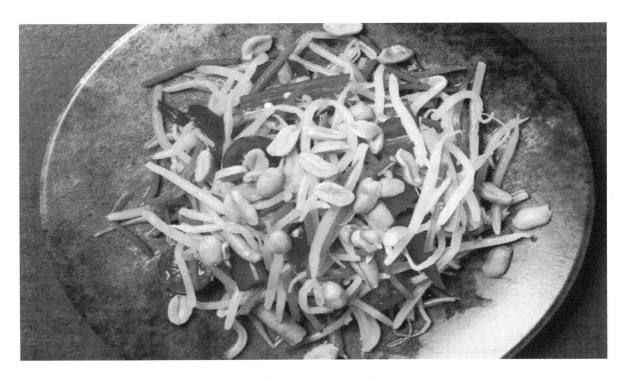

"It's not stress that kills us, it is our reaction to it." –Hans Selye

Stress is an inevitable part of modern life, affecting our physical, mental, and emotional well-being in profound ways. While some stress can be beneficial, motivating us to take action and overcome challenges, chronic or excessive stress can lead to a range of health issues, from anxiety and depression to weakened immunity and cardiovascular disease. Incorporating stress-reducing practices, natural remedies, and mindfulness techniques into our daily routines helps us manage stress more effectively, cultivate resilience, and promote overall well-being.

Topical Treatments

Stress-Relieving Citrus Spray

Ingredients:

- 1/2 cup (120ml) distilled water
- 1/4 cup (60ml) witch hazel
- 10 drops sweet orange essential oil
- 5 drops lemon essential oil
- 5 drops bergamot essential oil

Directions:

1. In a small spray bottle, combine the distilled water and witch hazel.
2. Add the sweet orange, lemon, and bergamot essential oils.
3. Secure the spray bottle lid and gently shake to mix the ingredients.
4. To use, mist the stress-relieving citrus spray into the air or onto surfaces, pillows, or fabrics when you need a refreshing and uplifting aroma.

Rosemary and Peppermint Aromatherapy Oil

Ingredients:

- 1/2 cup (120ml) carrier oil (such as sweet almond, jojoba, or fractionated coconut oil)
- 15 drops rosemary essential oil
- 10 drops peppermint essential oil

Directions:

1. In a small glass bottle or container, combine the carrier oil, rosemary essential oil, and peppermint essential oil.
2. Secure the lid and gently roll the bottle to mix the oils together.
3. To use, apply a few drops of the aromatherapy oil to your temples, wrists, or the back of your neck, and inhale deeply.
4. Alternatively, you can add a few drops to a diffuser or a warm bath for an aromatic experience.

Relaxation Herbal Bath Salts

Ingredients:

- 1 cup (240g) Epsom salts
- 1/2 cup (120g) coarse sea salt
- 1/4 cup (30g) dried lavender buds
- 2 tablespoons (14g) dried chamomile flowers
- 1 tablespoon (7g) dried rose petals
- 10 drops lavender essential oil (optional)

Directions:

1. In a large bowl, combine the Epsom salts, coarse sea salt, dried lavender buds, dried chamomile flowers, and dried rose petals.
2. If desired, add 10 drops of lavender essential oil for an additional calming aroma.
3. Mix the ingredients together until well combined.
4. Transfer the relaxation herbal bath salts to an airtight container or jar.
5. To use, add 1/2 cup to 1 cup of the bath salts to a warm bath and soak for at least 20 minutes, allowing the aroma and minerals to work their magic.

Herbal Brews and Drinks

Mint Chocolate Herbal Tea

Ingredients:

- 2 teaspoons (4g) dried peppermint leaves
- 2 teaspoons (4g) dried spearmint leaves
- 1 teaspoon (2g) dried cacao nibs
- 1 teaspoon (2g) dried licorice root (optional)
- 1 cup (240ml) boiling water

Directions:

1. In a teapot or heat-safe mug, combine the dried peppermint leaves, spearmint leaves, cacao nibs, and licorice root (if using).
2. Pour the boiling water over the herbs and cover the vessel.
3. Allow the tea to steep for 5-7 minutes.
4. Strain the tea into a cup or remove the tea infuser.
5. Sweeten with honey or your preferred sweetener, if desired.
6. Enjoy the refreshing and slightly chocolatey mint herbal tea hot or iced.

Calming Chamomile Tea

Ingredients:

- 2 tablespoons (6g) dried chamomile flowers
- 1 teaspoon (2g) dried lemon balm (optional)
- 1 cup (240ml) boiling water

Directions:

1. In a teapot or heat-safe mug, combine the dried chamomile flowers and lemon balm (if using).
2. Pour the boiling water over the herbs and cover the vessel.
3. Allow the tea to steep for 5-7 minutes.
4. Strain the tea into a cup or remove the tea infuser.
5. Optionally, add a touch of honey or lemon to taste.
6. Enjoy the calming chamomile tea hot or iced before bedtime.

Blue Moon Stress Tea

Ingredients:

- 1 tablespoon (4g) dried butterfly pea flowers
- 1 teaspoon (2g) dried lemon balm
- 1 teaspoon (2g) dried lavender buds
- 1 cup (240ml) boiling water

Directions:

1. In a teapot or heat-safe mug, combine the dried butterfly pea flowers, lemon balm, and lavender buds.
2. Pour the boiling water over the herbs and cover the vessel.
3. Allow the tea to steep for 5-7 minutes.
4. Strain the tea into a cup or remove the tea infuser.
5. The butterfly pea flowers will give the tea a beautiful blue hue.
6. Optionally, add a touch of honey or lemon to taste.
7. Enjoy the soothing and visually appealing Blue Moon Stress Tea hot or iced.

Strawberry Hibiscus Calmer

Ingredients:

- 1 cup (150g) fresh or frozen strawberries
- 2 tablespoons (6g) dried hibiscus flowers
- 1 cup (240ml) boiling water
- 1 tablespoon (15ml) honey or agave nectar (optional)
- Squeeze of fresh lemon juice (optional)

Directions:

1. In a heatproof jar or teapot, combine the dried hibiscus flowers and boiling water. Cover and allow to steep for 5-7 minutes.
2. Remove the hibiscus flowers by straining the tea.
3. In a blender, combine the strawberries and the hibiscus tea.
4. Blend until smooth and well-combined.
5. If desired, stir in honey or agave nectar for sweetness, and add a squeeze of fresh lemon juice for a tangy twist.
6. Pour the strawberry hibiscus calmer into a glass and enjoy chilled or at room temperature.

Stress-Busting Juice

Ingredients:

- 2 large carrots
- 1 cucumber
- 1 apple
- 1-inch piece of fresh ginger
- 1 lemon, juiced
- A handful of fresh spinach or kale leaves

Directions:

1. Wash and prepare all the ingredients by peeling the carrots, cucumber, and ginger if desired.
2. Feed the carrots, cucumber, apple, ginger, and lemon through a juicer.
3. Add the fresh spinach or kale leaves to the juice and stir gently to combine.
4. Pour the stress-busting juice into a glass and enjoy immediately for maximum nutrient benefits.

Cortisol Cocktail

Ingredients:

- 1/2 cup (120ml) unsweetened coconut water
- 1/2 cup (120ml) fresh orange juice
- 1 tablespoon (15ml) fresh lemon juice
- 1 teaspoon (5ml) apple cider vinegar
- 1 teaspoon (5ml) honey or agave nectar (optional)
- Pinch of ground cinnamon

Directions:

1. In a glass or shaker, combine the unsweetened coconut water, fresh orange juice, fresh lemon juice, and apple cider vinegar.
2. Add honey or agave nectar for sweetness, if desired.
3. Sprinkle a pinch of ground cinnamon on top.
4. Stir or shake the cocktail gently to combine all the ingredients.
5. Pour the cortisol cocktail into a glass filled with ice cubes.
6. Enjoy this refreshing and stress-relieving beverage.

Stress Relief Recipes

Kale Stuffed Sardines

Ingredients:

- 1 bunch kale, stems removed and leaves chopped
- 2 tablespoons olive oil
- 2 cloves garlic, minced
- 1/4 teaspoon red pepper flakes (optional)
- Salt and pepper to taste
- 1 can (4.4 oz) sardines in olive oil, drained
- Lemon wedges for serving

Directions:

1. In a large skillet, heat the olive oil over medium heat.
2. Add the chopped kale, minced garlic, and red pepper flakes (if using). Season with salt and pepper.
3. Cook the kale, stirring frequently, until it's wilted and tender, about 5-7 minutes.
4. Remove the kale mixture from heat and let it cool slightly.
5. Carefully stuff the cooked kale mixture into the cavity of each sardine.
6. Arrange the kale-stuffed sardines on a serving plate.
7. Serve with lemon wedges for squeezing over the top.

Rocket Pesto Pasta

Ingredients:

- 8 oz (225g) whole wheat pasta
- 2 cups (60g) fresh rocket (arugula) leaves
- 1/2 cup (60g) grated Parmesan cheese
- 1/4 cup (35g) toasted pine nuts
- 2 cloves garlic, minced
- 1/4 cup (60ml) olive oil
- Salt and pepper to taste

Directions:

1. Cook the pasta according to package Directions until al dente. Drain and set aside.
2. In a food processor, combine the rocket leaves, Parmesan cheese, pine nuts, and minced garlic. Pulse until roughly chopped.
3. With the food processor running, slowly drizzle in the olive oil until the pesto comes together.
4. Season the pesto with salt and pepper to taste.
5. In a large bowl, toss the cooked pasta with the rocket pesto until well coated.
6. Serve the rocket pesto pasta warm or at room temperature.

Mason Jar Asian Stress Salad

Ingredients:

- 1 cup (150g) cooked quinoa
- 1/2 cup (75g) shredded carrots
- 1/2 cup (75g) shredded red cabbage
- 1/2 cup (75g) edamame beans
- 1/4 cup (35g) sliced almonds
- 2 tablespoons (30ml) rice vinegar
- 1 tablespoon (15ml) sesame oil
- 1 tablespoon (15ml) low-sodium soy sauce
- 1 teaspoon (5ml) honey or agave nectar
- 1 teaspoon (3g) grated fresh ginger

Directions:

1. In a large mason jar or container with a tight-fitting lid, layer the cooked quinoa, shredded carrots, shredded red cabbage, edamame beans, and sliced almonds.
2. In a small bowl, whisk together the rice vinegar, sesame oil, soy sauce, honey (or agave nectar), and grated ginger.
3. Pour the dressing over the layered salad ingredients in the mason jar.
4. Secure the lid and give the jar a good shake to distribute the dressing throughout the salad.
5. Refrigerate the mason jar Asian stress salad until ready to serve, shaking it again before eating.

Tofu Summer Rolls

Ingredients:

- 8 oz (225g) firm tofu, drained and pressed
- 1 carrot, julienned
- 1 cucumber, julienned
- 1/2 red bell pepper, julienned
- 1/4 cup (35g) chopped fresh mint
- 1/4 cup (35g) chopped fresh basil
- 8 rice paper wrappers
- Dipping sauce (e.g., peanut sauce, sweet chili sauce)

Directions:

1. Cut the pressed tofu into thin strips or small cubes.
2. In a large bowl, combine the tofu, julienned carrot, julienned cucumber, julienned red bell pepper, chopped mint, and chopped basil.
3. Fill a shallow dish with warm water.
4. Dip a rice paper wrapper into the warm water for 10-15 seconds, or until it becomes pliable.
5. Transfer the softened rice paper wrapper to a flat surface.
6. Place a portion of the tofu and vegetable mixture onto the lower third of the wrapper.
7. Fold the sides of the wrapper over the filling, then tightly roll it up into a cylinder.
8. Repeat the process with the remaining wrappers and filling.
9. Serve the tofu summer rolls immediately, with your desired dipping sauce on the side.

Raw Pad Thai

Ingredients:

- 1 large zucchini, spiralized or julienned
- 1 large carrot, julienned
- 1 red bell pepper, julienned
- 1/2 cup (70g) chopped cashews
- 1/4 cup (35g) chopped cilantro
- 2 tablespoons (30ml) lime juice
- 2 tablespoons (30ml) almond butter
- 1 tablespoon (15ml) tamari or soy sauce
- 1 teaspoon (5ml) sesame oil
- 1 teaspoon (5ml) maple syrup or honey
- 1 clove garlic, minced

Directions:

1. In a large bowl, combine the spiralized zucchini, julienned carrot, julienned red bell pepper, chopped cashews, and chopped cilantro.
2. In a small bowl, whisk together the lime juice, almond butter, tamari (or soy sauce), sesame oil, maple syrup (or honey), and minced garlic.
3. Pour the dressing over the vegetable mixture and toss gently to coat evenly.
4. Let the raw pad thai sit for 10-15 minutes to allow the flavors to meld and the vegetables to soften slightly.
5. Serve chilled or at room temperature, garnished with extra chopped cashews and cilantro if desired.

Dark Chocolate Pots

Ingredients:

- 1 (14 oz) can full-fat coconut milk
- 6 oz (170g) dark chocolate, chopped
- 2 tablespoons (30ml) maple syrup or honey
- 1 teaspoon vanilla extract
- 1/4 teaspoon sea salt

Directions:

1. In a saucepan, heat the coconut milk over medium heat until simmering.
2. Remove the saucepan from heat and stir in the chopped dark chocolate until completely melted and smooth.
3. Whisk in the maple syrup (or honey), vanilla extract, and sea salt until well combined.
4. Pour the dark chocolate mixture into small ramekins or dessert cups.
5. Refrigerate the chocolate pots for at least 2 hours, or until set.
6. Serve chilled, garnished with fresh berries, whipped cream, or a sprinkle of sea salt if desired.

Sugar Regulation and Thyroid Function

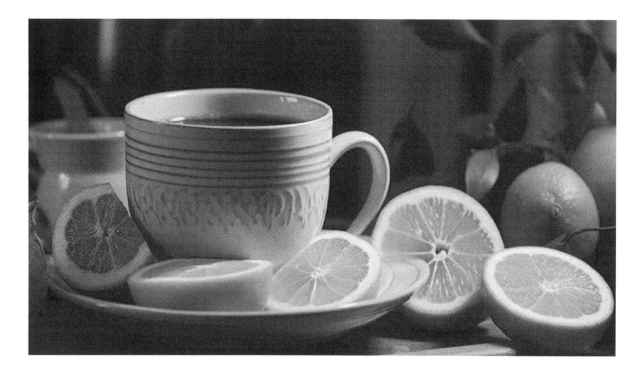

"What most people don't realize is that food is not just calories: It's information. It actually contains messages that communicate to every cell in the body." –Dr. Mark Hyman

Maintaining healthy blood sugar levels is crucial for overall health and well-being, as chronic high blood sugar can lead to a range of serious health issues, including type 2 diabetes, cardiovascular disease, and metabolic syndrome. Adopting a balanced, nutrient-dense diet, incorporating natural blood sugar-regulating remedies, and engaging in regular physical activity keeps our blood sugar levels in check, improves insulin sensitivity, and promotes optimal health.

Topical Treatments

Tea Infused Sugar Cubes

Ingredients:

- 1 cup (200g) granulated sugar
- 1/4 cup (60ml) strongly brewed tea (such as earl grey, jasmine, or chamomile)

Directions:

1. In a small saucepan, combine the granulated sugar and strongly brewed tea.
2. Heat the mixture over medium heat, stirring constantly, until the sugar has completely dissolved and formed a syrup.
3. Carefully pour the syrup into silicone molds or an ice cube tray.
4. Allow the tea-infused sugar cubes to cool and harden completely, which may take several hours or overnight.
5. Once hardened, gently remove the sugar cubes from the molds or tray.
6. Store the tea-infused sugar cubes in an airtight container at room temperature for up to several weeks.

Herbal Brews and Drinks

Soursop Leaf Tea

Ingredients:
- 1/4 cup (10g) dried soursop leaves
- 4 cups (960ml) boiling water

Directions:
1. Place the dried soursop leaves in a teapot or heat-safe pitcher.
2. Pour the boiling water over the leaves.
3. Cover the teapot or pitcher and let the tea steep for 10-15 minutes.
4. Strain the tea to remove the leaves.
5. Serve the soursop leaf tea hot or chilled, with or without a sweetener of your choice.

Chai Sugar Balancer

Ingredients:
- 1/2 cup (100g) granulated sugar
- 1 teaspoon ground cinnamon
- 1/2 teaspoon ground ginger
- 1/4 teaspoon ground cardamom
- 1/4 teaspoon ground cloves
- 1/4 teaspoon ground black pepper

Directions:
1. In a small bowl, combine the granulated sugar, ground cinnamon, ground ginger, ground cardamom, ground cloves, and ground black pepper.
2. Mix the ingredients thoroughly until well-incorporated.
3. Store the chai sugar balancer in an airtight container at room temperature for up to several months.
4. Use the flavored sugar to sweeten hot or cold beverages, such as tea, coffee, or smoothies, for a chai-inspired twist.
5. You can also sprinkle the chai sugar balancer over yogurt, oatmeal, or baked goods for an added flavor boost.

Butterscotch Sugar Regulator

Ingredients:
- 1 cup (175g) pitted medjool dates
- 1/4 cup (60ml) water
- 2 tbsp (30g) almond butter
- 1 tsp vanilla extract
- 1/4 tsp sea salt
- 1/2 tsp ground cinnamon

Directions:
1. Soak the dates in hot water for 10-15 minutes to soften, then drain.
2. In a blender or food processor, blend the soaked dates, water, almond butter, vanilla, salt, and cinnamon until smooth and well-combined.
3. The mixture should form a thick, caramel-like paste. If too thick, add a splash more water to reach a pourable consistency.
4. Transfer to an airtight container and store in the refrigerator for up to 2 weeks.
5. Use the date butterscotch sweetener to drizzle over oatmeal, yogurt, or as a dip for fresh fruit.

Orange Tea

Ingredients:
- 2 oranges, sliced (with peel)
- 1/4 cup (10g) dried hibiscus flowers
- 4 cups (960ml) water
- Raw honey or monk fruit sweetener (optional)

Directions:
1. Place the sliced oranges and dried hibiscus in a teapot or heat-safe pitcher.
2. Bring the water to a boil, then pour it over the oranges and hibiscus.
3. Allow it to steep for 10-12 minutes to infuse the flavors.
4. Strain the tea into another pitcher or pot, discarding the solids.
5. Sweeten with raw honey or monk fruit, if desired.
6. Serve warm or chilled over ice. Garnish with fresh orange slices.

Honeysuckle Iced Tea

Ingredients:

- 1/4 cup (10g) dried lemon balm leaves
- 2 lemongrass stalks, bruised
- 4 cups (960ml) water
- Raw honey or stevia (optional)
- Fresh lemon slices (optional)

Directions:

1. In a saucepan, bring the water to a boil.
2. Remove from heat and add the dried lemon balm and bruised lemongrass stalks.
3. Cover and let steep for 15-20 minutes to infuse the flavors.
4. Strain the tea into a pitcher, discarding the herbs.
5. Stir in raw honey or stevia to taste, if desired.
6. Refrigerate for 1-2 hours to chill completely.
7. Serve over ice, garnished with fresh lemon slices if desired.

Sugar Regulation Recipes

Overnight Date and Pine Oats

Ingredients:

- 1 cup (80g) old-fashioned rolled oats
- 1 cup (240ml) unsweetened almond milk or milk of choice
- 1/2 cup (75g) pitted medjool dates, chopped
- 1/4 cup (35g) pine nuts
- 1 tsp vanilla extract
- 1/2 tsp ground cinnamon
- 1/4 tsp sea salt
- Toppings: fresh berries, sliced bananas, honey, etc.

Directions:

1. In a medium-sized jar or bowl, combine the rolled oats, almond milk, chopped dates, pine nuts, vanilla extract, cinnamon, and sea salt. Stir well to combine.
2. Cover the jar or bowl and refrigerate overnight (or for at least 4-6 hours) to allow the oats to soften and absorb the flavors.
3. In the morning, give the overnight oats a good stir. If the mixture seems too thick, add a splash of almond milk or milk of choice to loosen it up.
4. Transfer the overnight oats to a serving bowl and top with fresh berries, sliced bananas, a drizzle of honey, or any other desired toppings.
5. Enjoy chilled or at room temperature.

Shrimp Tacos

Ingredients:

- 1 lb (450g) large shrimp, peeled and deveined
- 1 tbsp olive oil
- 1 tsp chili powder
- 1 tsp cumin
- 1/2 tsp paprika
- 1/4 tsp garlic powder
- Juice of 1 lime
- Salt and pepper to taste
- 8-10 small corn tortillas, warmed
- Toppings: shredded cabbage, diced avocado, pico de gallo, cilantro, etc.

Directions:

1. In a bowl, toss the shrimp with olive oil, chili powder, cumin, paprika, garlic powder, lime juice, and a pinch of salt and pepper.
2. Heat a skillet or grill pan over medium-high heat. Add the seasoned shrimp and cook for 2-3 minutes per side, or until opaque and cooked through.
3. Remove the shrimp from the heat and set aside.
4. Warm the corn tortillas according to package Directions or by heating them in a dry skillet for a few seconds on each side.
5. To assemble the tacos, place a portion of the cooked shrimp onto each tortilla.
6. Top with desired toppings such as shredded cabbage, diced avocado, pico de gallo, and cilantro.
7. Serve the shrimp tacos immediately, with lime wedges on the side for squeezing over the top.

Salmon Stuffed Avocado

Ingredients:

- 2 large avocados
- 1 (6 oz / 170g) can wild-caught salmon, drained and flaked
- 1/4 cup (35g) diced red onion
- 2 tbsp (8g) chopped fresh dill
- 2 tbsp (30ml) lemon juice
- 1 tbsp (15ml) olive oil
- Salt and pepper to taste
- Mixed greens or arugula for serving (optional)

Directions:

1. Cut the avocados in half lengthwise and remove the pits. Scoop out a bit of the flesh from the center of each half to create a larger cavity.
2. In a bowl, gently mix together the flaked salmon, diced red onion, chopped dill, lemon juice, olive oil, and a pinch of salt and pepper.
3. Spoon the salmon mixture evenly into the cavities of each avocado half.
4. If desired, serve the stuffed avocados over a bed of mixed greens or arugula.
5. Garnish with extra dill, lemon wedges, or a drizzle of olive oil before serving.

Raspberry Fish Tacos

Ingredients:

- 1 lb (450g) white fish filets (such as cod, halibut, or tilapia)
- 1 tsp chili powder
- 1 tsp cumin
- 1/2 tsp smoked paprika
- Salt and pepper to taste
- 2 tbsp olive oil
- 1 cup (150g) fresh raspberries
- 1/4 cup (35g) diced red onion
- 1 jalapeño, seeded and minced
- 2 tbsp chopped fresh cilantro
- Juice of 1 lime
- 8-10 small corn tortillas, warmed
- Toppings: shredded cabbage, diced avocado, etc.

Directions:

1. Pat the fish filets dry and season them with chili powder, cumin, smoked paprika, salt, and pepper.
2. Heat the olive oil in a skillet over medium-high heat.
3. Cook the seasoned fish filets for 3-4 minutes per side, or until opaque and flaky.
4. Remove the fish from the heat and gently flake it into chunks.
5. In a bowl, combine the flaked fish with fresh raspberries, diced red onion, minced jalapeño, chopped cilantro, and lime juice. Gently toss to combine.
6. To assemble the tacos, place a portion of the raspberry fish mixture onto each warmed corn tortilla.
7. Top with desired toppings like shredded cabbage, diced avocado, or extra cilantro.
8. Serve the raspberry fish tacos immediately, with lime wedges on the side.

Chicken and Broccoli Salad with Buttermilk Dressing

Ingredients:

- 2 boneless, skinless chicken breasts, cooked and diced
- 3 cups (300g) broccoli florets, chopped into bite-sized pieces
- 1/4 cup (35g) diced red onion

For the Buttermilk Dressing:

- 1/2 cup (120ml) buttermilk
- 1/4 cup (60ml) mayonnaise
- 2 tbsp (30ml) apple cider vinegar
- 1/4 cup (35g) dried cranberries
- 1/4 cup (30g) sliced almonds

- 1 tsp honey
- Salt and pepper to taste

Directions:

1. In a large bowl, combine the diced cooked chicken, chopped broccoli florets, diced red onion, dried cranberries, and sliced almonds.
2. In a separate small bowl, whisk together all the ingredients for the buttermilk dressing until well combined.
3. Pour the dressing over the chicken and broccoli salad mixture and toss gently to coat everything evenly.
4. Refrigerate the salad for at least 30 minutes to allow the flavors to meld.
5. Serve the chicken and broccoli salad with buttermilk dressing chilled or at room temperature.

Conclusion

We've come to the end of our herbal journey together and I hope that it has been as enlightening as my own introduction to Natural Healing Medicine. You have now been provided with the foundational tools needed to empower you through your natural journey but it's important that you understand how tailoring your own recipes to your needs is.

With your recipes on hand, you can now begin to develop a solid understanding of how to harness the power of herbs, plants, and natural remedies to support your health and well-being. Most importantly, I hope you realize that you have options when it comes to your health. Western pharmaceuticals don't have to be your only go-to. Nature has provided you with an incredible array of tools for healing—many of which have been copied and emulated by Western medicine.

Remember, this is just the beginning of your natural health journey. Keep exploring, experimenting, and listening to your body. And don't be afraid to share your newfound wisdom with others—the world could always use more natural health enthusiasts!

One last thing before you turn the last page. If you've enjoyed this book and found it helpful, I would be over the moon if you could take a moment to leave an honest review. Your feedback means the world to me and helps me to keep creating content that inspires and empowers others.

Simply scan the QR code below book, and you'll be able to share your thoughts.

Thank you, from the bottom of my heart, for joining me on this journey. I can't wait to see how you'll use this knowledge to transform your health and your life. Here's to a naturally vibrant, joyful, and abundant future–with love and green blessings!

Image References

8photo. (n.d.-a). Flat lay a cup of tea with tea herbs on dark textured background. horizontal [Image]. https://www.freepik.com/free-photo/flat-lay-cup-tea-with-tea-herbs-dark-textured-background-horizontal_8111256.htm#fromView=search&page=1&position=32&uuid=5e8fe1f8-d8dc-426b-97fd-618ba9fbe906

8photo. (n.d.-b). Fruit infused water in teapot with tea, dried apricots, wood, kitchen towel, container side view on stone tile and wooden surface [Image]. https://www.freepik.com/free-photo/fruit-infused-water-teapot-with-tea-dried-apricots-wood-kitchen-towel-container-side-view-stone-tile-wooden-surface_8756266.htm#fromView=search&page=2&position=2&uuid=406ed937-1d48-4ee7-b1b4-659dfdb220e5

Astrid Alauda. (n.d.). Astrid Alauda Quotes. Www.goodreads.com. Retrieved May 8, 2024, from https://www.goodreads.com/author/quotes/7340883.Astrid_Alauda

Chandlervid85. (n.d.). Green Papaya Salad som tam thai on black slate background [Image]. https://www.freepik.com/free-photo/green-papaya-salad-som-tam-thai-black-slate-background_135516071.htm#fromView=search&page=1&position=28&uuid=f1d54ca7-9f59-4f-8f-90f7-01a3a44439201

DemandDeborah. (n.d.). Vegetable chickpea sandwiches [Image]. https://demanddeborah.org/resource-type/recipes

Ededchechine. (n.d.). Chashushuli Traditional Georgian dish of veal stewed with onions and peppers the dish lies [Image]. https://www.freepik.com/free-photo/chashushuli-traditional-georgian-dish-veal-stewed-with-onions-peppers-dish-lies_135385182.htm#fromView=search&page=1&position=35&uuid=30b4f987-ade2-48de-b76f-faf15a205f76

Freepik. (n.d.-a). Cupcake; cookies and chocolate truffles made with coffee beans and chocolate on black background [Image]. https://www.freepik.com/free-photo/cupcake-cookies-chocolate-truffles-made-with-coffee-beans-chocolate-black-background_3652365.htm#fromView=search&page=2&position=35&uuid=5a9646c3-8795-4fba-afd7-35c858b82f77

Freepik. (n.d.-b). Delicious banana bread on table [Image]. https://www.freepik.com/free-ai-image/delicious-banana-bread-table_65618840.htm#fromView=search&page=2&position=4&uuid=968957ff-c6db-474c-be60-a43a503407d3

Freepik. (n.d.-c). Delicious high protein meal assortment [Image]. Retrieved 2024, from https://www.freepik.com/free-photo/delicious-high-protein-meal-assortment_18003165.htm#fromView=search&page=2&position=0&uuid=92fdc193-3a46-4fd2-a57a-10f98f449342

Freepik. (n.d.-d). Delicious nougats on tray top view [Image]. https://www.freepik.com/free-photo/delicious-nougats-tray-top-view_31124698.htm#fromView=search&page=2&position=2&uuid=4c9f5ada-932b-449a-b8dc-e4e6b34c6a6d

Freepik. (n.d.-e). Delicious tacos on table [Image]. https://www.freepik.com/free-ai-image/delicious-tacos-table_65628474.htm#fromView=search&page=1&position=21&uuid=1b14ded2-98fa-42a6-8a0e-94944409d7b8

Freepik. (n.d.-f). Front view of strawberry milkshake with copy space [Image]. https://www.freepik.com/free-photo/front-view-strawberry-milkshake-with-copy-space_10556913.htm#fromView=search&page=1&position=38&uuid=e4d347e7-8c56-4c1f-9313-884e42ffa344

Freepik. (n.d.-g). Modern kitchen composition with healthy ingredients [Image]. https://www.freepik.com/free-photo/modern-kitchen-composition-with-healthy-ingredients_3362230.htm#fromView=search&page=1&position=0&uuid=af43daa2-e9f1-415b-9232-68bc1c5e55b5

Freepik. (n.d.-h). Salmon fishcakes [Image]. www.freepik.com

Freepik. (n.d.-i). Top view cream soup and autumn leaves [Image]. https://www.freepik.com/free-photo/top-view-cream-soup-autumn-leaves_10067940.htm#fromView=search&page=1&position=9&uuid=329bc1a0-e134-49f4-acba-1db2e99c598c

Freepik. (n.d.-j). Top view of winter broccoli soup with spoon and bread [Image]. https://www.freepik.com/free-photo/top-view-winter-broccoli-soup-with-spoon-bread_10554428.htm#fromView=search&page=1&position=2&uuid=7fbacba2-184a-485b-8265-4d563f9262a9

Get Started Today | Cove. (n.d.). Www.withcove.com. https://www.withcove.com/learn/best-migraine-headache-recipes

Gibson, B. (2023, April 8). The Best Herbal Tea Blend for Headaches. The Homestead Challenge. https://thehomesteadchallenge.com/the-best-herbal-tea-blend-for-headaches

GRMarc. (n.d.). A homemade dessert fresh and sweet on a wooden table generated by artificial intelligence [Image]. https://www.freepik.com/free-ai-image/homemade-dessert-fresh-sweet-wooden-table-generated-by-artificial-intelligence_80536318.htm#fromView=search&page=2&position=16&uuid=968957ff-c6db-474c-be60-a43a503407d3

Grmarc. (n.d.). Freshness and green color of leafy vegetables in a healthy meal generated by artificial intellingence [Image]. https://www.freepik.com/free-ai-image/freshness-green-color-leafy-vegetables-healthy-meal-generated-by-artificial-intellingence_77071959.htm#fromView=search&page=1&position=24&uuid=16dabd4a-ed33-48a8-96d3-8a5a513b4296

Kamran Aydinov. (n.d.). Close up view of yummy breakfast with strawberries in a bowl on the right side on dark color background with free space [Image]. https://www.freepik.com/free-photo/close-up-view-yummy-breakfast-with-strawberries-bowl-right-side-dark-color-background-with-free-space_22290719.htm#fromView=search&page=1&position=28&uuid=5a81f36e-b842-47a1-86a4-a8a8a070184c

KamranAydinov. (n.d.). Top view beet salad with sour cream and garlic on dark desk [Image]. https://www.freepik.com/free-photo/top-view-beet-salad-with-sour-cream-garlic-dark-desk_13537464.htm#fromView=search&page=1&position=9&uuid=1b0a4890-e-96a-4e04-a099-b27ec2612ddb

Maria Edgeworth. (n.d.). Maria Edgeworth Quote. Lib Quotes. Retrieved May 8, 2024, from https://libquotes.com/maria-edgeworth/quote/lbq1x8g

Naturedoc. (n.d.). Cranberry hormone balancer [Image]. https://naturedoc.com/spiced-cranberry-hibiscus-mocktail/

Timolina. (n.d.-a). Home made fish cake cod [Image]. https://www.freepik.com/free-photo/home-made-fish-cake-cod_6582101.htm#fromView=search&page=1&position=1&uuid=e772d737-89c0-4f5c-ad40-4b578e9c61a1

Timolina. (n.d.-b). Vegetarian stew eggplants, bell peppers, onions, garlic and tomatoes with herbs [Image]. https://www.freepik.com/free-photo/vegetarian-stew-eggplants-bell-peppers-onions-garlic-tomatoes-with-herbs_6933492.htm#fromView=search&page=1&position=8&uuid=02d0b19d-eeef-4fa8-a3b9-13855b2464d2

Toptnpt26. (n.d.). Mulberry juice [Image]. https://www.freepik.com/free-photo/mulberry-juice_1240021.htm#fromView=search&page=2&position=27&uuid=968957ff-c6db-474c-be60-a43a503407d3

Vecstock. (n.d.-a). A bowl of lentil soup with a slice of bread on the side [Image]. https://www.freepik.com/free-ai-image/bowl-lentil-soup-with-slice-bread-side_41483621.htm#fromView=search&page=1&position=1&uuid=ee332fed-984f-4f39-9682-e78862ba5aae

Vecstock. (n.d.-b). Fresh lemon slice in hot tea on wooden table generated by artificial intelligence [Image]. https://www.freepik.com/free-ai-image/fresh-lemon-slice-hot-tea-wooden-table-generated-by-artificial-intelligence_79687923.htm#fromView=search&page=3&position=50&uuid=28ea388f-4f68-43d4-8bc0-f19b7aca21f1

Vecstock. (n.d.-c). Fresh lemonade on rustic table perfect summer refreshment generated by AI [Image]. https://www.freepik.com/free-ai-image/fresh-lemonade-rustic-table-perfect-summer-refreshment-generated-by-ai_42212362.htm#fromView=search&page=1&position=20&uuid=5550e069-0718-4b40-a2c0-c4e574d181b8

Vecstock. (n.d.-d). Freshly baked homemade pizza with mozzarella tomato and savory sauce generated by artificial intelligence [Image]. https://www.freepik.com/free-ai-image/freshly-baked-homemade-pizza-with-mozzarella-tomato-savory-sauce-generated-by-artificial-intelligence_122382832.htm#fromView=search&page=1&position=27&uuid=1a555638-ee6f-4d82-9a4b-d0114317fd3b

Vecstock. (n.d.-e). Freshness of summer berries on a rustic wooden table refreshing cocktail generated by artificial intelligence [Image]. https://www.freepik.com/free-ai-image/freshness-summer-berries-rustic-wooden-table-refreshing-cocktail-generated-by-artificial-intelligence_89236358.htm#fromView=search&page=2&position=14&uuid=4cbfc837-684a-4c6f-9936-249a7566c9a3

Vecstock. (n.d.-f). Freshness of summer fruit in a gourmet dessert generated by artificial intelligence [Image]. Retrieved 2024, from https://www.freepik.com/free-ai-image/freshness-summer-fruit-gourmet-dessert-generated-by-artificial-intelligence_122367684.htm#fromView=search&page=1&position=34&uuid=812d0baa-9470-4fe9-b850-c653c95e1d0a

Vecstock. (n.d.-g). Grilled beef and vegetable plate ready to eat generated by AI [Image]. https://www.freepik.com/free-ai-image/grilled-beef-vegetable-plate-ready-eat-generated-by-ai_42663453.htm#fromView=search&page=1&position=2&uuid=13db8a-ab-1db9-42e6-a2bf-298d6409daf3

Vecstock. (n.d.-h). Grilled beef burger with tomato on bun generated by AI [Image]. https://www.freepik.com/free-ai-image/grilled-beef-burger-with-tomato-bun-generated-by-ai_41312024.htm#fromView=search&page=1&position=3&uuid=0fdefbf2-b252-4dac-8a9e-b-7d8418308f6

Vecstock. (n.d.-i). Grilled chicken fillet with fresh vegetables a healthy gourmet meal generated by artificial intelligence [Image]. https://www.freepik.com/free-ai-image/grilled-chicken-fillet-with-fresh-vegetables-healthy-gourmet-meal-generated-by-artificial-intelligence_126499554.htm#fromView=search&page=1&position=0&uuid=5150e32a-622e-429b-b534-9a8b6c176da7

Vecstock. (n.d.-j). Hot tea on wooden table a cozy and refreshing drink generated by artificial intelligence [Image]. Retrieved 2024, from https://www.freepik.com/free-ai-image/hot-tea-wooden-table-cozy-refreshing-drink-generated-by-artificial-intelligence_79684722.htm#fromView=search&page=1&position=28&uuid=fedfcb6f-8810-4c87-869e-950e43ccace0

Vecstock. (n.d.-k). omemade vegetable soup fresh and healthy meal generated by AI [Image]. https://www.freepik.com/free-ai-image/homemade-vegetable-soup-fresh-healthy-meal-generated-by-ai_41214027.htm#fromView=search&page=1&position=27&uuid=a22d35dd-efcd-4610-b54a-4721549140d7

Vecstock. (n.d.-l). Stack of homemade pancakes with honey syrup drop generative AI [Image]. https://www.freepik.com/free-ai-image/stack-homemade-pancakes-with-honey-syrup-drop-generative-ai_47211130.htm#fromView=search&page=1&position=13&uuid=968957ff-c6db-474c-be60-a43a503407d3

Verywell. (n.d.). The Health Benefits of Migraine Tea. Verywell Health. https://www.verywellhealth.com/migraine-tea-5198811

Made in United States
Orlando, FL
16 September 2024

51575777R00117